# Yoga for the Three Stages of Life

# Yoga for the Three Stages of Life

Developing
Your Practice
As an Art Form,
a Physical Therapy,
and a Guiding
Philosophy

Śrīvatsa Rāmaswāmi

Inner Traditions
Rochester, Vermont

Inner Traditions International
One Park Street
Rochester, Vermont 05767
www.InnerTraditions.com



LIBRARY OF CONGRESS CATALOGING-IN-PUBLICATION DATA

Rāmaswāmī, Śrīvatsa.
Yoga for the three stages of life : developing your practice as an art form, a physical therapy, and a guiding philosophy / Śrīvatsa Rāmaswāmī
p. cm.
Includes index.
ISBN 0-89281-820-4
1. Yoga, Haòha. 2. Yoga. I. Title.

RA781.7 .R34 2000
613.7'046—dc21

00-059781

Printed and bound in The United States

10 9 8 7 6 5 4 3 2 1

Text design and layout by Virginia L. Scott-Bowman
This book was typeset in Times with Bauer Bodoni as the display typeface

OM

*Śrī Rāma Jayam*

THIS BOOK IS DEDICATED TO the memory of my mother, who said early in my life "There is more to life than making a living"; to my father, who encouraged me in all my endeavors; to my guru, who had so much to give, and from which I could take so little; and to Lord Almighty—Śrī Kriṣṇārpaṇamastu.

# Contents

# Acknowledgments

I WISH TO THANK my wife, Dr. Umā Rāmaswāmī, for her encouragement and her help, especially with the technical details of writing this book.

I also wish to state my sincere appreciation and thanks to several people who have directly or indirectly helped me to teach yoga and write this book. To my sons Prasanna and Badri, who encouraged me, sometimes like buddies, in the writing of this book and in other yoga activities. They have been a great source of joy.

To the late Rukmini Devī and Śankara Menon, former directors of Kalākṣetra Institute, and Mr. Rajaraman, its present director, for the opportunity afforded me to teach there for two decades. To the late M. C. Subramanian of the Public Health Centre for the opportunity to introduce yoga in the hospital. My thanks are due to C. S. Sampath of Public Health Centre Hospital, Professor Janardhanan of Kalākṣetra, S. Chitra of Padma Seshadri Schools, and K. Gopalakrishnan for studying this system and teaching for more than twenty years. To John Coon, the dynamic director, and other senior students and teachers of Yoga Center of Houston, Texas, for studying the *vinyāsakrama* in depth and teaching in Houston and elsewhere in the United States, I am grateful. Many students and their students have helped in the development of the book by contributing several of their yoga pictures. They ranged in age from ten to seventy-five and comprised schoolchildren, medical students, physiotherapists, a renowned artist/painter, an athlete, classical Bharatnatyam dancers, teachers, corporate executives, and, of course, a couple of yoga teachers. Girija Menon has done exquisite but difficult postures for the chapter on women and yoga. Pam Johnson, Hilary Nixon, and John Coon have portrayed several *āsana* sequences artistically and with vigor. R. Soundrarajan, M. Parvati, and S. Ramya have done several other yoga sequences beautifully. Others whose pictures appear in the book are C. S. Sampath, Jaya Reddy, Jayashree Soundararajan, R. Sowmya, C. Vidya, Maanasaa, A. Yamini, and Prentis Fatherree. Śrīmān Srinivasan of Krishna Photos shot all the pictures done in Chennai and made special prints of all pictures in this book. To them all, my sincere thanks. To the late Śrī Harigopal Agarwal for the tremendous enthusiasm, encouragement, and opportunities given to me to teach in the huge free yoga camps conducted for nearly ten years at the yoga brotherhood; to Mr. H. M. Mahesh of Sangeetha and Mr. Murali of HMV for producing and marketing my audiocassettes; and to M. Gopalakrishnan, my always optimistic and cheerful cousin, for all his work and support.

To the respected *paṇḍit* Śrī Rājamaṇiji for the opportunity to give introductory lectures on yoga and workshops and classes at the Himalayan Institute at Honesdale, and also for the great support; to Sandy Anderson, Mary Gail, and Rolf Sovik, and to Nishit Patel and Virat Xavier for offering introductory programs and workshops and classes in yoga at the Himalayan Institutes in Buffalo, New York, and Chicago; to my cousin Dr. Ambujam, my niece Chitra, and other cousins; to Dr. M. Subramaniam and Mr. M. Hariharan; and to Dr. Sundara Gandhi, Dr. Senthamarai Gandhi, Dr. Sundaraman, Dr. J. L. Sarma, and Dr. Sethuraman, many thanks for hosting and helping me talk about this system of yoga to selected groups. To Professor T. K. Parthasarathy, vice chancellor, and Professor S. Rangaswamy, head of the Holistic Health Center, Śrī Ramachandra Medical University, Chennai, for their efforts to introduce yoga as a program of optional study for both faculty and students of the university, and for the opportunity afforded me to teach there.

My sincere thanks are due also to Kala for the beautiful line sketches she prepared; to Sujayā, a senior teacher of the Kriṣṇamācārya method of yoga, for her critical input in the writing of this book; to my nephews Dinesh, my Internet provider, and Kartik, my software consultant, for their ready and sustained assistance; and to Professional Touch for their services in having the whole manuscript typed.

My sincere thanks are due to Dr. Nagalakshmi Narayanan of Osmania University, India, for reading through the manuscript and making valuable suggestions, especially in the chapter on Patañjali. My thanks are also due to Dr. Laurel Smith for her help and suggestions in making useful changes to the manuscript. Again my thanks are due to Ehud Sperling, president, and Rowan Jacobsen, managing editor, Inner Traditions, for their efforts in publishing the book. I am much beholden to Cannon Labrie for bringing his vast experience and knowledge of Indology and Sanskrit to bear on the editing of the book.

# Introduction

MORE BOOKS ON YOGA HAVE BEEN WRITTEN in the past twenty years than ever before, perhaps since Vedic times. It might seem that there would be no need for yet another book on the subject, but I felt that I had something to add to the discussion. My goal is to portray the three aspects of yoga—as art, physical therapy, and philosophy—that are appropriate for the young, for the middle-aged, and for retirees, in that order. The physical therapy aspects are not discussed separately from various *āsanas*, *vinyāsas*, *prāṇāyāma*, and chants. It should be mentioned that this book is not a substitute for a teacher or a physical therapist; it is written for general information.

In *Yoga Rahasya*, Nāthamuni refers to the need to take into consideration the individual's stage in life while practicing yoga. The general rule is to follow *vṛddhi*, *sthiti*, and *laya kramas* (methods) during, respectively, youth, midlife, and old age. When one is young, the body is known as *deha*, because it grows. At that stage of life, practicing *āsanas* as an art *(vinyāsa)* is appropriate. The various *āsanas* and the myriad *vinyāsas*, with proper breathing, help the young person grow *(vṛddhi)* with good physical and mental health. This aspect is dealt with extensively in several chapters in this book.

During midlife, when there is neither growth nor decay *(sthiti)*, the yoga practice would include important *āsanas* with a few *vinyāsas*, good yogic breathing exercises and *bandhas* (locks), meditation, mantra chants, and so on. These aspects also are covered in this book. In midlife the main requirement is to maintain mental and physical health and ward off diseases. This is the stage when one has to achieve results, discharge heavy responsibilities, and make progress in life. As one gets old, when the body is called *śarīra* because it decays, yoga practice will be directed to maintain reasonable mobility, through *āsana* and *prāṇāyāma* practice. The *laya krama* will consist primarily of intense meditation, along with study of, and reflection upon, the philosophy of Yoga. These aspects, too, are given extensive treatment.

But the yogi's life is a long journey to *kaivalya,* or liberation, and could take several life cycles to achieve. While ordinary mortals would cherish the desire to defy death, the yogi wants to defy rebirth. Classical Yoga defines a yogi's spiritual evolution as comprising three stages, or levels, and this book is structured accordingly.

This book follows the thought progression of Patañjali, author of the *Yogasūtras,* but it adds material gathered from my guru and from other authentic yoga texts, as well as from my own understanding of the subject. Chapter 1 is about my studies with my teacher, Paṇḍit Śrī T. Kriṣṇamācārya, and a few other elders. This chapter may be read first to get a better appreciation of my treatment of the subject. Chapter 2 tells the story of Patañjali from folkloric sources, compiled by a Sanskrit scholar some three hundred years ago. Chapter 3 discusses the definitions of the word *yoga* and gives the essentials of some ancient yoga systems. This chapter may provide a good introduction for those with a general interest in Indian philosophies, and also for those who have been studying yoga, especially *haṭhayoga,* for a long time and who would like to now move on to other aspects of yoga. *Mantrayoga* is the subject of chapter 4, and it is treated as part of the *kriyāyoga* of Patañjali. My teacher placed considerable emphasis on chants *(pārāyaṇa* of the *mūla granthas)* and on the study of scripture, and hence I would recommend this to all students of yoga. Part 1 concludes with chapter 6, which gives all the dos and don'ts for practicing *aṣṭāṅgayoga* and is universally applicable to all forms of yoga. In part 2, chapters 7 to 13, different important groups of *āsanas,* along with their variations or *vinyāsas* and health benefits, are presented in detail.

This book is addressed not to absolute beginners, but to those who have been practicing *yogāsanas* for some time, or to those who have come to yoga for health reasons. It should also be useful to *haṭhayoga* teachers and physical therapists, who should know as many *vinyāsas* on the various *āsanas* as possible so they can design a regimen for their students and those who come to them for help. *Vinyāsakrama,* the art of linking together related sequences of *āsanas,* brings the entire scope and depth of *āsana* practice into focus, and if one studies it, it will help the teacher or physical therapist to tailor a program for the student according to his or her individual needs. In Sanskrit, *viniyoga* means "individual distribution," and the teacher should be well equipped with *vinyāsakrama* in order to give what should be given to whom. Chapters 14 to 16 are for those who want to go beyond *āsanas* and *prāṇāyāma.* Anyone who feels stuck in his or her routine *haṭha* practice may find these last three chapters opening up a different dimension to the practice of yoga.

# PART ONE

# *Yoga Siddhānta*, or Theory

# 1 My Studies with Śrī T. Kriṣṇamācārya and Others

*The purpose of life is to understand the meaning of the*
*śāstras (scriptures).*

—Paṇḍit T. Kriṣṇamācārya

MY FAMILY HAILS FROM A SMALL, picturesque village known as Kari-suzhnda-mangalam ("a serene place surrounded by elephants") in deep south India. It is situated along the southern bank of the Tāmrabharaṇi River and boasts several native sons who were great saints and spiritual scholars. Śrī Nāthamuni, the famous Vaisnavite yogi and the inspirational beacon for my guru, Paṇḍit T. Kriṣṇamācārya, in the writing of his *Yoga Rahasya* (Secret of Yoga), was one of them, as was Śrī Sadāśiva Brahmendra, an Advaita yogi of the Śaṅkara school of Vedānta who wrote a succint and independent commentary on the *Yogasūtras* of Patañjali.

I was born in a Tamil *smārta* family. *Smārtas* are those who follow the religious and ethical codebooks called Smṛtis that were written by different ṛṣis (sages) and that closely adhere to the Vedas. Sage Āpastambha's books are followed by most families in south India. Our family deity *(kula devata)* is Lord Venkaṭācalapati, the same presiding deity as in the famous hill temple of Tirumala. My great-grandfather was a priest in the village temple and was himself an *upāsaka* (worshiper) of Lord Narasimha, the man-lion incarnation of Lord Viṣṇu.

My *upanayana* (thread ceremony or religious initiation) was performed when I was nine in the Tirumala hill temple. The *brahma upadeśa* (Vedic initiation) was done by my grandfather, as my father was, at the same auspicious time *(muhūrta)*, performing an initiation ceremony for my older brother, and thus my grandfather became my first guru. Over a period of about two months, he taught me to do *sandhyāvandanam,* the oblation to the sun and other deities performed thrice daily, at dawn, at midday, and at dusk.

One day a few months after my initiation, at about five o'clock in the morning, I heard Vedic chanting in my house. My father, because he was not able to learn Vedic chanting *(pārāyaṇa)* when he was young, having moved in his teens to the city of Madras for work, had decided to learn Vedic chanting at the young age of forty-five. His teacher was a scholar from the renowned Sanskrit college at Madras. The method of teaching involved the teacher speaking a manageable portion of the Vedic mantra that was then repeated twice by the student, followed by the same process with the next portion, and so on. This would go on for a few days, with maybe twenty-five to thirty portions learned each day, until the student could perfectly chant a section along with the teacher. In ancient times no books were used, but in the past one hundred years or so, books with notations of the *svara* (notes), which make it easier to learn chanting, have appeared. Purists frown on the practice of learning from such books rather than committing the notes to memory. That morning I quickly performed my ablutions and sat with my father and started learning to chant with him. He was well into the chapter on the *sūryanamaskāra* (sun salutation), which is the first chapter in the Yajur Veda of the Taittirīya delineation, Āraṇyaka (forest chants) portion. We completed it in about six months; the chanting of this chapter normally would take about one hour. Being young (about ten years old), I was able to listen intently and pronounce clearly all the mantras. I was happy doing this exercise, and I still believe that youngsters like to chant. This learning of Vedic chanting went on almost every morning for about four years, and by the end of that period we had completed, apart from the *sūryanamaskāra,* the five *sūktas* (stanzas); three chapters of Taittirīya Upaniṣad and the Mahānarayaṇa Upaniṣad, which together from the last four chapters of the Kṛṣṇa Yajur Veda; and Rudram and Camakam from the Taittirīya Saṃhitā of the same Veda. I then had some lessons in Sanskrit grammar, Sanskrit being the third language I had to study in school, in addition to Tamil, my mother tongue, and English.

I was fortunate to go to a school run by the renowned Rāmakriṣṇa Mission. Even as I was receiving instruction in Vedic chanting, the school afforded the necessary atmosphere for religious studies. For a few days every week, in the morning hours, we would listen to discourses by a *paurāṇika* (an expert in Purāṇa, or Hindu mythology), Kallidaikurici Rāmakrisṇa Śāstri, on the two great epics *(itihāsas),* the Rāmāyaṇa and Mahābhārata. In the afternoon, during lunch break, a few of us would gather for informal lectures on the Bhagavad Gītā, given by the principal of the school, Anna Subramania Iyer. Many in south India knew the principal as a great scholar and a devotee of Śakti. His Friday prayers to the goddess Devī and the group recitation of the Lalitā Sahasranāma (One Thousand Names of Lalitā) were well attended. He translated several Hindu classics, including the 108 Upaniṣads and Purāṇic works such as Devī Māhātmya (the Glory of Devī) and the *Soundarya Laharī* (Wave of Beauty), for the Rāmakriṣṇa Mutt, which published them; these books are read by thousands of devotees, even today. In my house, at that time, my mother organized *pūjā* for Mīnākṣī (the presiding deity of the famous Madurai temple) with the recitation of the Lalitā Sahasranāma. All other religious functions were faithfully followed in our house. Frequent *homas* (fire worship) and *pūjās* (religious rites) were also conducted at home. I also had *yogāsana* lessons in school taught by a teacher there. We used to give *āsana* demonstrations on special occasions such as parents' days and other school days.

I went to junior college in 1954. The institution was known as Vivekānanda College, named after the outstanding Hindu spiritual master, and it was also run by the Rāmakriṣṇa Mission. I studied mathematics, physics, and chemistry, and, of course, Sanskrit.

One afternoon, as I was coming out of class, I saw an elderly man pass by. Wearing a pure white dhoti and the upper loose cloth, he seemed to have an arresting personality. I thought from his looks that he had come to the college to initiate someone and perform some *pūjā.* But I was later surprised to find that he was a yoga teacher engaged by the college to teach a few interested students. I always thought that yoga teachers wore shorts and were dry, skinny, and hungry-looking—at least that was what all the yoga teachers and yogis I had come across looked like.

A few days later, at about 7:30 A.M., the same person came to my house in a rickshaw. He was stern-looking. My father received him and took him upstairs to start some physical therapy lessons for my elder brother. The man left an hour later and then started coming five days a week. Soon enough, my father and mother joined the yoga lessons, followed by my sister and myself. He used to teach each of us different āsanas at the same time: inverted postures for me, the desk pose for my mother, a lengthy stay in *pascimatānāsana* for my brother, and exquisite back-bending *āsanas* and *vinyāsas* like *uṣtrāsana* for my little sister. What struck us even on the first day was the introduction of breathing with the movements, something that we had never known. "Inhale with a hissing sound, or exhale with a rubbing sensation in the throat," he would say in English, even as he would talk to us in general in his accented Tamil. We all loved those classes. He was known to us in the family as *āsana vādyar* (teacher of *āsanas*). One day I learned his name was Paṇḍit T. Kriṣṇamācārya. He would keep on changing the routine of *āsanas* and *prāṇāyāma,* and each class would be different and interesting.

One day, I did not attend the class because of some stomach cramps. As he was going out, he stopped by and asked me why I did not attend. When I said sheepishly that I had stomachache, he asked me to lie down, checked my *nādī* (pulse), and then examined my abdomen. He then dug his strong fingers and thumbs into the rectus abdominus below the navel and gripped the muscles with both hands. He slowly but firmly pulled up the muscles, held them for a few seconds, and then let go. He did that a couple of times more and the feeling was very pleasant. I felt the taut muscles relax, and the cramps disappeared momentarily. With a smile he left, asking me not to eat spicy food for a couple of days and to take periodically small quantities of gooseberry and ginger. His fingers were thick and firm, and his touch, sure.

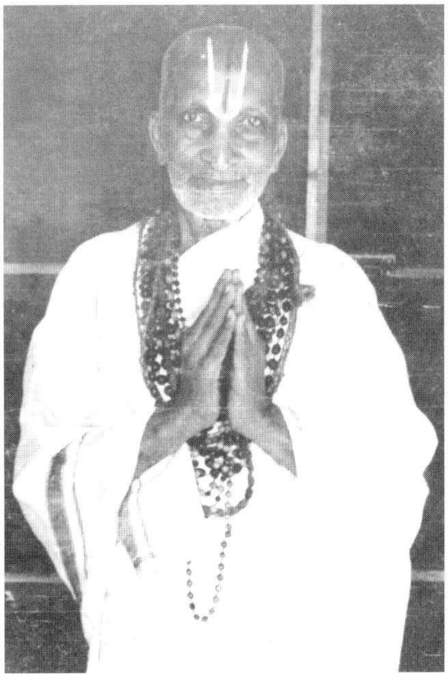

*Photo by the author.*

Śrī T. Kriṣṇamācārya in his nineties

The next four years, I was in Coimbatore for my undergraduate studies in electrical engineering. But every summer and during interterm holidays, I used to join the group for more yoga classes. It is fun doing very difficult postures, especially when one is young, but I had other interests like playing tennis, acting in stage plays, and so on. He used to correct all the movements, sometimes holding one's legs or the arms or supporting the body, as in shoulder stand or headstand. At the beginning of each class he would sit erect in an *āsana* and recite the appropriate prayers. He would repeat this at the end of class. He had a very deep voice, but it was very pleasant. He had a magnetic personality. Anybody who passed by would involuntarily turn and take a second look at him, a young, handsome, sixty-five-year-old.

In 1960, after graduating, I got a job in a mining company's electrical generation plant, about 150 miles from Madras. I had wanted to continue to study with my teacher, but the only way was to find a job in the city itself, and this was difficult. One day I told my teacher that I had to leave Madras. He immediately talked to my father and suggested to him that he get me a job in Madras. My father was a leading stockbroker who had helped in the formation of a few industrial undertakings. Soon enough, I got a junior-level job in a company that was manufacturing motorcycles.

During this period, only my father and myself from our family were studying with him. My job required that I be at the factory at 7 A.M. and I needed to catch the factory bus at 6 A.M. Śrī Kriṣṇamācārya by then had many more students, and he had asked us to come to his house for the classes.

We knew that Śrī Kriṣṇamācārya used to be up at 2 or 3 A.M. to do his yoga practice and his *pūjā,* and used to be in his room to receive his first student at about 7 A.M. It was then decided that both my father and I would be at his home early enough to have an hour-long class. So we used to get up at 4:00 A.M., have a bath, and drive to his home by 4:45. After an hour's class, my father would drop me at the bus stop by 6 o'clock and return home. Every morning for six days a week we would be at his house at the appointed hour, when, having completed his morning workout, we would find him ready and waiting for the early-bird students. God knows how he managed to do it all.

Proper breathing was given equal or more importance than the postures. After a few *vinyāsas,* if a student appeared to be tired or having difficulty breathing, Śrī Kriṣṇamācārya would ask him to lie down and rest, during which time the student would be asked to follow the breath rather than allow the mind to wander. Sometimes he would recite a passage from the Rāmāyaṇa or Mahābhārata, or another great work, and explain an idea or two. *"Anabhyāse viṣam vidyā,"* he would say and then explain the meaning: Anything one studies must be put into practice or else it will produce undesirable results. Never did I hear him discuss politics or indulge in small talk. He was always kind and pleasant, and would inquire occasionally about the welfare of family members but never say anything flippant. It would appear that his mind was always attuned to imparting his vast knowledge of the *śāstras* and the tradition to which he proudly belonged.

The early-morning classes went on for about a year before I left to attend Oklahoma State University for graduate study in industrial engineering and management. I returned home in 1962, after completing the requirements for a master's degree. I had the option, like many other Indian students, to go on for a Ph.D. or take a job in the United States, but I decided to return home, as I was convinced more than ever that I wanted to continue my studies with my teacher. Looking back, I feel that this was one of the best decisions I have ever made. It would have been a shame if I had not made use of this God-given, golden opportunity.

My studies became more intensive, and I learned more *vinyāsas* and *āsanas.* Sometime in 1965, about ten years into my studies with him, it was decided that some of his long-term students should learn more theory and study the original texts. He started *svādhyāya,* or Vedic recitation. Even though I had done quite a bit of Vedic chanting when I was young, I resumed chanting classes with him. His chanting was clearer and slower. He would not put up with even minor mispronunciations or mistakes in the *svara* (notes). Once again I started with the Taittirīya Upaniṣad and the Mahānārāyaṇa Upaniṣad, which are the last four chapters of the Kṛṣṇa Yajur Veda. One day Śrī Kriṣṇamācārya explained the last portion of *śikṣā valli* (on

Vedic chanting) of the Taittirīya Upaniṣad and the interesting paragraph containing what may be termed a convocation or commencement address *(anuśāsana)* of the teacher to the graduating *(sāmavartana)* students. He suddenly looked up and said to me, "You have studied English. Why don't you translate this paragraph, make copies, and distribute them to as many people as you can?" I did the translation and got it printed with some money I had and distributed it free to as many of my friends as possible. I do not know how many read it, but I was happy at that little exercise. It slowly dawned on me that he was not just another *āsana* teacher, but also a great scholar of our scriptures. As we chanted, he might stop in the middle, explain a few passages or mantras, and go on. In India, many people who chant (there are exceptions) do not always know the meaning of what they chant, so it was a great revelation to me that I had stumbled onto an *ācārya* without even having made an attempt to find one. Who could be luckier?

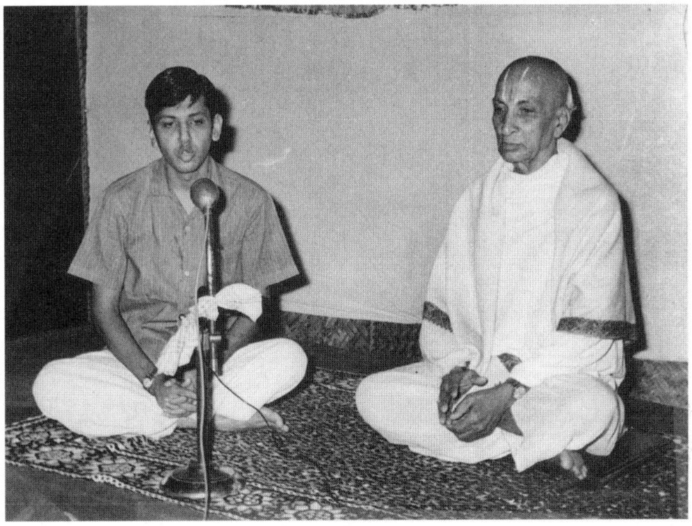

The author with Śrī T. Kriṣṇamācārya, 1968

My mother, who was married at the age of fourteen and had lost her mother when she was a child, was a very religious person. Her daily routine included cleaning the *pūjā* room, lighting the lamp in the morning and at dusk, and doing *pūjā*, prayers, and meditation. She observed festival *pūjā* rites scrupulously. She was an ardent devotee of the divine Mother, and every Friday she would perform *pūjā* for the goddess Mīnākṣī, with the Lalitā Sahasranāma performed by family priests in our home. My mother also started taking specific *vratas* (religious vows), and she made my father perform several Vedic functions in our home. In short, there was some religious activity or other taking place in our house all through the year.

When we were children my mother also used to tell us religious stories (like most mothers did in India), and we were quite familiar with Hindu mythology. She gave me, when I was very young, children's books on the Mahābhārata, Rāmāyaṇa, and Bhagavad Gītā, three monumental works. She had a steadfast belief in the grace of the divine Mother. Additionally, my paternal grandmother was a voracious reader of the original Purāṇas written in Tamil, which she read aloud and to which we children used to sit around and listen. In addition, my parents quite often took us to religious discourses on the great epics and Purāṇas, which contain many educational and morally uplifting stories and which form the bedrock of Hindu *dharma*, or law of piety.

One day Śrī Krisṇamācārya said that we would begin study of some important texts in order to reinforce our understanding of yoga. He started with the *Yogasūtras* of Patañjali. First we learned how to chant the sūtras and then took up the meaning of the words. To explain the sūtras he referred to the commentary of Vyāsa. As a practicing yogi, his explanations of the sūtras were lively and very profound. Simultaneously, I started reading the commentary on the *Yogasūtras* written by Śrī Sadāśiva Brahmendra and the *vivaraṇa* (elucidation) by Śrī Śaṅkarācārya on Vyāsa's commentary. I should confess that by then I had started getting into studying independently some of the preliminary works *(prakaraṇa grantha)* of Ādi Śaṅkara. Being from deep south India, our family was affiliated with the Śaṅkara Maṭh of Śrīngeri. I had *darśan* of the Śaṅkarācārya of Śrīngeri during my visits to south India. During one of the visits of the *ācārya,* my father invited him to visit our home and bless us all. It used to be the custom to invite great *sannyāsis* (spiritual mendicants) to visit one's home, host them, and pay homage to them. It was a great experience to watch the *ācārya* perform *pūjā,* and also hear him speak about Hindu *dharma* in general and Advaita philosophy in particular. After listening to him, I became more interested in Advaita literature. The Śrīngeri Maṭh had at that time undertaken to translate into Tamil and publish the great Sanskrit works of Ādi Śaṅkara on Advaita, such as his *Aparokṣaṅubhūti* (Direct Experience of the Self), *Ātma Bodha* (Knowledge of the Self), and so on. My father subscribed to them, and over the course of a few years these books, about twenty-eight in number, arrived one by one, and I studied them very closely. Fortunately, a friend of my father's, Śrī S. V. Harihara Iyer, who was about forty years older than I, worked near my office, and almost every day, during lunch hour, I used to ask him questions on the transcendental nature of Advaita. He himself had attended several lectures in the early 1930s and 1940s given by the renowned pontiff of Kāncīpuram, the Śaṅkara Maṭh, who was *paramācārya* (the highest teacher). He helped me understand many intricate questions contained in Advaitic parlance and explained and helped me reconcile many apparent contradictions.

Thus, even as I was engrossed in the *Yogasūtras,* I was studying with equal interest the Advaita works of Ādi Śaṅkara. This helped me to make a comparative study of the two important sister philosophies derived from the Vedas. Further, I also found that since my teacher was a staunch Vaiṣṇavite, there was a definite orientation toward theism in his teaching of the *Yogasūtras,* whereas Ādi Śaṅkara's commentary on Vyāsa's commentary on the *Yogasūtras* tended to highlight the common features of the *puruṣa* (individual soul) and Īśvara (the supreme soul) and hence their identity. One could see what great thinkers the earlier *ācāryas* were.

At the rate of two or three classes per week, it took nearly two years to go through the whole of Vyāsa's commentary. Śrī Krişṇamācārya would explain every word in the commentary, give the etymological derivation, quote extensively from other texts and narratives, and give examples that were entirely traditional, often with some unusual insights. As a rule I never asked him questions, but on one occasion when I asked a question without much reflection, he was clearly annoyed and told me bluntly that I was not being attentive. I soon realized that my mind had wandered while he was lecturing. Thereafter, if I had any doubt, I would keep it to myself, and sure enough the explanation would come in another session, but come it would. As Śrī Krişṇamācārya lectured, his eyes would be closed, but occasionally he would open them and stare at the attentive student in front of him with his penetrating gaze. Day after day I would attend private class and return home very happy. There was always something new or unusual he would say each day. I never would interrupt him, for the flow of his words were like honey—sweet and continuous. Whenever he was teaching from a text, it would be wonderful. But I also found that when he gave a general talk in public to a more heterogeneous audience, he tended to go off on tangents, skipping from topic to topic, because he wanted to cover a lot of ground within a short period of time. He would visit our home on special occasions at the invitation of my parents and spend some time talking to all of us. He was the chief guest at the function arranged to celebrate the sixtieth birthday *(śaṣtiabdapūrti)* of my father in 1968. During the evening reception, to an audience of two hundred strong, he gave a talk on Hindu *dharma,* which was well received.

Along with my study of the *Yogasūtras,* I continued to take chanting classes. Again we took up the chapter on the Sūryanamaskāra (sun salutation), the largest in the Yajur Veda, and every Sunday I attended his joint chanting session, which took about an hour. His pronunciation was clear; the flow, effortless. I never failed to feel a sense of peace and satisfaction after one of those sessions; God knows how many Sundays we did this chanting.

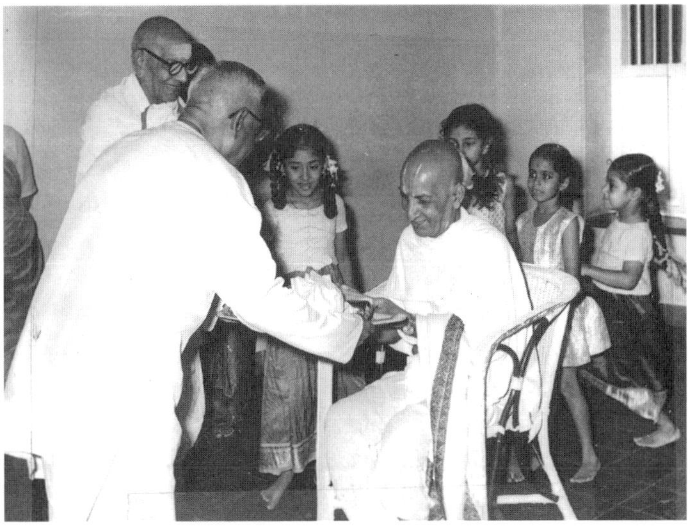

Śrī T. Krişṇamācārya being received by Śrī H. Subramaniam, the author's father and Krişṇamācārya's student, on the sixtieth birthday of Mr. Subramaniam in 1968

The next chapter we learned to chant was the one on *svādhyāya,* which contains *kuşmāṇḍa homa* mantras. This chapter follows the *sūryanamaskāra* chapter and takes about thirty-five minutes to chant. It exults the greatness of the *gāyatrī* mantra and Vedic chanting in general. We also completed the following chapter on *caturhotra*, which starts with the mantra *citti sruk*, and the next two on *pravargya* and *pravargya brāhmaṇa*, respectively, which take about two hours between them to chant. Then we learned the three chapters of Taittirīya Kāṭhaka, the chanting of which takes about two hours. As the years rolled by, my studies with Śrī Kriṣṇamācārya were more open-ended—I let him take care of me and he did, thank God, like a cat takes care of its kittens.

His method of teaching Vedic chanting consisted of dividing the mantras into smaller, more manageable portions, so that when he spoke the mantra, the student would be able to hear and say it twice, correctly and with the correct note *(svara)*. In one sitting, a fifteen-minute passage would take about an hour, allowing time for the gaps between repetition and correction. This process would be repeated for a number of days, and when the teacher was satisfied, the entire passage would be chanted by teacher and student together another five to ten times. Then we would move on to the next portion. Chanting is an integral part of yoga. *Svādhyāya* is a Vedic word used by Patañjali in both *kriyāyoga* and *aṣṭāṅgayoga*. Among other benefits, chanting also helps one's breathing and concentration. My teacher used to say that since each Sanskirt syllable is connected to a different *cakra*, the Vedic mantras were designed in such a way that auspicious vibrations are produced in the various *cakras* when one chants Vedic passages. Also known as Veda *pārāyaṇa*, this practice is considered a sacred part of any religious activity and yoga practice.

Śrī Kriṣṇamācārya also started teaching us to chant a chapter called "Ekāgni Kāṇḍa," which contains mantras for *upanayana* (Vedic initiation) and *vivaha* (wedding). He explained the meaning of the vows, prayers, and rituals in great detail. He also explained that *sannyāsa*, or the life of a renunciate, is neither desirable nor even possible in the Kali Yuga. That being the case, except for a very small number of people, nobody can choose to remain unmarried. The Veda and its related Smṛtis say that marriage is a necessary *saṃskāra* (cleansing ritual) for the individual. The scriptures do allow for a few, who, remaining in *gurukula* (a guru's house), being absolutely desireless and having complete control over their senses, to remain a *naiṣṭika brahmacāri* (absolute bachelor) all their lives and then attain salvation without going through the other stages of life. According to Mīmāṃsā, which is one of the six *darśanas* (Vedic expositions), remaining a bachelor is permitted only in the case of one who has the temperament and physical capacity to maintain celibacy in the stictest sense, and anyone who does not meet this requirement has no option to remain unmarried. Śrī Kriṣṇamācārya would be very disparaging about institutions or religious practices where a large number of people take to the celibate life, say, in an *āśram* or a monastery-like setting. And to attain salvation, he would say, celibacy was not an absolute necessity; one can, if one matures spiritually, take to *sannyāsa* after leading the life of a householder and discharging one's duties to one's family, one's forefathers, and society at large. Soon enough, I got married, and, touch wood, I have remained happily married to date.

I had not entertained any idea of teaching myself, being perfectly happy to continue my studies. My desire to study with that ocean of knowledge and experience continued unabated. So in 1967, when I was selected to do a two-year graduate program at the Harvard School of Business—after considerable deliberation—I decided to forgo that opportunity. By then I had joined my father's business, both to make a living and to ensure that I would not be required to leave Madras, whether for travel or work, so that I could continue my studies with my teacher.

At this time, in order to prepare me to be a teacher, Śrī Kriṣṇamācārya said that I should start studying other, sister philosophies. A series of Upaniṣad studies started in earnest even as I was attending regular practice classes on *prāṇāyāma, āsana,* and chanting. I started having more classes every week. There were periods when I would have two sessions in a day, one in the morning on practice and the other in the evening on theory. First we took up the Māṇḍūkya Upaniṣad, which gives an esoteric interpretation of the *praṇava* syllable (OM), the only mantra mentioned in the *Yogasūtras.* I simultaneously started private study of the classic commentary on the same Upaniṣad, which is along the lines of Advaita philosophy, Gauḍapāda's *Māṇḍūkya-kārikā* (in which *asparśayoga* is explained). It was a great revelation to study the different approaches to the same Upaniṣad.

For several years thereafter, I had the privilege of studying other Upaniṣads to gain a better understanding of Vedānta, in addition to learning more about yoga. We studied *sad-vidyā* (study of the essential being) from the Chāndogya Upaniṣad of the Sāma Veda, one of the ten best-known Upaniṣads. This contains the great saying *(mahāvākya), "Tat tvam asi"* ("That you are"), which *vakya* itself is interpreted differently by the three renowned schools of Vedānta, Advaita, Viśiṣtādvaita, and Dvaita. We also studied *bhūma vidyā* (the study of the greatest) from the same Upaniṣad. The Upaniṣads, through different *vidyās* (skillful study), explain the same ultimate truth from different viewpoints, answering different questions arising in different minds at different times. All students who study yoga as a discipline would do well to study other *darśanas,* especially Vedānta, and students of Vedānta would appreciate Vedānta more if they studied its sister philosophies, such as Sāṃkhya, Yoga, and so on. Śrī Kriṣṇamācārya had mastered all these Vedic philosophies, as could be seen from the various titles and diplomas he had received from respectable institutions: Nyāyācārya, Sāṃkhya Siromaṇi, Vedānta Vagīsa, Yogācārya, Vedakesari, are some of the titles he had been given in recognition of his scholarship.

As I mentioned before, I had never thought of teaching. So when it was suggested that I could start teaching, with the blessings of my guru I took on a few patients with bronchial asthma who were referred by physicians in the nearby hospital. Their therapy consisted of yoga *āsana vinyāsas* for the auxiliary chest muscles, slow and deliberate *ujjāyi* breathing, and in some cases a gradually introduction to *viparīta karaṇī* (inverted postures) with varied degrees of assistance. The preferred training period was during the summer months, when the attacks were at a minimum. I learned that most of the people I taught showed considerable reduction in the frequency and severity of their attacks in the following year, especially if they continued with the yogic exercises. Many expressed a better sense of well-being, and some even started learning more *āsanas* and breathing routines.

But I could never take to full-time teaching. Except for a very few, yoga teachers in India in those days—and even now—had a very difficult time making both ends meet. The pecuniary needs of my family were taken care of by working in my father's office. I decided to teach during my spare time—late evenings, early mornings, and on holidays and weekends. Teaching would help me clear my mind and allow me to study a subject from various angles.

Kalākṣetra is a renowned institution of Indian arts, founded by Mrs. Rukmini Devī. One day I was directed to meet her, and what followed was a twenty-year association with the institution. I started teaching yoga for about a dozen people, half of whom were dance teachers. The others were senior *bharatanātyam* (dance drama) students. Kalākṣetra is a college of arts (now a university) teaching classical *bharatanātyam* and *kathakali,* another form of native classical dance, separate from Carnatic music. I used to teach about twice a week. The classes would run from 6:00 A.M. to 7:00 A.M., and I used to leave home by 5:30 A.M. Being dancers, my students were very supple, sensitive, and graceful, and it was a great pleasure and a unique opportunity to teach them, even though their breathing required much work in order to do the sequences called for in *vinyāsakrama* yoga. In a few years, yoga was included in the curriculum and all the students were obliged to study it.

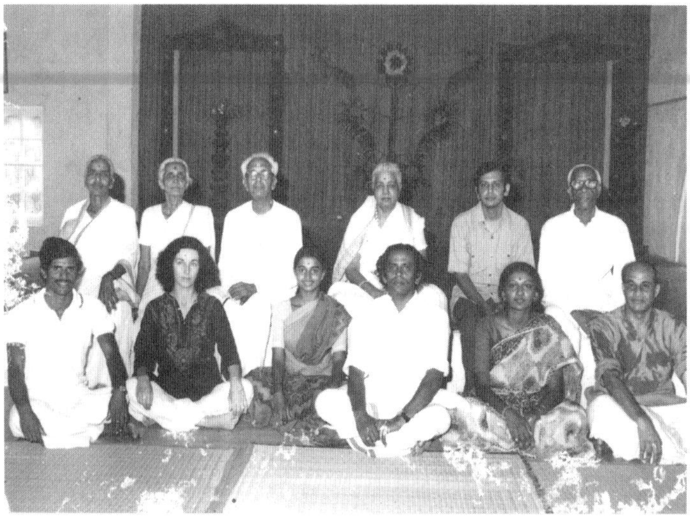

The author (back row, second from right) with Rukmini Devī (third from right), founder-director of the Kalākṣetra Institute, and the institute's first group of yoga students

One day I told my teacher that I had been teaching the students what I had learned from him, which, by and large, was what was required of me. He had taught me several *āsanas* with many *vinyāsas* that, while quite useful to me in my own practice, I felt I was not doing full justice to in my own teaching. Some of the students were so good that their potential was not being brought out. When I expressed my views that as a teacher I needed to have a deeper understanding and know a wider range of *āsanas,* he smiled.

Then he gave me more in-depth instruction in the *vinyāsakrama* way of doing *yogāsanas.* Step by step he showed me all the variations in each of the main postures, the order in which the various *vinyāsas* could be strung together, and the type of breathing to accompany each movement. It took several months to learn all the *vinyāsas,* or at least all those that he taught me. This method of doing *āsanas* is most appropriate for youngsters and is an important part of *vṛddhi* or *śruṣtikrama,* the method of practice for youngsters. I also knew that even though my teacher was teaching me on a one-to-one basis, in his earlier years he had taught yoga in groups. Every teacher should learn the *vinyāsakrama,* especially when teaching children. It brings out the art form of yoga, which is considered one of the sixty-four ancient arts of India. Furthermore, when one learns the *vinyāsakrama,* one will be able to pick and choose some of the appropriate *vinyāsas* and string them together, so that the adapted version can be tailor-made to individual conditions, be it for an elderly person or for someone who requires yoga for physical therapy.

Once in a while, Śrī Kriṣṇamācārya used to say that we should all spread *śāstrīyayoga* (traditional yoga), as many unsavory practices were creeping in. Some of his better-known students had started spreading his yoga far and wide, and yoga students and teachers started taking a deep and critical look at his system as it was taught by his students. There are significant differences in approach among many of his disciples who became teachers. It is hard to explain, but then he taught differently to different people (as I could vouch from what I have seen among my own family members), taking into consideration the temperament, requirements, and capabilities of each person. This is what was unique about his system—that is, his capacity to tailor programs to his students, which was made possible because of his vast experience and deep understanding of the traditional Vedic philosophies.

I soon started offering several free yoga programs with the blessing of my teacher, even though he frowned on the idea of teaching for free. For about seven years, I did these yoga camps for the Yoga Brotherhood, which took care of all the arrangements including publicity. The large hall where I taught, which could accommodate more than one hundred people doing yoga, was given free by the Gītā Bhavan or the AVM charities, and I taught the class with the help of a few of my students from Kalākṣetra and the Public Health Centre, a charitable hospital with about one hundred beds. I was also teaching at the health center as part of the hospital's efforts to promote health using a traditional, indigenous system.

I continued my studies with Śrī Krişņamācārya, both on practice and on theory. We plunged into study of *pañcāgni vidyā* (five fires or five transformations) of the individual self between death and birth from the Bṛhadāraņyaka Upanișad, as well as the Praśna, Muņḍaka, and Kena Upanișads. The first eight sūtras of the Brahma Sūtras (on Vedānta) were also covered in great detail. My teacher even volunteered to teach the Brahma Sūtras, according to the Advaitic interpretation. We also worked through the Śvetāśvatara Upanișad and *Haṭhayogapradīpikā*. The study of all of these works took several years to complete.

For a better appreciation of the *Yogasūtras*, we then took up, in some detail, one of the most clearly written works and a classic in Sanskrit literature—the *Sāṃkhya Kārikā*. This masterpiece describes the Sāṃkhya system of philosophy on which yoga heavily relies. I feel strongly that a better appreciation of the *Yogasūtras* becomes possible by the study of the *Sāṃkhya Kārikā* and the commentaries of Gauḍapāda and Vācaspatimiśra. Patañjali's *Yogasūtras* presuppose an understanding of the essentials of Sāṃkhya. In the meantime, with the blessings of my guru, I also started contributing articles on yoga *āsanas* and other systems of philosophy to some Indian journals both in Tamil and in English. In all, I wrote about fifty articles.

My own private practice boiled down to about a half hour of *vyāyāma (āsanas* and *prāṇāyāma)*, followed by a half hour of Vedic or other chanting, which I used to do in our *pūjā* room. One day our neighbor, Mr. Jayaraman, husband of Mrs. Vani Jairam, a renowned singer, was sitting in the drawing room waiting to meet my father. As I came out of the *pūjā* room, he said that my Vedic chanting was very pleasing and clear. This strengthened my desire to make a recording of the *Yogasūtras*, as at that time a number of yoga students were becoming interested in chanting the *Yogasūtras* as part of their yoga studies.

A couple of my friends volunteered to talk to some audiocassette producers. When I finally got my recording of the *Yogasūtras* heard by a leading recording company, the producers said that they were satisfied with the rendition, but because I was an unknown entity, marketing would be a problem. It was suggested that I try to do a few programs for the national radio network, All India Radio.

At that time television had not made much headway into the countryside, and the smaller towns and villages were still served by radio. After some effort, I managed to get a fifteen-minute program in AIR's Sanskrit slot in which I discussed and recited a few of the *Yogasūtras*.

Before going into the studio, I told Śrī Krişņamācārya about the program and asked him if he would like to listen to the tape I had made. He asked me to close the door and play the tape. He listened to it intently and said that it was clear and nice and blessed me with a beaming face. Naturally, I felt elated. The program was well received and led to further programs in Sanskrit on various topics, such as *prāṇāyāma,* Upaniṣad *kāvya* (literature), the Sūryanamaskāra, *āsana* practice, *haṭhayoga,* wedding mantras, and the story of Patañjali. My teacher encouraged me in preparing for several of the radio programs and also other talks I was invited to give. In fact, he would even dictate part of the text for some of these talks. For the one on Upaniṣad *kāvya,* he composed a masterly survey in Sanskrit, tracing the Upaniṣadic tradition from Vedic times up through the Purāṇas, the Smṛti, the Sūtras, and into the modern period; it was an outstanding essay.

About three years later, a fledgling recording company agreed to record and release a cassette entitled *Yoga of Patañjali and Ādi Śaṅkara,* which contained a synopsis of all four chapters of the *Yogasūtras* as well as chanting and a rendition of Ādi Śaṅkara's *Yoga Taravali.* Because of the general interest in the *Yogasūtras,* I thought that it would be well received, but it bombed. I offered to make good on the losses to the producer. But he in turn offered to do another program. He had received positive feedback about my rendition and thought that things might turn out differently with a more popular topic. He asked if I would record a recitation of the Lalitā Sahasranāma from the Brahmāṇḍa Purāṇa. Though this particular version of the Sahasranāma used to be performed by my mother, I was not familiar with the text. I took a couple of months to study it and then recorded the whole text. It met with good reception. Because of the chanting training I had received from my guru, Śrī Kriṣṇamācārya, the rendering was unhurried and clear, which made it easy for listeners to follow the text and be able to recite it by themselves after listening to the tape a few times.

I was able to record almost all of the Vedic chanting I had learned from my guru, including the Sūryanamaskāra (together) with Varuṇapūjā, which ran for ninety minutes and was one of the earliest, and the Āditya Hṛdayam from the Rāmāyaṇa and the Svādhyāya Prakaraṇa (the chapter on Vedic chanting and *kuṣmāṇḍa homa*). The Taittirīya Upaniṣad, which is one of the earliest chants taught and an Upaniṣad that gives the definition of Brahman and discusses shades of bliss and ultimate bliss, was another important work. The Mahānārāyaṇa Upaniṣad, the last chapter of Yajur Veda, containing the mantras recited daily, like *sandhyā, prāṇāyāma,* and so on, was also released, as was the *aśvamedha,* the famous mantra recited during the highest Vedic rite, and which ran for three hours. The third chapter in Taittirīya Āraṇyaka, along with Śiva Kavacam (Protection by Lord Śiva), was yet another popular subject. I also recorded and released several other Purāṇa and Smṛti works in Sanskrit that are regularly recited by Hindus. They included the *sahasranāma* of all the deities popularly worshiped, such as Viṣṇu, Subrahamaṇya, Āñjaneya, Rāghavendra (a saint), Gaṇeśa, and Hariharaputra, in addition to the seven-hundred-stanza work on Devī, the Devī Māhātmya (in three volumes) from the Mārkaṇḍeya Purāṇa, all of which texts form part of the yoga of worship *(mantrayoga).*

I also released a recitation of the five-hundred-stanza work called the

*Mukapancaśati* on the goddess Kāmākṣī of Kāncīpuram. The *paramācārya,* Śaṅkarācārya of Kānci Maṭh (who lived for one hundred years), listened to the cassette and blessed me with a shawl. These readings, which run for three hours, contain an introduction by the present Śaṅkarācārya of Kānci Maṭh, Śrī Jayendra Sarasvatī. The Bala Rāmāyaṇa (History of Lord Rāma), a classic of over two hundred verses, is a condensed version of the whole of the Rāmāyaṇa, the text taught to beginning students of Sanskrit in schools in India. It also contains an introduction by the Kānci pontiff. In all, twenty-five cassettes were released on many Hindu classics that are normally used for *pārāyaṇa* (chanting or prayer). I have also completed the recording of the Sundara Kāṇḍa, the fifth chapter of the Vālmīki Rāmāyaṇa. This work, which contains about three thousand verses (including the coronation of Śrī Rāma in Yuddha Kāṇḍa), is contained in a set of ten, one-hour cassettes. *Svādhyāya,* or chanting, is an important aspect of the *kriyāyoga* and *aṣṭāṅgayoga* of Patañjali. In the course of my training, my guru spent perhaps as much time on chanting and theoretical studies *(svādhyāya)* as on the physical aspects of yoga.

During the early years, Śrī Kriṣṇamācārya used to quote often from the *Yoga Rahasya* of Nāthamuni, many of which quotes I noted down. For instance, he quoted the following passage to emphasize the importance of finding means for contraception and family planning *(mitā santāna).* This *sloka, Pāśāsanam yoganidrā garbhapiṇḍañca bhadrakam | Matsyendrāsanākhyete, sarva garbha nirodhakāḥ,* mentions the *āsanas* (noose posture, yogic reclining posture, fetus posture, auspicious posture, kingfish posture) that prevent conception. But when I asked him where the text was available, he said with a chuckle that it used to be available at Sarabhoji Māhāraja of Tanjore and that he had seen the text, which was written on palm leaves and kept in an ivory box. He even suggested that I write to the Sarasvatī Mahal library in Tanjore and ask for a copy. I did write to them, and received a reply that no such text existed. I subsequently learned from a Vaiṣṇavite friend that Nāthamuni had intended to transmit the knowledge of yoga, the *Yoga Rahasya* (Secret of Yoga), to his grandson, but he passed away before he could do so. I sort of figured out that *Yoga Rahasya* was the work of my own guru, inspired by his *upāsana* (devotion) to Nāthamuni. The work contained several of the instructions Śrī Kriṣṇamācārya used to give while teaching yoga. But there were variations in the same *slokas,* when he quoted them on different occasions, which is further evidence that *Yoga Rahasya* may have been the masterpiece of my own guru, inspired by tradition and devotion.

In the early days of my studies, I accompanied Śrī Kriṣṇamācārya to several temples. I remember vividly our visits to temples of Śrī Rāma at Madurantakam, Tiruvallur, Sṛperumpudur, Kāncīpuram, and others. He climbed the steep steps at Sholingar for almost an hour to reach the shrine of Lord Narasiṃha. He was always respectfully received by the temple authorities, and visitors to the temple would pay their respects to him in the traditional way.

During the last four or five years of his life, from 1985 until his death, my visits to him became infrequent, as he was exceptionally busy and much sought after by scholars from abroad and from within India. His movements also became rather restricted due to a fall. He managed to overcome the problem to some extent and was able to sit up for long hours to instruct his disciples. I again went to him for lessons in 1988, a year before he passed away. He gave me voluminous notes in Sanskrit on some of the Upaniṣads, marriage mantras, and other subjects, but most of our time together was spent in chanting various Vedic texts. Sometimes he would even lie down in bed and recite from memory, while I followed with the help of a book. One morning when I went to see him, he was sitting up in bed and preparing for his daily *pūjā*, the icons in position in front of him on the table. He was applying *tiruman* (holy dust) to his forehead with all the care and attention in the world. For ten minutes I watched him doing the *pūjā*, totally concentrated, absolutely oblivious to my presence at his doorstep. He was concentration and devotion personified while doing *pūjā* alone at the age of ninety-nine. One could feel the depth of his faith and devotion.

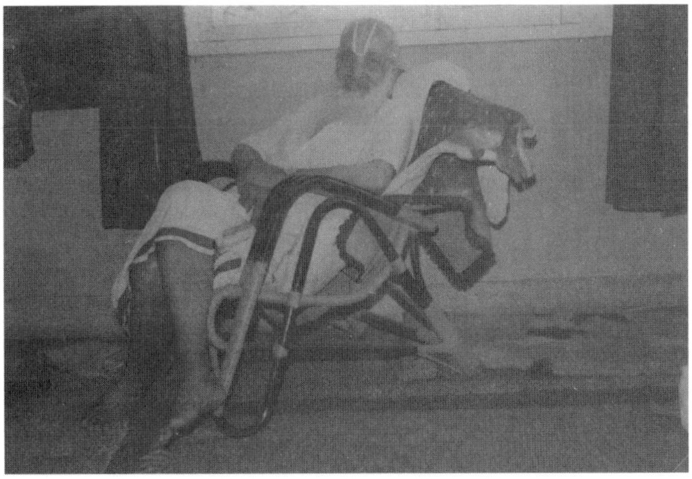

Śrī T. Kriṣṇamācārya, age ninety, in the room where he taught yoga for several years. (Photo by Professor T. Radakrishnan)

One day as we completed a session, I heard him, at least I thought I heard him—perhaps I imagined it—say that I should try to become like him *(yenna mathiri varanum).* I was choked with emotion as I walked out of his room. Thereafter, I stopped going for his classes, since there was a lot of activity with his centenary approaching—TV crews, journalists, biographers, scholars, foreign yoga experts, publicity people, and several others were all over his Spartan little abode.

One morning I heard that he was seriously ill, and I went to see him with my parents. He was attended by some of his senior students. When later that afternoon I heard that he had reached the lotus feet of the Lord (Ācārya Tiruvadi), we went again to pay our last respects. Appropriately, on his chest were the sandals *(pādukā)* of the icons he had worshiped. I felt a lump in my throat; I had enjoyed a long association with him. Although I was not intimately close to him, there was always an undercurrent of goodwill and affection. Ours was the optimum student-teacher relationship for more than three and a half decades.

At sixty, one tends to look back rather than forward. One thing that appealed to me throughout my studies with him was his unshaken faith in, and devotion to, God and the authenticity of the *śāstras* (scriptures). One day he would ask a question, "What is the purpose of life?" He himself would answer, "The purpose of life is to study the *śāstras,* understand their meaning, and abide by it." I was drawn to him and continued to study under him for perhaps longer than anyone outside of his family, because one feels the confidence and conviction that the *śāstras* are authentic in the presence of his transparent sincerity. In hearing him talk and explain the texts or do yoga, one got the feeling that he was 100 percent genuine and brutally honest. With how many gurus can one get that feeling?

I was fortunate to stumble onto a guru like Śrī Kriṣṇamācārya. Would you not agree?

# 2 The Story of Patañjali

*"My prayers to Patañjali, hailing from a family of sages, who by his work on yoga, grammar, and therapy, helped mankind eradicate defilements of mind, language, and body."*

***—Sanskrit prayer***

PATAÑJALI WAS A *ṚṢI*, a word that means "one who sticks to truth" *(ṛṣayaḥ satyavacasaḥ* and *ṛtey Īṣaṇāt ṛṣiḥ).* The *Amarkośa*, a thesaurus of Sanskrit roots, says that *ṛṣis* and truth speakers are synonymous. A civilization is at its best when the people enjoy good health, express themselves well and meaningfully, and have clarity of thought. Bhartṛhari, a great Sanskrit grammarian and philosopher, emphasizes the need for purity in the three human activities *(kāraṇa)*: mind, speech, and body *(mano, vāk,* and *kāya).*

Maharṣi Patañjali is believed to have written treatises on these three subjects, and evidence for this can be found in eulogies about him in ancient Sanskirt literature. Legend has it that once people suffering from the corruption of the above-mentioned *kāraṇas* prayed to Īśvara (the Lord) for guidance. In response to their prayers, Īśvara sent Ādiśeṣa, the divine serpent king, to incarnate as Patañjali, who then wrote three important texts—on medicine *(cikitsā),* on Sanskrit grammar *(pāda),* and on mental health (yoga).

Patañjali's yoga treatise is written in cryptic statements and contains four chapters *(pāda)*. Being written by a grammarian, the sūtra-like (aphoristic) language of Patañjali is of a very high order and his choice of words immaculate. Patañjali's yoga system, complete unto itself, shows the place and practice of many subsystems such as *jñāna* (wisdom), *bhakti* (devotion), *karma* (action) *kriyā* (purification), *haṭha,* and mantra yogas. An authentic commentary on the sūtras was written by the sage Vyāsa, believed from time immemorial to be the author of the Brahma Sūtras and also the compiler of the Vedas. Further elucidations have also been written by such well-known commentators as Śaṅkarācārya, Vācaspatimiśra, Rājabhoja, and Sādāśiva Brahmendra. Swāmi Vivekānanda also has written a detailed commentary on the *Yogasūtras*.

About Patañjali, an outstanding devotee of Lord Śiva, and an incarnation of Ādiśeṣa (on whom Lord Viṣṇu rests), there are several references in many ancient works. Only a few, however, give his life story, and of them, only Rāmabhadra Dīkṣita's *Patañjali Caritra* is written with Patañjali as the main character *(nāyaka)*. Composed in the style of the great poet *(mahākāvi)* Kālidāsa, this Sanskirt work is considered a *mahākāvya* (a great work of literature). When comparing references to Patañjali in other works, there are a few differences. But written with great poetic beauty and artistry, this work tells, in coherent fashion, the life story of Patañjali. Let us see the drama unfold.

The Lord, with his bewitching smile, is resting on Ādiśeṣa, floating on the milky ocean. The Lord's incarnations as Matsya (fish) and Kūrma (turtle) have been completed. The milky ocean has been churned, and the unique, priceless objects, such as the Airāvata (the white elephant of Indra), have come out of the ocean, and Mount Mandara, which was used to churn the milky ocean by the *devas* and *asuras* using Vāsuki as the rope, has been put back in its original position. The various creatures in the mountain, such as the serpents—the garlands of Lord Śiva—drink the milk remaining in the crevices and caves of Mount Mandara and are ecstatic.

All of a sudden, Lord Viṣṇu's weight rapidly increases. Ādiśeṣa, as the couch of the Lord, struggles to maintain his balance owing to the increased heaviness of the Lord; he breathes heavily through his thousand hoods. Sanatukmāra the *nityāsūri* (who permanently directs his gaze toward the Lord) himself is disturbed and withdraws a little from his usual fixed position. Garuḍa, the divine aerial vehicle of Viṣṇu, moves toward Ādiśeṣa to help him out, offers him a word of encouragement, and asks about the cause of this sudden change in the weight of the Lord. Ādiśeṣa wonders anxiously if the Lord might be testing him because of a possible lapse on his part. The goddess Śrī Lakṣmī is also shaken. Just then the Lord opens his eyes, waking up from his *yoganidrā* (yogic sleep), and with tears of joy in his eyes. His weight is back to normal and Ādiśeṣa is able to bear the weight of the Lord as before. Ādiśeṣa asks, "My Lord, why this unbearable heaviness?"

With his bewitching smile back on his face, the Lord began to explain the wonderful spectacle he saw when he was in *yoganidrā*. He describes the ecstatic divine dance *(tāṇḍava)* of Lord Śiva in the *ponnambalam* (the golden chamber) to the accompaniment of various musical instruments played rhythmically by several *devas* (celestial beings). It was on account of the infinite bliss *(ānandaghana)*, he experienced that he became heavy, he says. Hearing that, Ādiśeṣa, himself a loyal servant of Lord Viṣṇu and also a great devotee of Lord Śiva, expresses spontaneously his desire to witness the divine dance of Lord Śiva and requests the Lord to give him the boon.

Viṣṇu says that this is exactly what Śiva had ordained Ādiśeṣa to do. By way of background, the grandson of Paṇi, known as Pāṇini, performed severe penance and surrendered to Lord Śiva, once upon a time. Śiva, with great compassion toward Pāṇini, played his small drum *(ḍamaru)*, and from the sound created by the drum was born the Māheśvara Sūtra, the basis of Sanskrit grammar. Based on Māheśvara's aphorisms, Pāṇini wrote a sūtra that became the basic text for Sanskrit grammar. Further, Kātyāyana, again with the grace of Lord Śiva, wrote a detailed commentary on Pāṇini's aphorisms. Then Pāṇini's student Vyāghrabhūta and Kātyāyana's pupil Svabhūti taught the *vārtika* (commentary) to several others. Lord Parameśvara, however, was satisfied neither with the quality of these works nor with the pace of propagation of Sanskirt grammar, which resulted in very unsatisfactory communication among people and a poor understanding of the *śāstras* (scriptures). Hence Lord Śiva desired that Ādiśeṣa take birth as a human being, witness the dance of Śiva, and then write a detailed and authentic commentary on Sanskirt grammar. "Thus the Lord Parameśvara has ordained," Viṣṇu informed the eager Ādiśeṣa. He was overwhelmed with joy at the prospects of witnessing the celestial dance of Naṭarāja (the Lord of the dance, Śiva) and of writing the authentic commentary, the *Mahābhāṣya* (the great elucidation).

In due course, Ādiśeṣa, desiring to reincarnate as a human being, moves around in space looking out for a suitable family to be born into, and reaches a *tapovana* (serene forest). There, as he would later define *ahiṁsā* (nonviolence) in his *Yogasūtras*, he finds *ahiṃsā* fully manifested. Natural malefics are found to live in harmony in one another's company. In that forest, the daughter of a sage, called Goṇikā, was performing penance, desiring a *satputra* (a worthy son). Śeṣa decides to bless Goṇikā by being "born" to her as a child. As she offers oblations to Sūrya (the sun), the *pratyakṣa* (manifest) god, and with her hands kept in *añjali mudrā* (folded), Śeṣa enters into the *arghya* (oblation) water in her hands and falls to the earth as a child along with the water of oblation. Goṇikā, pleased immensely with the birth of the divine child, showers her love on the baby and names him Patañjali, meaning "one who falls out of folded *(añjali)* hands." As years pass by, Patañjali, with a preponderance of the *sattva guṇa* (quality of *dharma*, or order and piety), has a deep desire to do *tapas* (intense meditation) on Śiva. Promising his mother that he would be at her side anytime she needed him, he moves toward the southern seashore to commence his intense meditation on Lord Śiva.

As is his wont, Indra, the celestial king, uneasy with the prospects of the spiritual success of Patañjali, dispatches several celestial damsels to distract the attention of Patañjali and frustrate his yogic attempts to have a vision of Lord Śiva. Patañjali, however, who is to write an authentic text on yoga, remains steadfast in his meditative endeavors, and the damsels *(apsarās)*, sensing defeat, retreat to the abode of Indra. Afraid that Patañjali may curse them later for their *adharmic* (improper) advances, the celestial dancers praise the yogic prowess of Patañjali to Indra.

Subsequently, Lord Maheśvara (Śiva), pleased instantly with the unwavering *sāmadhi* (absorption in yoga) and the intense *tapasya* and *ekāgrya* (one-pointedness) of Patañjali, presents himself, along with his consort, Umā, and seated on his bull, Nandi, in a divine vision to Patañjali. He is ready to grant the boon of the vision of the celestial dance to Patañjali, which was the very purpose of Ādiśeṣa's birth as a human being.

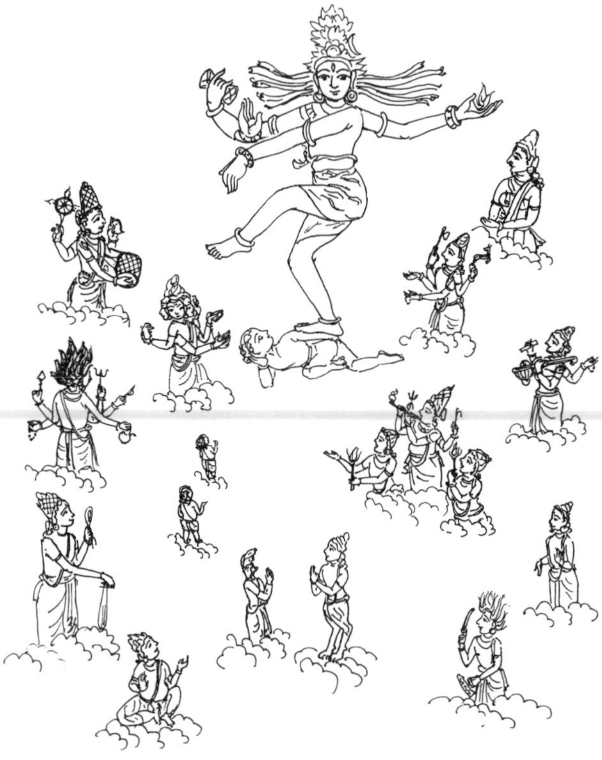

The *ānanda tāṇḍava* of Śiva witnessed by Patañjali

The cosmic vision of the moon-crested Parameśvara brings out the poet in Patañjali. Prostrating himself in front of Him, he eloquently and poetically describes the Lord's immaculate form from foot to head *(pādādi keśānta varṇanā)*. Reminding Patañjali, who because of nescience *(avidyā)* had forgotten his original form of Ādiśeṣa, his true nature and also his mission on earth, the Lord orders him to come to Cidambaram and witness the *ānanda tāṇḍava* (dance of bliss) in order that he may have firsthand knowledge of the original Maheśvara Sūtras and write the Mahābhāsya, or great commentary, on the grammar aphorisms and reconcile the differences and iron out the confusion that had arisen in the work of subsequent authors and teachers. So saying, the Lord disappears.

Journeying along the landscape and forests full of natural beauty and peace, Patañjali reaches the holy place of Cidambaram. There, the *bhūta gaṇās* and other Śiva devotees are waiting, with great expectation, to witness the dance of Śiva. Patañjali, along with another devotee, Vyāghrapāda (tiger-footed), and other sages, reaches the golden theater *(ponnambalam)* to witness the dance. Several celestial gods, among them Agni, Yama, Niruruta, Varuṇa, Marut, Kubera, and, of course, Indra, are already present. Patañjali is overwhelmed by the grand assembly of renowned figures, ordinary mortals, and others expressing their joy by blowing conches and beating drums.

Taking the aerial route, Lord Candraśekhara ("moon-crested"), in all his divine splendor and accompanied by the goddess Umā, arrives at the theater riding the great Nandikeśvara (bull vehicle of Śiva). The celestial dance is about the start. To maintain decorum and to conduct the dance, Nandikeśvara takes the baton. Viṣṇu becomes the percussionist, Brahma plays the chime, Indra the flute, and Sarasvatī the *vīṇā*. Umā, the Lord's consort, oversees the arrangement with her bewitching smile. Specifically asking that Patañjali and Vyāghrapāda carefully and intently watch the dance for all the details, the Lord gives the necessary *divyadṛṣṭi* (divine vision). The great *tāṇḍava* starts with a slow rhythm and in time reaches a crescendo. Engrossed completely in the divine dance, the great sages lose their separate identities and merge in the great oneness *(paravaśa)* created by the *tāṇḍava*. They then realize that this was precisely the experience of *advaita* (oneness with the only essential principle of conciousness). It is said that one gets the *advaita* experience as a result of the grace of Lord Parameśvara. The *tāṇḍava* slowly comes to an end. Asking Patañjali once again to write a commentary on Sanskirt grammar and then return to his divine abode, Śiva disappears from mortal vision. Both Vyāghrapāda and Patañjali, desiring that other devotees not as fortunate as they were also have the bliss of seeing the *tāṇḍava*, engrave in stone the dance of Śiva in Cidambaram. Patañjali, concentrating fully on the divine vision he had of the celestial dance of Śiva, writes a detailed commentary called the *Mahābhāṣya*. Several students, hearing about the greatness of the masterly work, flock to him from all directions. Patañjali, desiring to teach them all simultaneously, but individually as well, withdraws behind a curtain and orders the students not to open the screen; he takes his original form as the thousand-hooded Ādiśeṣa and starts teaching all of them. As is the custom, the students chant the invocatory and ending prayers dutifully and study in an orderly fashion. This goes smoothly up to the point of their studying the sūtra known as the Vasu Sūtra.

Several of his students, unable to control their bewilderment as to how a single person can teach so many of them simultaneously on a one-to-one basis, withdraw the curtain. They are stunned to find Ādiśeṣa instructing them individually with his myriad heads. But the students have committed an offense and have broken the law.

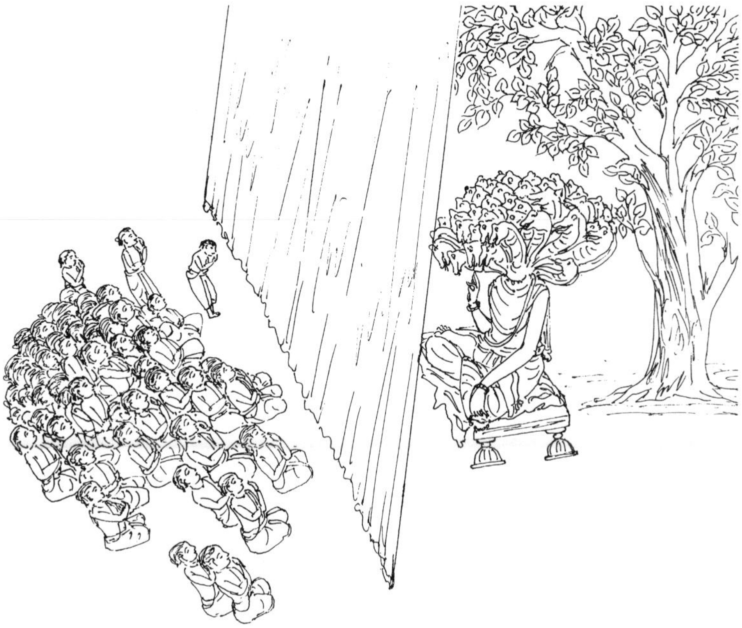

Patañjali teaching Sanskrit grammar to his students in the form of the thousand-headed Ādiśeṣa

It suddenly dawns on one of them, Gauḍapāda, that what has happened is a sacrilege, and everyone will have to pay for this unpardonable indiscretion.

Desiring to save his mates, he ventures to suggest to the furious Patañjali that this unfortunate incident happened because he (Gauḍapāda) had left when the discourse was only half through, Gauḍapāda being the one ordained by Patañjali to guard the screen from being tampered with by the students. Patañjali, angry that a student left class without chanting the *uttara* (ending) *śānti pāṭha* (peace invocation), curses him as a *rākṣasa,* or demon. A *rākṣasa* is one who accumulates wealth but gives away little. Gauḍapāda was cursed to become a *brahma rākṣasa,* one who accumulates knowledge but keeps it to himself. In the olden days, scholars always looked for students to whom they could impart their knowledge, lest they become a *brahma rākṣasa.* Gauḍapāda, like a lightning rod, takes the wrath of the teacher and becomes a *brahma rākṣasa.* Regaining his composure quickly, Patañjali, taking the form of an old man, suggests an antidote for his own curse to his student *brahma rākṣasa.* The curse will be exorcised, he says, "if you are able to find one who could tell him [Gauḍapāda] the *nista* (past participle) of the Sanskrit root *pac,*" a grammatical peculiarity. "After giving full instructions in the *Mahābhāṣya,* Patañjali writes the *Yogasūtras,* a classic on conventional yoga, and another work, a commentary on the science of medicine. He then meets his mother and, after obtaining her blessings and being satisfied that he has accomplished his mission, assumes his original form of the countless-hooded Ādiśeṣa. The *brahma rākṣasa,* sitting on the top of a banyan tree, asks all and sundry who pass by the question posed by Patañjali. Everyone, instead of saying that the *nista* conjugation of *pac* is *pakva,* gives *pacita* for an answer, thinking it like any other root. Promptly they are all gobbled up by the ghost, *brahma rākṣasa.*

With Gauḍapāda as a *brahma rākṣasa* and thus unable to propagate, the

*Mahābhāṣya* (Sanskrit grammar) is not being taught properly and the Sanskrit language starts to suffer corruption. After a considerably long time, Ādiśeṣa, finding that his work had not spread far and wide as expected, takes another human birth. He straightaway goes to the *brahma rākṣasa* and answers the vexing grammatical question himself. The *rākṣasa,* getting down from the tree, and having had his curse and spell removed, volunteers to teach the *Mahābhāṣya* to the traveler.

The traveler says that he is from Ujjain and that his name is Candra. He also says that he came to him only to learn the *Mahābhāṣya.* Even though Candra Śarmā was an *avatāra* of Ādiśeṣa, as is the custom he had to learn the subject from a guru to remove his *ajñāna* (covering veil) to bring out the hidden knowledge in him. Without food or sleep the traveler Candra learns the text of the *Mahābhāṣya* in just two months. He writes down the complete notes on dry banyan leaves, using his fingernails as a pen. Having disburdened himself of the knowledge, the *rākṣasa* assumes his divine form, bids Candra to propagate the text faithfully, and then disappears. Candra collects the leaves and starts walking through the forest.

Upon reaching a beautiful spot in the forest, and having quenched his thirst with the flowing river water, Candra sits down under a tree to spend the night. As he falls asleep, a goat pulls at the bundle of dry leaves containing his notes. Waking up immediately, he collects all the leaves, but finds that in certain places where the teeth of the goat had made an imprint there are marks, making the letters at these places unclear. Because the words were not clear in these places, there could be some doubt about the exact letters used.

Without food and water, Candra travels hither and thither, and falls down unconscious. Then a damsel approaches and gives him some butter to eat. She informs him that she had dutifully served several sages, and they had indicated to her that Patañjali, in the garb of a Brahman scholar—after studying the *Mahābhāṣya* with the *brahma rākṣasa*—would be spotted by her and would marry him. Thereafter Candra Śarmā, on getting the approval of his mother, marries her and takes her to Ujjain. Candra then marries women belonging to other sects, and he fathers four sons, Vararuci, Kātyāyana, Vikramārka, and Bhartṛhari. All of them study the *Mahābhāṣya* with Candra Śarmā. After marrying off all his children, Candra takes to *sannyāsa,* the fourth order of a renunciate, thanks to the grace of his guru Gauḍapāda, and stays in Vārāṇāsī, the renowned abode of learning, for some time. A true Advaitin, he then reaches Badrikāśrama in the Himālayas, establishes a *maṭh* (hermitage), and remains in the experience of *advaita* (oneness with the absolute). He becomes known as Govindaswāmī.

Vararuci, the first son of Candra, was well versed in all the *śāstras* (scriptures) and became proficient in mathematics and astronomy. Vikramārka, later known as Vikramāditya, became a pioneer in law and justice. It is believed that Indra, finding the legal acumen and sense of justice of Vikramāditya superior, gave him a *simhāsana* (throne) made of high-quality gems. He also received Indra's boon to rule the country for a millennium. The other brother, Bhatti (Kātyāyana), becomes his minister. Bhartṛhari, taking his father's profession as a Sanskrit scholar and a grammarian, wrote a grammatical masterpiece called the *Rāvaṇavadha*. He also wrote three well-known works called *satakas* (100 verses) on love *(sṛṅgāra)*, justice *(nītī)*, and dispassion *(vairāgya)*. Then, after going through his father's work in great detail, he prepared a commentary of 125,000 verses. It is said, however, that he became conceited over time and, according to legend, his work became obsolete and without followers.

Enter Śaṅkara, the great Advaita exponent. Śaṅkara, after escaping from the jaws of a crocodile, takes to *sannyāsa* at a very young age and proceeds to Badrikāśrama in the Himālayas to get an audience with Govindaswāmī. One night at Vārāṇāsī, Śaṅkara offers prayers to Śiva in the form of a *liṇga*, and Lord Śiva confers on him the boon to write a detailed commentary on the Brahma Sūtras (aphorisms on Vedānta philosophy). Eating only fruits and drinking plain water, Śaṅkara reaches Badrikāśrama after traveling through many forests. At Badri, Śaṅkara gets a *darśana* with Govindaswāmī, who was in a trance in the caves of the *āśram*. Thereafter, praising him as an incarnation of Ādiśeṣa, Śaṅkara asks that he be taken on as his student. Govinda asks Śaṅkara who he is, and Śaṅkara, with great alacrity, answers that he is "just Śaṅkara" *(kevalah Śaṅkaraḥ aham)*. Realizing that Śaṅkara was an *avatāra* of Lord Śiva himself, Govindaswāmī, as the custom demands, takes on the role of a formal guru to teach Śaṅkara the sciences of the eternal *(brahma vidyā)* and how to attain salvation. Śaṅkara, who writes a commentary *(bhāṣya)* on the Brahma Sūtras in the tradition of Advaita, becomes known all over the world.

This story of Patañjali was written by Rāmabhadra Dīkṣita over three hundred years ago. For a community of people to prosper, richness of language, pure hearts and minds, and good health are all necessary, says Bhartṛhari. For attaining these, the disciplines of grammar, yoga, and life sciences (Āyurveda) developed. Patañjali wrote three authentic texts on these subjects, and that is the most significant part of Patañjali's life. Lord Śiva is also known as Yogeśvara (lord of yoga) and Bhaiṣajaya (great healer). Śiva also gave the original Sūtras the Māheśvara Sūtra, which form the basis of the Sanskirt language, perhaps the oldest one. Thus Patañjali wrote texts on all three subjects by the grace of Lord Parameśvara. The Kaivalya Upaniṣad says that the experience of oneness with the supreme, the *advaita* experience, is possible owing to the grace of Śiva, as the great sages who saw the divine dance of Lord Śiva realized. Thus Patañjali and his later incarnation Govindaswāmī also realized the state of *advaita*. Then the Lord himself became the *avatāra* Śaṅkara and, as was the custom, took initiation from Govindaswāmī (Govinda Bhagavatpāda), an *avatāra* of Ādiśeṣa. Thereafter, Śaṅkara taught the great Advaita through his numerous works, and we know this from studying the story of Patañjali as propounded by Rāmabhadra Dīkṣita.

Scholars may find some historical inaccuracies in the narration of Patañjali's history by Dīkṣita. But he put together the story from the folklore available in different parts of India into a *mahākāvya*. Students of the *Yogasūtras* may want to read this legend of Patañjali compiled and written by Dīkṣita.

# 3 What Is Yoga?

*If a man does not know to which port he is sailing,*
*No wind is favorable to him.*

***—Seneca***

IT IS COMMON KNOWLEDGE that the Sanskirt word *yoga* is derived from the root *yuj,* "to unite." Based on this derivation, the term *yoga* encompasses a variety of practices with different ends. If the word *yoga* means "union," then there will have to exist at least two distinct principles, with some commonality existing between them, prior to the actual union. Furthermore, there has to be some activity in either or both of the principles prior to yoga, so that there is movement toward each other, culminating in union. And a system of yoga that facilitates such a union should not only specify the principles but also detail the relevant activity required for union. It should also define and describe the actual state of union and the resultant experience thereof. It may, as a system, also describe the inferior or subsidiary results.

Perhaps the most important system of yoga based on this interpretation is the one describing the union between the individual soul and the Supreme Being. This system of yoga describes the nature of the individual and the supreme souls, the action necessary for the union, and the subsequent results. *Yoga Yājñavalkya,* an important text on yoga, describes it as: *Saṃyoga yoga ucyate! Jīvātma paramātmanoḥ!,* which means that "total integration between the individual and the supreme souls is called yoga."

The individual soul, or *jīvātma*, depressed at seeing and experiencing unending mundane existence, birth after birth, turns its attention toward the supreme soul. All the efforts toward achieving this ultimate integration between the two souls will come under the yoga. The ultimate experience of the *jīva* in this union is unsurpassed bliss—the Vedas and other texts such as the Smṛtis and Purāṇas describe this in great detail. In the present context, when we define yoga, we are interested in knowing where the activity takes place. Who acts, the individual soul, the supreme soul, or both? There are differing views on that. According to one school, the effort is like that of either a monkey or a cat in taking care of its offspring. A baby monkey, when it wants to be taken care of by its mother, clings to the mother's belly as the mother monkey moves about from branch to branch, tree to tree, wall to wall, going about its activity. The effort and care is on the part of the baby monkey. In this same way, the individual devotee, the *jīva*, should constantly cling mentally to the supreme soul (God), so that in the course of time the merger with the supreme soul takes place. By and large, the effort is on the part of the devotee-soul. This is the essence of *bhaktiyoga*. There is a constant endeavor on the part of the devotee to keep the thought or image of the deity constantly in the mind's eye. After such intense devotion, the mind is nothing but the unwavering thought of the Supreme. In the other view, the god-soul relationship can be likened to that of a cat *(mārjāla)* and its kitten. According to this school, when the individual surrenders completely to the will of God, then He, owing to His immense love for the yearning soul, takes care of it completely and facilitates the emancipation of the *jīva* through its integration with Him. Here the effort emanates entirely from the Supreme Being, and the individual makes the initial move of total surrender, like a kitten that completely lets the mother take care of it—the cat carries the kitten with its teeth as it moves around, keeping its offspring out of harm's way. This initial and total move to surrender oneself to God is called *śaraṇāgati* or *prapatti*. The Lord in the Bhagavad Gītā (18.66) describes this concept as *Sarva dharmān parityajya, māmekaṃ śaraṇaṃ vraja! Ahaṃ tvā sarva pāpebhyo, mokṣayiṣyāmi mā śucaḥ,* "Surrender yourself completely to me, leaving out all concern about your emancipation. I shall remove all the impediments and obtain your release (from mundane existence)."

While *sāyujya* (complete integration, *yuj*, "unity") is the ultimate end of yoga, the inferior ends will include *sāloka* (living in the same world of heaven as the Lord), *sārūpya* (having the same or virtual image of the Lord), *sāmīpya* (constant proximity to the Lord). These goals are described in the Vedas and discussed extensively in the Purāṇas.

Which of the two subsystems is more efficacious—to be constantly engaged all through one's life until the desired, constant vision of the Lord is obtained, as Nārada would say in the *Bhaktisūtras* (Aphorisms on Devotion), or to surrender totally to God and go about doing one's duties properly?

Nārada was a great devotee of Lord Nārāyaṇa. His *Bhaktisūtras* are a classic. He constantly sang the praise of the Lord and held his form in his mind's eye. He became known as an embodiment of devotion. But then, the story goes, he became slightly conceited, thinking that he was the best among all the Lord's devotees. Wanting to bring to Nārada a home truth, the Lord told Nārada that if he wanted to see the best devotee, he should go down to earth *(bhūloka)* to a particular village, where a laborer would toil all day long. After a day's keen observation of the laborer, Nārada returned to see the Lord. "But then he muttered your name just twice in the day, once in the morning as he woke up and again as he retired to bed, and the rest of the day he was going about doing his day's mundane duties. What is so great about that, for a devotee of the Lord?" queried Nārada.

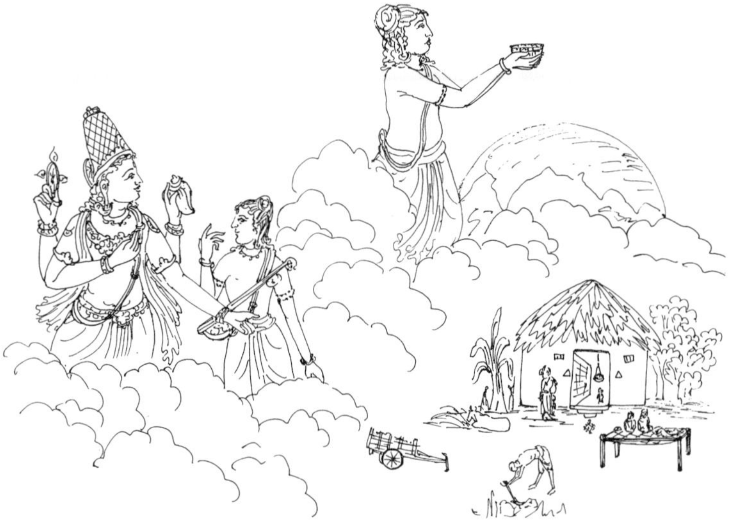

The story of Nārada

The Lord then gave Nārada a small cup filled to the brim with oil and asked him to go around him once *(pradakṣina)*, the only condition being that not a single drop of oil should spill to the ground. Concentrating, Nārada completed the task without spilling a drop. Beaming with joy and pride, Nārada looked up to Nārāyaṇa for appreciation. "But then how often did you think of me, my dear Nārada?" asked the Lord. "Not once," said the great devotee, "not even once." With a mischievous smile the Lord said, "Look at the ordinary man, my other unpretentious devotee. In spite of all the cares of several exacting problems, he never failed to remember me at least twice each day." Nārada was put to shame, but he became a greater devotee, without the conceit.

Suffice it to say that action is needed in yoga. What effort is to be put in by the devotee, and how much ground is covered by the Lord in this yoga or unity of *jīvātma* and *paramātma*, is a matter of lively discussion in several faiths. One may ask one's teacher for more details.

Another classic yogic system involves the union (yoga) of the primordial energy (Śakti) with the supreme principle of auspiciousness (Śiva) in the microcosm itself. The Śiva principle is in the *sahasrāra* (center of thousand petals) in the head and is pure consciousness, or bliss. It does not move. The Śakti in the form of *kuṇḍalinī* (coiled serpent) is at the bottom of the spine, dormant and not moving. Thus, normally there is no movement between the two principles *(tattvas),* Śakti and Śiva, separated, as it were, by the entire spine *(merudaṇḍa)* consisting of six other *cakras* (wheels) and three *granthis* (knots). Arousing *kuṇḍalinī* and guiding its movement all along the *suṣumṇā nāḍī* (fine pathway), piercing through the six *cakras* and cutting asunder the *granthis,* and finally integrating it with the Śiva *tattva* are the components of this yoga. How the Śakti is aroused and guided by the practitioner forms the essence of this system. All the Śakti-worship texts (Tantras) describe in great detail this Śakti principle and the means of achieving its movement and integration with Śiva. The Lalitā Sahasranāma (a text important in the cult of Śakti worship) of the Brahmāṇḍa Purāṇa describes the oneness, or yoga, of Śakti and Śiva (Śiva-Śakti-aikya). So in this system of yoga, the *sādhaka,* or yoga practitioner, follows the procedures given in the texts and by the guru (initiator) and slowly arouses the dormant Śakti in the *mūlādhāra* (the base *cakra*), guides it along the right path to facilitate her union with Śiva, in *suṣumṇā,* all within his own organic being. What does he get by facilitating that union, or yoga? According to Śrīdhara, the commentator on Śaṅkara's *Soundarya Laharī* (Wave of Beauty), the merger produces unsurpassed bliss, which the practitioner experiences permeating all his *nāḍīs* (energy pathways). These methods also describe the experiences that a yogi gets in the intermediate stages, as the *kuṇḍalinī* Śakti moves through the different *cakras* and cuts asunder the three *granthis.*

The unity between the sun and the moon principles, *ha* and *ṭha,* is *haṭhayoga* (the word *haṭha* is usually mispronounced as *hatha,* its *th* as in *feather;* the *t* should be pronounced as it is in *matter,* a strong *t,* with the letter *h* being added to indicate that the *t* is strong). The sun and moon principles in practical terms are *prāṇa* and *apāna,* two aspects of the physiological forces in the body. The union of these two is the objective of this system of yoga, achieved mainly through *āsanas* (postures) and more especially *prāṇāyāma* (breath control). Brahmānanda, a commentator on the *Haṭhayogapradīpikā,* states that the unity of *prāṇa* and *apāna,* or *prāṇāyāma,* is *haṭhayoga.* It is rather strange that many people who practice *haṭha* spend so little time on yogic breathing exercises, choosing instead to do rather involved *āsanas* without proper breathing. In an hour's practice of *haṭha,* they spend the entire time on *āsanas,* ending the session profusely sweating and breathing heavily.

If *prāṇa* and *apāna* are to be united, which should be the more active principle in achieving the union? In *antaḥ-kumbhaka* (internal retention of breath), the *prāṇa,* whose position is in the chest, is pushed down, whereas in *bāhya* (external) *kumbhaka,* the *apāna* is free to move upward with the help of *bandhas* (locks) to facilitate the union. These two *haṭhayoga* practices are identified by Lord Kṛṣṇa in the

Bhagavad Gītā (the Song of God). "Some say that *prāṇa* is to enter *apāna (prāṇam apāne juhavati),* and others say *apāna* entering *prāṇa (apānam prāṇe juhavati)* is yoga." Suffice it to say that the word *yoga,* when interpreted to mean "unity" by a system of practice, should contain the following:

1. A description of the principles *(tattva)* between which unity or yoga is to take place;
2. the method of achieving such union;
3. the intermediate benefits, or milestones;
4. the nature of ultimate unity;
5. the benefit that arises out of such a yoga.

It might also be mentioned that while the term *yoga* is normally used to mean integration between any two principles, in spiritual parlance it refers to unity with a higher principle: *Aprāpya prāpaṇam yogam,* "Yoga is achieving or uniting with the extraordinary." The methodology of yoga is quite involved, prompting Lord Kṛṣṇa to say that a minuscule portion of mankind takes to yoga and a very much smaller portion reaches the ultimate goal.

A variant of the root *yuj* for unity is *yuñj.* The *Dhātupāṭha,* an authoritative work on the meaning and usage of roots, indicates that *yuñj (yuñj-bandhane)* is used to indicate binding. Thus in *mantrayoga,* the unity between the mind of the practitioner and the mantra itself is called yoga. The yogi prepares his mind first, completely removing all distraction by following the preliminary practices *(aṅga)* so as to become a *sāmahita citta* (one with a balanced and serene mind). He then concentrates on the mantra in its entirety, that is, on both the sound and its import. The fourth chapter of Taittirīya Āraṇyaka of the Yajur Veda starts by asking the performer and the priest of the sacrifice *(yajña)* first to prepare the mind with yoga: *Yuñjate mana uta yuñjate dhiyaḥ, viprāḥ viprasya,* "The performer of the *yajña* should unite his mind completely with the mantra."

Sanskirt words are derived from roots. Sometimes, different roots can give rise to the same word; conversely, a word can be considered as derived from one or more roots, giving rise to different meanings for the same word, depending on the origin chosen. For instance, the well-known word *ātman,* generally meaning "self," can be derived from different roots. It could mean "one who consumes" *(att iti ātma)* or it could mean "that principle that permeates" *(āpnoti iti ātma).* It can also mean "one who gathers or collects" *(ādatte iti ātma).* Though the word indicates the same priniciple here, depending on the root from which it is derived it will indicate a different functional entity. In this way the word *yoga* can also be derived from the root *yuja* and mean *samādhi* or *samādhāna,* "to put in place perfectly" (*sum,* "completely," *ādhāna,* "to place"). The *Dhātupaṭha* puts it as *yuja samādhou,* or *yuja* in the word *samādhi.* Thus yoga, by this definition, would mean putting all mental energies in place, or harnessing mental energies without any dissipation. This definition is different from the earlier derivation of the word *yoga* from the root *yujir,* meaning "unity" *(yujir yoge).*

Based on this interpretation, the yoga of Patañjali is a system of practices that lead to the total harnessing of mental energy without any dissipation whatsoever (*nirodha*, "completely contained"). One can note that ultimately it is not unity with a higher principle that is aimed for in this form of yoga, but, rather, the removal of all the distractions of the mind. When such a feat is achieved, the *puruṣa,* the indwelling consciousness principle, remains alone *(kaivalya),* free from the distractions created by the mind. Thus we have two classical approaches to yoga—the one, unity with the higher, supreme principle, and the other, the regaining of the pristine stature of the innermost principle, the *puruṣa,* or soul. One system talks of unity, the other of freedom. In the yoga *darśana* of Patañjali, all the methods necessary to bring about a completely contained *(nirodha) citta* are prescribed. The ultimate goal in Patañjali's yoga is *kaivalya,* the freedom resulting from the cessation of *saṃsāra,* or transmigration. The intermediate benefits, or the necessary by-products, are the various *siddhis,* or supernatural accomplishments. The means of achieving *kaivalya* varies from individual to individual, depending on the number or types of holes to plug (to prevent the outflow of *citta*), and Patañjali, recognizing this, talks of different *adhikāris* (levels of evolution) and the appropriate yogic practices for each group of yoga practitioners.

# 4 Advanced Yoga

*"No! No!" said the queen,*
*"sentence first, verdict afterwards."*
***—Alice in Wonderland***

WHEN I CIRCULATED THE FIRST draft of this book among some friends, all of them kept it for a long time. When I asked for their opinions, some chuckled and some were silent, and I could see that something was bothering them. One friend said that it had lots of interesting information, but that a number of changes would have to be made (apart from editorial ones), and that he was unable to decide where to begin making them. It all fell into place when this friend said that I seemed to start with, and dwell in, the final picture, filling in the details slowly rather than building up the concept from the fundamentals.

This is true, and it is also the way Patañjali has presented his whole treatise on yoga, which many people find overwhelming, jolting, and rather disconcerting. The achievable and ultimate goal *(sādhya)* is described fully at the outset, and the author attempts to complete the subject by assuming that the yogi whom he addresses is so evolved that it is not necessary to explain the preliminaries and the means in any great detail. Then, having finished with the evolved ones, and as if they were an afterthought, the requirements of the less evolved are taken up. The subject is then dealt with in great detail, and the means *(sādhana)* are explained.

This method of presentation is common to treatises on the ancient philosophies of India. The Taittirīya Upaniṣad, a classic in Vedānta, starts with the goal, which is to obtain the highest knowledge, the knowledge of Brahman, the ultimate and only reality. The text defines Brahman almost immediately. But the means of attaining the ultimate are taken up in a later chapter, where a step-by-step approach is described. Of course, many find considerable merit in this approach of first describing the *sādhya* (goal) and then the *sādhana* (means). It is useful because one can keep the goal in the back of one's mind even as the beginner starts with the first step in the long spiritual journey.

The first important point to be noted in traditional yoga as propounded by Patañjali is that his yoga faithfully follows thoughts about yoga contained in Vedic tradition. By using the word *anuśāsana* (exposition) in the very first sūtra, Patañjali drives home the point that his treatise is written so that authentic yoga could be properly understood and practitioners could refrain from doing all other yogic practices that are not in conformity with traditional yoga. Over a period of time, every religion or philosophy becomes corrupt or degenerates and requires a cleansing process, and Patañjali has performed that task following the directive of the Lord. The first sūtra thus affirms that the treatise is *the* work on traditional yoga. My teacher used to point out several unacceptable practices in latter-day yoga texts and systems and would ask his yoga students to keep the teachings of Patañjali as a beacon to steer clear of the mire of discordant practices propounded under the banner of yoga.

*Anuśāsana* would also indicate that yoga follows Vedic tenets. There are five other philosophies or *darśanas* that purport to convey the essence of the Vedas. The six *darśanas* are Nyāya, Vaiśeṣika, Mīmāṃsā, Sāṃkhya, Yoga, and Vedānta. These sister philosophers betray considerable sibling rivalry, but never deviate from their obedience to the mother scripture, the Vedas. They implicitly subscribe to the basic traits of the Vedas. That every effect has a cause, and the elaborate theory of *karma* based on this premise, is faithfully followed by all the *darśanas* or *śāstras.* "As you sow, so shall you reap" is the basic refrain of the karma theory. The Vedas prescribe what the activities are that will bring happiness here and hereafter, and one's present birth is one link in the chain of lives one goes through. Hence the karma theory is the cornerstone of all the Vedic philosophies, including Yoga.

Having said that Yoga is a *śāstra* or a system of philosophy based on the authority of the Vedas, it follows that Yoga's goal should be consistent with those of the Vedas. The Vedas are a body of texts that contain knowledge about what is favorable and what is unfavorable, about activities that, when performed, give the desired results, and about activities that are to be avoided so that undesirable consequences do not occur *(anukūla prāpti, pratikūla parihārayoḥ, aloukikam upāyam yo grantho vedayati, sa vedaḥ).* The *śāstra*s (the system of knowledge based on the Vedas) also have the same goal. A *śāstra* or an *anuśāsana darśana* is defined as

*Pravṛtir va nivṛttīrvā nityena kritakena vā! / Pumsām yenopadiśyate tat śāstram abhidhīyate!* ("All the *śāstras,* including Yoga, should show the means of attaining happiness or avoiding unhappiness").

At this point one might inquire about what the Vedas have to say regarding in what happiness, or bliss—which is beyond the human conception of happiness—consists. The whole range of happiness is presented in great detail. Take the case of a young person *(yuvā),* well versed in all the *śāstras (yuvā adhyāyikaḥ).* He is pious *(āśiṣtah),* and all his senses function perfectly *(dṛḍhīstaḥ).* He is physically strong *(baliṣtaḥ),* and he may be endowed with extensive properties and wealth *(pritvī vittasya pūrnasyāt).* Such a fortunate person's happiness can be taken as the maximum of possible human happiness. In contrast, the happiness of *manuṣya gandharva* (celestial man) is one hundred times more perfect than this human happiness. Continuing on in this ascending Vedic scale of happiness or bliss of beings, in multiples of one hundred, are the *devagandharva* (celestial musicians), *pitru* (inhabitants of the celestial world of ancestors), then *ājānājana devas* (those who reach the higher world because of charitable acts), then *karma devas* (those who have become angels through righteous deeds), then the *devas* (the celestial beings), Indra (the leader of the *devas*), Bṛhaspati (the preceptor of the *devas*), Prajāpati, and Brahma (the four-faced creator of the phenomenal universe). These various levels are achieved by performing the various prescribed actions that are mentioned in the Vedas during one's human existence.

On the other hand, by performing forbidden *(niṣiddha)* activities, one falls into births that are more and more painful. Human unhappiness reaches its maximum in a person who is old, ignorant, and immoral, and who has lost his faculties, is physically weak, and is poor. One hundred times more pitiable is the life of cattle, and the graduated scale of unhappiness increases one hundredfold in each order of animals, birds, reptiles, ants, worms, trees, shrubs, stones, and lumps of clay (or dust). The Mīmāṃsā and other *dharma śāstras,* based on the ritualistic portions of the Vedas, detail the karmas necessary to reach the higher levels of bliss, even as they catalog activities that are reprehensible, apart from the daily *(nitya)* and special *(naimittika)* duties, the performing of which can prevent one from falling into abysmal misery. Thus, in great detail, bliss, or happiness, is described along with the means of achieving it. Two questions that may arise will need to be answered. The first is, how does one know for sure or prove that such worlds and beings exist at all? To this the karma theory, which is inferential, is introduced as an answer. This will be taken up in greater detail later, following Patañjali. Sāyaṇa, who has written an elaborate commentary on the Vedas, says dismissively that such premises as the existence of hell and heaven, and whether the various Vedic rites would give rise to experiences in such worlds, can neither be proved nor disproved by logicians, even if they would debate and argue for a billion years *(śata koti varṣam).* The second question concerns the experience of pain by such inanimate objects as stones and dust. According to Vedānta, pure consciousness, or Brahman (or God, from another viewpoint), pervades the universe and that consciousness manifests as awareness or intelligence wherever there is life; otherwise it is dormant. There are some popular myths that discuss the concept of an all-pervading consciousness (or God).

Hiraṇyakaśipu was a demon king, but his son Prahlāda (the blissful one) was pious and a great devotee of Lord Nārāyaṇa, the Supreme Being. The demon king had acquired such great supernatural powers, because of his *tapas* (penance), that he declared himself as God. But he was horrified to find that his son would not accept him as God, even though, out of fear, the celestial beings were prepared to worship Hiraṇyakaśipu as they would worship their Lord. Prahlāda, so the story goes, was subjected to all kinds of torture, including being thrown into fire and drowned in deep sea, but he came back unscathed, thanks to the grace of his benefactor Lord Nārāyaṇa. With impotent rage, and unable to find his son's Lord, the demon king asked his son where his benefactor Nārāyaṇa was. The serene, smiling devotee, with tears of joy in his eyes, said, "Father, don't you see? He is everywhere. He is in this pillar in front of us and in the dry grass blade that floats around here." The story goes on to say that the furious king then hammered his mace against the pillar. The Lord, in his famous Narasimha (man-lion) form, split open the pillar, came out, and destroyed the demon king, Hiraṇyakaśipu. This particular story is told, as are others, to stress the truth about the all-pervasiveness of Brahman (consciousness/God) and that all objects are thought to have consciousness.

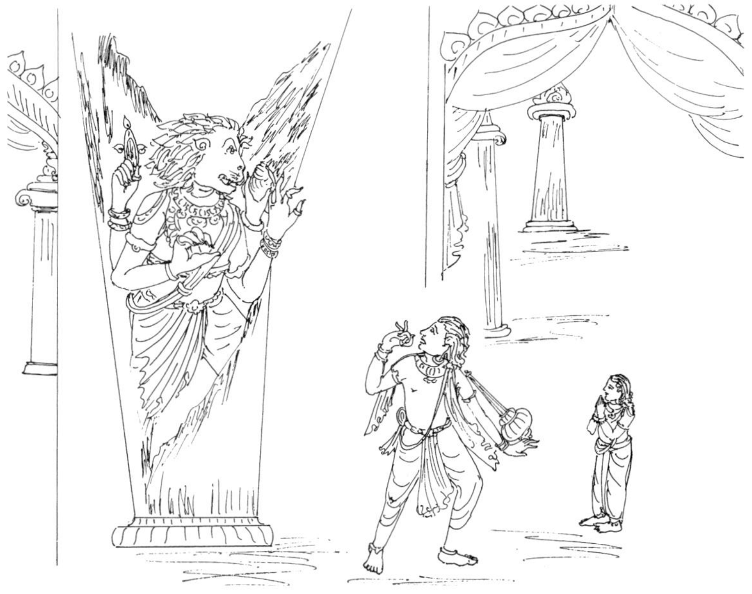
Hiraṇyakaśipu's day of reckoning

Yet another story from the great Rāmāyaṇa indicates that stone could be a stage an individual self may experience, the result of doing forbidden karmas or of performing *adhārmic* actions. It would appear that Ahalyā, the chaste wife of the great sage Gautama, was tricked into committing adultery by Indra, the celestial king, who assumed the form of the sage. Gautama, who came to know about the treachery through his yogic powers, not only condemned Indra to a pitiable state, but also cursed his unsuspecting, victimized wife to the inert state of a stone to suffer insurmountable pain for the transgression. After a long period of suffering in the inert state, Ahalyā was rescued when the divine feet of Lord Rāma brushed by her while she was in her inanimate state. This story implies that a stone is also believed to have consciousness.

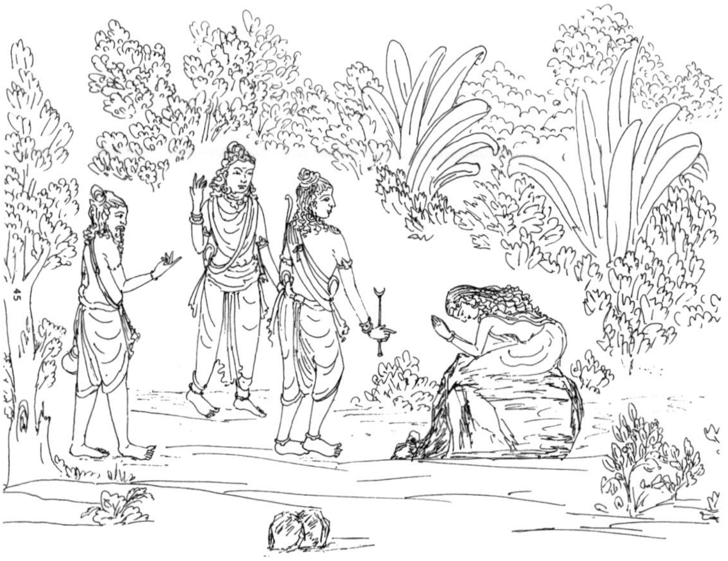

Ahalyā's curse exorcised by Lord Rāma's grace

The truths, morals, and messages contained in the Vedas are thought to be understood better through the stories, anecdotes, and narratives in the Purāṇas (mythology) and *itihāsas* (epics). The Vedic *vākya* (injunction), *satyāt na pramaditavyam* (never deviate from the path of truth) is driven home in the "Hariścandra Upākhyāna" (Story of Hariścandra) in which the triumph of truth against all odds is described. The Rāmāyaṇa, through the conduct of Śrī Rāma, shows what right conduct, or *dharma,* is by depicting Rāma as the embodiment of virtue *(ramo vigrahavān dharmaḥ).* The same is true of the Mahābhārata.

The Mīmāṃsā philosophy of actions that follows the Vedic directives and injunctions will help the individual achieve greater happiness and avoid pain. The Vedāntins, on the other hand, point to the limitations of time for all the fruits of pious actions and achievements. As long as the karma in store is able to provide the highest states, then such happiness continues, but on the exhaustion of the *puṇya* (effects of meritorious deeds), one falls back to the cycle of huge ups and downs. They point out that by the realization of the identification of the soul with Brahman, unsurpassed bliss *(paramānanda)* occurs, and this state being final and permanent, they urge the aspirant to follow the thought process contained in the Upaniṣad portion of the Vedas to attain permanent supreme bliss and avoid the cycle of birth and death *(mokṣa).* Sāṃkhya and Yoga philosophers, on the other hand, take the approach that they are not concerned about happiness, but would like to avoid pain, or *duḥkha,* since the so-called happiness or bliss discussed by the Mīmāsakas is always limited and tinged with sorrow. The philosophers belonging to the Nyāya school would say that happiness tinged with sorrow is like a sweet dessert *(pāyasa)* contaminated with a drop of poison. The Sāṃkhyas point out that human beings suffer as the result of three kinds of causes: those arising from within *(adhyātmika),* such as disease, and depression; those triggered by natural phenomena (or acts of God, as they are commonly known), called *ādhidaivika;* and those caused by other creatures, including fellow human beings *(ādhibhoutika).* All the known methods used by human beings to ward off the attendant pain suffer from two deficiencies, because the efficacy of the methods is neither permanent nor definite—like taking medicines to cure a disease (as suggested by Āyurveda). Sometimes medicines seem to work, but the cure may not be permanent. Similarly, worldly efforts to obtain what is desirable, whether it be wealth or a spouse, may or may not result in success or unalloyed happiness on succeeding in the endeavor. In the same vein, the Sāṃkhyas find fault with Mīmāṃsākas' advice on how to reach different *lokas* (heavenly abodes detailed in the *śāstras*) in the life hereafter for being fraught with the same deficiencies. The activities are mixed with some *pāpa* (sin), because some of the rituals, for instance, the violence involved in sacrificing life in the *aśvamedha,* will produce their own undesirable effects in the future, even as one may enjoy the celestial worlds. Thus the Sāṃkhyas conclude that all human effort will produce mixed and impermanent results, and they recommend deep introspection aimed at finding out the nature of one's own self. They propose that a thorough understanding of the various aspects of nature *(prakṛti)* and the immutable state of consciousness of the soul, and the direct perception of their distinction *(prakṛti-puruṣa viveka),* will permanently remove the cause of the threefold pain. The *citta* thus becomes free of all pain. Thus the Sāṃkhya *śāstra* is a *nivṛtti śāstra* (an antidote to unending pain). Yogis follow the same line of reasoning and proceed to lay out a detailed methodology to attain the state of *kaivalya* of the soul from the mind.

So what does Yoga have to offer? What is its goal? What are its benefits? These questions will have to be answered, for who would subject him- or herself to the various disciplines, restrictions, and difficult practices of Yoga, unless, at the outset, the goal and the various ways and means leading to it are clearly laid out. There is a saying that no one, not even a dimwit, would make an effort unless he or she knew what the benefits of the effort were. If one accepts the contention that for a discriminating person *(viveki)* the entire range of human and superhuman happiness is pain *(duḥkham eva sarvam),* then Yoga becomes meaningful, and the *Yogasūtras* proceed to address, among other things, four questions.

1. What is it that one should escape from or avoid *(heyam)*? The answer is *saṃsāra,* or phenomenal existence.
2. What is the cause of this *saṃsāra,* which is to be avoided? The cause *(heya-hetu),* according to Yoga, is the wrong thinking (ignorance) that the

observer, the Self *(puruṣa),* and the observed self-locus, or ego, are one and the same. The subject is unaware or ignorant of the two distinct principles, Self *(cit)* and self-locus *(citta).*

3. What are the means of attaining the release *(hānopaya)* of the Self from being constantly required to toe the line of *citta?* The release is attained by first knowing and then maintaining an unwavering awareness that they are in fact different. This is direct perceptive knowledge *(yougika).*
4. What is the nature of the destruction of ignorance *(hāna)* that is the benefit of the yogic exercise? It is called *kaivalya,* or freedom, or a state of aloneness (*kevala,* "alone," "only").

Patañjali, in his treatise on yoga, recognizes three distinct principles, called *tattvas.* They are *puruṣa, prakṛti,* and Īśvara. It is necessary to expand on these to have a proper appreciation of Patañjali's yoga. *Puruṣa* means "the indwelling principle." It is the observer, pure and simple in every being. It is total consciousness/intelligence *(dṛśi mātra)* and is nonchanging. But it is constrained to observe and oversee the continuous activity and presentations of the *citta,* which may be taken to mean the brain or the principle that receives and collates all sensory impressions, feelings, moods, and so on, and presents them to this Self *(puruṣa).* Thus, even though the *puruṣa* is different from the engulfing *citta,* it is not entirely free of it. This ceaseless mental activity *(citta vṛtti),* and the necessity of the observer or Self to identify with it, is the cause of bondage. *Prakṛti* is that which evolves, the evolution itself taking place in stages, producing twenty-four principles in all. The first stage, or the irreducible level, is known as *aliṅga,* the nonmanifest, nonspecific. This stage, also known as *mūlaprakṛti,* or root of the universe, has its three fundamental constituent characteristics, namely, *sattva,* whose main characteristic is clarity; *rajas,* which gives mobility; and *tamas,* which restrains. All are in perfect equilibrium *(sāmya avasthā).* Evolution itself starts with the disequilibrating of these three basic *guṇas,* or constituents. Even though they are opposed to one another, the *guṇas* mutually support one another in the process of evolution. *Prakṛti* itself is made up of the three *guṇas,* and Patañjali refers to the evolution of the *guṇas* as the cause of experience for the *puruṣa.* The second stage is called *liṅga,* the stage of primary or indicative manifestation. It is also known as *mahat,* or universal mind. The third stage is known as *aviśeṣa,* or nonspecificity. In this, *mahat* evolves into six distinct aspects, that is, *ahaṃkāra,* or the individualized existence (ego), and the five sensations, sound *(śabda),* touch *(sparśa),* form *(rūpa),* taste *(rasa),* and smell *(gandha).* These five are known as *tanmātras,* or the pure forms of sensation, which require further instruments *(indriyas)* for being perceived and media *(bhūtas)* for their manifestation. The individualized existence and the five *tanmātras* hence require the means of perception, and thus we have the next stage of evolution of *prakṛti,* which is the mind *(manas)* and the five instruments of perception: the organs of hearing, touching, seeing, tasting, and smelling. Then there are the five instruments of action: legs, arms, speech organs, and secretory and generative organs. Finally, there are the five basic gross aspects of the phenomenal universe: space *(ākāśa),* matter in the form of energy *(agni),* air *(vāyu),* fluid *(ap),* and solid *(pritvī).* These are the media by virtue of which objects, in terms of their *tanmātras,* move. The things we observe consist of the various combinations of these five gross aspects, and following from them are innumerable other objects with different names and forms. Patañjali describes the entire creation as it is observed by the individual soul *(puruṣa).* The instruments of perception receive signals from the gross elements, which the mind collects and, with the coloring of the "I"-feeling, presents to the *puruṣa,* or observer. It could be noted that even the *citta,* an aspect of which is mistaken for the Self, is actually part of the observed, since all the mental modifications *(citta vṛtti),* including the I-exist feeling *(asmitā),* are observed by the *puruṣa. Prakṛti* can be of no use except to the *puruṣa* (since without it, *prakṛti* will not be seen to exist), and the ego makes use of this principle for a variety of experiences *(bhoga)* or for renunciation *(apavarga).* The distinction between *puruṣa* and *prakṛti* is the greatest revelation of the Vedic philosophies, especially Sāṃkhya, Yoga, and Vedānta. *Prakṛti,* which consists of three *guṇas* (aspects), permeates the twenty-three evolutes. And all three *guṇas* are discernible. *Sattva* is order *(dharma); tamas* is disorder *(adharma);* and *rajas* is energy. At the individual level, the three aspects are recognizable as follows: *Sattvam laghu prakaśakam, iṣṭam, upaṣṭambhakam calam ca Rajaḥ / Guruvaraṇakam etat tamaḥ, pradīpavat cartato vṛttiḥ* ("*Sattva* is lightness at the physical level and clarity at the mental level, which is the most desirable quality; *rajas* is restless physical activity and instability at the mental level; and *tamas* is heaviness at the physical level and complete inertia at the mental level").

The third principle apart from *prakṛti* and *puruṣa* is Īśvara. The inspirational basis of Yoga is Sāṃkhya. But unlike Nīrīśvara Sāṃkhya philosophers, Yoga also recognizes the principle of Īśvara, the cosmic or universal Lord. According to Patañjali, God is one special *puruṣa,* but unlike individual souls, it is unaffected by affliction *(kleśa),* actions (karma), results of actions *(vipāka),* and accumulation of karma *(āśaya).* In Him is contained all potential knowledge (omniscience). He is the first spiritual preceptor, and transcends space and time. He responds and manifests Himself to the devotee in the repetition of His name, the most sacred mantra, the *praṇava* (OM). *Praṇava* literally means "highest praise." The repetition of OM (pronounced AUM) is known as *japa,* which is to be done while contemplating the secret meaning of the sacred syllable. Such contemplation helps in the removal of all obstacles in a yogi's quest for self-realization.

The second sūtra defines the essence of Patañjali's yoga. It contains the words *citta, vṛtti,* and *nirodha.* Even as he goes on to describe the *vṛttis* in a later sūtra, this succinct definition is sufficient for the evolved yogi, whom Patañjali addresses in this sūtra. Several commentators have taken the trouble to explain these words in great detail for the benefit of a varied audience.

What is *citta? Cit iva bhāvayati iti cittam.* In this explanation, *citta* is that which acts as if it possesses consciousness, or *cit.* In a limited way, *citta* may be compared to a highly complicated and extraordinary robot that is wired and appears to have intelligence when electricity passes through the different circuits. In this theory, the *citta* whose circuitry is evolved according to one's *saṃskāras* has no consciousness of its own, but appears to when *prāṇa,* the life energy, passes through it. The distinction between it and *cit* needs to be understood by the yogi; the word *cit* is synonymous with *puruṣa,* the indwelling, nonchanging, pure consciousness principle. What are the characteristics of *citta?* The Sāṃkhyas use the term *antaḥkaraṇa* to describe this internal organ/instrument, which can be called the brain, for want of a better word. This "organ" has three different aspects: *buddhi* (intellect), *ahaṃkāra* (self-locus or ego), and *manas* (mind). At any particular moment, one of the aspects appears to function predominantly. When active, the *buddhi* aspect *(buddhi vṛtti)* is able to analyze *(adhyavasāya)* various things presented to it—like a plow that breaks down the hard soil, making it fit for agriculture (*adhyavasayo buddhiḥ*). But this *buddhi* can be pure *(sattvic)* or corrupt *(tamasic).* When *buddhi* is *sattvic,* it may analyze all the aspects of the universe (*prakṛti* and its evolutes) and lead the ego in the direction of *dharma* (law of piety), *jñāna* (spiritual knowledge), *vairāgya* (extreme dispassion, after proper analysis), and *aiśvarya* (supernatural powers and ethical leadership). In effect, the *buddhi* in its *sattvic* mold makes a proper analysis and directs the individual mind in any of the four uplifting paths. On the other hand, if the *buddhi* is in a *tamasic* mold, it leads the individual to act immorally or unlawfully *(adharma);* or with *ajñāna,* or spiritual ignorance, about the nature of self or *cit;* with *avairāgya,* or a lack of dispassion; or with *anaiśvarya,* that is, as a slave to the senses. In short, when *buddhi* is *tamasic,* the capacity to discriminate what is good from what is not *(dharmādharma)* is blunted. The next *vṛtti* is *ahaṃkāra vṛtti* (ego-locus preponderance), which leads to an extreme attachment to the body, senses, and worldly possessions and pleasures. *Manas,* the other aspect *of citta,* coordinates the senses.

The next word in the definition of yoga is *vṛtti,* which means "activity" or "function" *(vṛtti jivane).* The *citta* constantly thinks, plans, and acts to achieve what it believes is desirable (if the *citta* is *sattvic*) and to avoid what is not. Endeavoring to achieve what is desirable is *pravṛtti,* and avoiding and eradicating what is not is called *nivṛtti.*

*Nirodha* is the third word in the definition. It means "to prevent both streams" of mental functioning, that is, both *pravṛtti* and *nivṛtti.* This prevention does not come from outside, but has to be evolved by a thought process called *jñāna,* mentioned earlier. *Jñāna* is the correct knowledge of the *puruṣa,* as distinct from the virtual self, the one experienced as a self-locus or ego by all of us.

If *nirodhaḥ* is to prevent all the functions of the *citta* from within, will it not lead to death? In this regard Patañjali talks about the *viśeṣa vṛttis* (specific functions) pertaining to each individual brain. What keeps life going is another form of *vṛtti* (function) called *sāmānya* (general) activity, which helps maintain the physiological functions of the individual through the five *prāṇas,* or vital forces. Sāṃkhya indicates this as follows: *Sāmānya karaṇā vṛttiḥ, prāṇādhāyaḥ vāyavaḥ pañca,* "The five vital forces are the general function of the internal organ (brain)." Nyāya also says that effort is of three kinds—proactive, reactive, and life sustaining: *Prayatnam trividam proktam, pravṛtti, nivṛtti, jīvanaprayatnaḥ.* The notion of *nirodhaḥ* entails the complete cessation of the activities of the *citta* and the containing of its energies within itself. *Nirodha* comes from *ni* or *nitarām,* "always," and *rudhirāvaraṇe: rudhi* is *āvarana,* which means to encircle an object completely so that it does not move or flow out (here, through the senses). The *citta,* by a special process called "yoga," contains its own energies within itself. In short, the sūtra says that the study and practice of "yoga" will facilitate the complete stopping of the *citta,* by the *citta* itself. This is what has been explained earlier as *samādhāna,* or harnessing the whole mental energy without dissipation. And this level of *nirodha* is to be distinguished from all other levels. Vyāsa and other commentators explain them so that one may be able to distinguish *nirodha* from other mental states (levels or *bhūmi*) even though Patañjali takes it that the evolved yogi will be able to attain the ultimate goal of yoga without any further elucidation.

In his commentary on the *Yogasūtras,* Vyāsa classifies the mental levels *(citta bhūmi)* into five, from the viewpoint of a yogi. At one extreme is the group of people who could be deemed to have *kṣipta citta,* or a demented state. This group, lacking concentration, cannot even comprehend yoga and its benefits. The next group is in the level of *mūḍha* (totally covered or infatuated). Such people cannot reconcile themselves to the separate existence of a distinct indwelling intelligence principle (*puruṣa,* or Self), or inwardly to the all-pervading cosmic principle. They live by the dictates of the senses and the undifferentiating mind, rolling with the punches and riding with the tide, and as such are afflicted. The third, the restless level, is called *vikṣipta.* It is a state of evolution in which the individual yearns toward realizing his true nature, but is constantly distracted by the senses and recollection of earlier disturbing experiences. He intellectually recognizes the true nature of the self when it is pointed out by the treatises of Yoga and Vedānta, but is constantly distracted, the distraction itself arising out of acquired habits, a result of beginningless previous karmas (residues of action). Our *citta* is made up of the remainder of tendencies arising out of past karmas *(saṃskāra śeṣam hi cittam).* For many of us, it is first of all difficult to accept the distinction between the Self and the most fundamental cognitive focus, or *citta vṛtti,* which is the I-feeling. Even if one mentally accepts that view, since the mind is used to different activities, this discriminating knowledge *(viveka)* itself is fleeting. Thus, such persons in whom a faint spiritual restlessness is discernible are dissatisfied with mundane and phenomenal existence. They occasionally do achieve a state of total absorption *(samādhi)* in a higher principle, but such experiences are few and far between. According to Vyāsa, those experiences are not to be categorized under yoga as such, which requires a total transformation of the *citta.* Yoga is the science that helps one achieve such a transformation of *citta,* by the appropriate practices of the *citta* on the *citta,* so that the prevailing distracting *saṃskāras* (formed habits) are replaced, as it were, by nondistracting or concentrating habits. When a person thus takes to the practice of yoga with a view to achieving the objective of mental transformation leading to self-realization, he is known as *āruruksu,* or one who is desirous of treading the path of yoga. Even here practitioners vary and are known as mildly, moderately, or totally involved, depending on their dedication to practice.

The last two mental levels really come under yoga. In the fourth, called *ekāgra* (one-pointed), the same object is kept by the *citta* in successive moments. The object could be a gross object grasped by the senses or an eternal idea, a subtle feeling, or bliss. In *ekāgra,* there is only one idea, and even the feeling of "I exist" is absent, or at least dormant. The *citta* is completely absorbed in the particular thought to the exclusion of all others. Obviously a *citta* that is habitually one-pointed should have developed the *ekāgra saṃskāra* by prior *abhyāsa* (practice), either in this birth or heretofore. *Ekāgra* and *nirodha* are the two deep mental states that yoga is interested in. In both cases the yogi is said to be in *samādhi. Nirodha* means "to prevent the movement" of the mind, or *citta,* "always and completely"; *nitarām* (always) *rudhyata* (stops) is *nirodha.* My teacher sometimes explained *nirodha* differently, taking the preposition *ni* as meaning "not," in which case *nirodha* would mean "not preventing" rather than "always preventing"; *nirodha,* then, is not preventing the mind from being free from involvement in *saṃsāra.*

Patañjali's *Yogasūtras* contains four chapters. The first is *samādhi pāda,* or the chapter on *samādhi. Samādhi* is not an end in itself but a means of thorough understanding, or *prajñā.* The objective knowledge attained by a yogi is unambiguous and is naturally different from the understanding arrived at in a distracted state *(vikṣipta).* The first chapter deals with both kinds of *samādhi,* the one used for *prajñā* or yogic knowledge, and the other, objectless *samādhi,* arising out of *nirodha* practice, leading to the absolute quietude of *citta.* When *citta* becomes absolutely quiet, without any active state or feeling *(pratyaya),* then the Self *(puruṣa),* which is pure consciousness, remains in its true form or state, undistributed. It is unlike the other stage when it is invariably required to observe the various states of *citta*—acquisition of knowledge *(pramāṇa),* confusion *(viparyaya),* imagination *(vikalpa),* sleep *(nidrā),* and remembering *(smṛti).* These mental levels can be explained by an analogy. Take the case of a cloudburst. All the water that falls from the sky is scattered over a wide area. If some of this water flows down a drain, this can be compared to the mental energies in the state of *kṣipta* (wasted). When the water seeps into the ground and cannot be utilized, it can be compared to *mūḍha* (covered). Then think of the rainwater collecting in small puddles at different places. Some of this water can be utilized, and this can be compared to a state of *vikṣipta,* a state in which the mental energies are put to proper use only partially. In the case of the rainwater slowly collecting and flowing along the path of a river (toward the ocean), the flow is controlled by the banks, guided as it were, and it is unidirectional. This can be compared to *ekāgra,* being one-pointed or unidirectional. The case of the river being blocked by a dam or an anicut so that the water is held in a huge reservoir, the case of water flowing into a large lake embanked all around by bunds, the case of a whole river stopping or freezing because of intense cold—these are examples that may help to understand the state of *citta* in *nirodha.*

How does the adept attain the state of mind in which he or she can habitually refuse to entertain any thoughts, refuse to react to any stimulus? People in the first three stages of mind will not be able to experience that stage, merely because their *cittas* are habituated to distraction. But one in a million may be born (possibly owing to previous *saṃskāras*) who is not habitually distracted. Such a born yogi is said to have a *samāhita citta,* a balanced and contented mind. The first chapter gives the necessary theoretical background so that the *samāhita citta*'s already pure mind will develop *ekāgrata* or *nirodha,* as the case may be. The ultimate aim is to attain self-realization. How does a *samāhita citta* attain the state of *nirodha,* leading to *kaivalya?* As mentioned earlier, *citta* can flow in two different directions—toward good and toward evil. According to Yoga and Sāṃkhya, that which flows in the inward direction of discrimination (of *puruṣa* and *citta*) ending in the Self, remaining in its true, pure conscious nature, which is also known as independence *(kaivalya),* is said to lead to a favorable goal. On the other hand, if the *citta* runs in the direction of *pravṛtti,* arising out of a nondiscrimination *(aviveka),* it leads to evil, rebirth, the threefold sorrows, and it could go on endlessly birth after birth. While *mūḍha* and *kṣipta* people are invariably inclined toward *pravṛtti,* the *vikṣipta citta* is at a crossroads. The *samāhita citta,* however, already has in place the tendency toward discrimination and subsequent self-realization. To strengthen that tendency, practice *(abhyāsa)* and renunciation *(vairāgya)* are the widely suggested means throughout the Vedic philosophies and *śāstras.*

A *samāhita citta* has already acquired a state of tranquillity through previous karma or by the grace of Īśvara. Absence of the commonly experienced states of mental distraction known as *citta vṛitti* is called *sthiti* (stationary) or absolute tranquillity. If the *citta*, moment after moment, remains in this state, it is called *praśānta vāhitā* (flow of peace). This is the most desirable state in which the yogi's *citta* may exist, and the yogi practices in order to remain in that state continuously. Since his mind remains in that state habitually, further practice is not only easy but also desirable, which is difficult for ordinary mortals without considerable effort and willpower. This practice *(abhyāsa)* is the attempt to remain habitually in the state of mental tranquillity. This practice, when done continually for a long time and without interruption, and supported by the requisite reverent and authentic study of the scriptures on yoga, will result in the *citta* getting a firm foundation for proceeding along the path of self-realization.

What are these *citta vṛttis* that Patañjali expects the yogi to transcend? Can the *citta* remain in the state that is beyond the stage of *vṛttis?* The five *vṛttis* are (1) *pramāṇa* (acquiring correct knowledge); (2) *viparyaya* (active state of wrong impression or mistaken knowledge); (3) *vikalpa* (mental activity of the imagination); (4) *nidrā* (dreamless sleep); and (5) *smṛti* (remembering). What are the means of obtaining correct knowledge? According to Pātañjala yoga, they are *pratyakṣa* (direct perception through the senses), *anumāna* (inference), and *āgama* (scriptural testimony). Other philosophical schools have different views about obtaining correct knowledge. Cārvākas believe in only one means of right knowledge, direct perception. Vaiśeṣikas rely almost entirely on perception and inference, though they are an *āstika* school. Bauddhas also believe in perception and inference and not on scriptural testimony. Sāṃkhyas and followers of Yoga add verbal testimony or the scriptures. The Nyāya school of philosophy adds comparison *(upamāna)* as well to obtain correct knowledge. The Mīmāṃsās' *prābhākara* school also admits presumption, while the Bhātta school and the Vedāntins add the sixth category of nonexistence *(abhāva)*. Those who follow mythology (Purāṇa) add two more, probability and traditional belief *(aitihya)*.

Even as Patañjali would expect the yogi to transcend all the *vṛttis* to attain *apavarga*, or total release from *saṃsāra*, he also acknowledges some aspects of *vṛttis* as favorable *(akliṣṭa)* to obtain *apavarga* and others unfavorable *(kliṣṭa)*. In the case of *apavarga*, the most favorable *vṛtti* will be *āgama pramāṇa*. While *pratyakṣa pramāṇa* may be the most valid as far as sensory perceptions and worldly knowledge are concerned, spiritual knowledge cannot be obtained by ordinary sensory perception or inference. Hence, for spiritual knowledge, scriptures are the starting point. Having studied and understood the scriptures, yogis make use of inference or *anumāna* to confirm by logic the validity of spiritual teachings. For instance, Patañjali uses *anumāna* to show that the *puruṣa* has to be immutable by stating that since all the *vṛttis* of the individual *citta* are constantly experienced, there has to be a conscious nonchanging principle, which is *puruṣa*. Then by deep meditation and absorption *(samādhi)* of a yogic practice, the yogi's *citta* directly experiences or "sees" the true nature of the Self. That knowledge, valid knowledge, is also called *pratyakṣa* (direct perception). But it is special because of its unique nature; it is called yogic (direct) perception *(yougika pratyakṣa).* Thus true knowledge of the spirit starts from the scriptures and is reinforced by *anumāna,* and the yogi, by the methodology detailed in the yoga *śāstra,* is able to experience directly the spirit within. The same approach is advocated by the Vedāntins. In the Bṛhadāraṇyaka Upaniṣad, the call is to directly perceive *(draṣtavyaḥ)* the *ātman* (indwelling spirit) by first studying the scriptures *(śrotavyaḥ),* then by deep meditation and contemplation infer *(mantavyaḥ),* and finally by yogic *samādhi (nidhidhyāsitavyaḥ)* directly experience, the spirit.

*Viparyaya* is the mistaken impression about an object. In spiritual matters, the impresson that the ego (the I-locus in the *citta*) is the Self, even as they are two distinctly different principles *(tattvas),* according to the *śāstras,* is a mistaken impression. There are several other instances in the day-to-day observations that indicate one's *citta* is in a state of misapprehension. Here the main purpose is to point out that one does not have the correct knowledge about the nature of one's own self. *Viparyaya* is a misconception *(mithyā),* and it can be removed by the correct perception of the self through the practice of *samādhi.* Except for those who are spiritually awakened, the refrain is that everyone is in a state of *viparyaya* so far as the knowledge of one's own self is concerned. Like the dream self that vanishes as a nonself when one wakes up, the wrong identification *(viparyaya)* of the *citta* with regard to the nature of the Self (that is, as ego) vanishes when the correct knowledge of the Self dawns in the mind. *Vikalpa,* the third *vṛtti,* is different from *pramāṇa* and *viparyaya* in that it depends on words and impressions, or words without an object. Many poets can be faulted on this account.

Once a destitute, dimwitted devotee of Lord Śiva came to know that the author of the best piece of original poetry in a competition at the king's *darbar* (assembly) would be honored with a bag full of gold coins. He prayed to the Lord for help, and Lord Śiva wrote an exquisite poem, which, among other things, praised the beauty and natural fragrance of the divine Mother's tresses. Our destitute friend recited the stanzas, and the king, himself a great devotee of the Lord, was immensely pleased and decided to honor the poet with the prize money. Kīra, the palace poet, sprang to his feet and objected to the decision of the king, stating that the poem was flawed because even though it was grammatically correct, to state that hair would have a natural fragrance was not factual, and thus the poem suffered from an objective flaw. In effect, Kīra said that it was only in the imagination of the poet that such a fragrance existed. This is an example of *vikalpa.* The story goes on to say that Lord Śiva became furious at the impertinence of Kīra, and challenged him as to whether he dared say that about the hair of the divine Mother, whom he worshiped dearly.

Kīra is said to have remarked firmly that a flaw is a flaw even if the Lord would open his third eye and direct his wrath on Kīra.

*Nidrā,* or sleep, is the next function of the *citta.* Many people object to categorizing *nidrā* as a *vṛtti,* saying that *vṛtti,* or a function, requires movement or change. But when something is restrained, or when an object is stationary requiring effort to remain at a place, this is evidence of a function. Hence, sleep is considered a *vṛtti* of *tamas,* one of the three *guṇas.* It restrains other *vṛttis. Smṛti* is remembering. This could be beneficial or otherwise, depending on whether it is going to help or hinder one's spiritual progress. Remembering the sayings of the scriptures or the inferences based on the *śāstras* is beneficial. Other memories may not be beneficial, as they may not help in *kaivalya,* or *apavarga,* of the *citta.* The cessation *(nirodha)* of all these functions of the *citta* is the ultimate good. Except for the most evolved, it will not be possible. Patañjali adds a rider that some of the functions *(vṛttis)* are favorable to achieving *nirodha* and others are not.

A young man once lost a precious possession. He did not know where or when he had lost it. He went out of his house and went on searching day in and day out. He continued his search for many days and years, and became a tired old man. One day during his clueless search, he met an old well-wisher who inquired after his welfare. He narrated his plight. The friend told him that the priceless object could be found only in his home, and that he should return there to find it. Even though his search had ended, he had to return to his house and take possession of his dear treasure. Since he had lost his way, the old man gave him directions for the return journey, mentioning all the milestones he would find on the way. The story holds that he completed the return journey as advised and found his treasure. Thereafter, he did not have any other function in the matter of finding the lost treasure. Here the wise old man is the *anuśāsana* (scripture, *śāstra*). It gives all the direction necessary to find the *puruṣa,* the treasure. The return journey is akin to the *akliṣṭa* (favorable) function of the *citta.* The *anumāna* (inferences) are the milestones, and the direct seeing of the treasure is the direct perception of the *puruṣa,* the priceless and unique treasure.

*Abhyāsa* and *vairāgya* are the means that facilitate the return journey *(apavarga).* The Sāṃkhyas refer to *abhyāsa* (practice) as the practice of deep inquiry into the twenty-five principles *(tattvas)* such as "this is *prakṛti,* those are the four subsets of five principles (five *tanmātras,* five *bhūtas,* five *karma indriyas,* and five *jñana indriyas*), and the three internal instruments (the mind, intellect, and ego-locus). The deep inquiry referred to here is known as *samādhi* in yogic parlance. When such an inquiry is made, the correct, direct perception of the twenty-fifth *tattva,* the *puruṣa,* or the indwelling consciousness principle, takes place in the *citta* without any error *(viparyaya)* whatsoever. The Sāṃkhyas say that the three erroneous impressions about the self are overcome and in the *citta* what is not the self becomes clear, as this passage from the *Sāṃkhya Kārikā* illustrates: "The twenty-four principles, other than the Self, are not mine *(na me)*. I am not *(nāham)* the twenty-four *tattvas*, they are not 'me.' I do not exist *(na asmi)* in the twenty-four *tattvas* (because as pure consciousness I am different from them)."

When clear knowledge dawns in the *citta*, consequently the *citta* withdraws from all its *vṛttis* (functions). According to Sāṃkhyas, the only way by which a *citta* can attain a state of *nirodha* is by the correct understanding of the twenty-five principles. A person with such understanding is known as one with the knowledge of the twenty-five principles *(pañca vimśati tattvājñāḥ)*. The means to this end is *abhyāsa* on the principles *(evam tattvābhyāstāt)*. Hence, *abhyāsa* is to be taken as a technical word. To drive home the point that correct *abhyāsa* is the key to self-realization, Sāṃkhyas say the external appearances or the stages in life have no relevance. It does not matter if one has a tuft of hair *(śikhī)*, a shaved head *(muṇḍī)*, is long-haired *(jaṭī)*, or in any of the four stages of life, only the exact knowledge of the *tattvas* will get permanent release *(kaivalya)* from the threefold sorrows. The word *samādhi* here is used in the sense of deep unwavering contemplation *(samyak adhīyata iti samādhiḥ)*.

*Vairāgya*, or dispassion, is the next means of *apavarga*. Having known all the principles, and having known that all the twenty-four *tattvas* of *prakṛti* are neither I nor mine, the *citta* develops dispassion toward all the twenty-four principles, and that is called *vairāgya*. The terms *vairāgya* (renunciation) and *viveka* (discrimination) are such common household terms in many Hindu families that they are almost taken for granted. In fact *vairāgya*, which should be done in a positive spirit, is commonly but mistakenly thought of as a willful or even perverse negation of all wants. *Vairāgya*, or desirelessness, is difficult to practice, but for a *samāhita citta*, it is a natural and enlivening state of mind and practice. When the mind becomes indifferent (a) to worldly things observed through the senses and the pursuit of material objects, status, power, etc.; (b) to those things promised in the karma portions of the Vedas that result from performing such rites as *aśvamedha*, such as reaching the height of the heavens; (c) to remaining in the subtlest states, including reducing to *tanmātra* bodies, becoming a celestial being, and so on; (d) to achieving the various *siddhis* mentioned in the texts; (e) to finding, owing to deep study, every acquisition to be ephemeral and causing pain, resulting in repeated births and deaths, pleasure, and sorrow, then such a detachment is called *vaśikāra vairāgya*, or thorough detachment. Naturally, this *vaśikāra* state of *vairāgya* of the *citta* is not reached in one stroke. The ancients, to aid this practice and also by way of milestones to ascertain progress in *vairāgya*, mention three preceding levels of desirelessness. The first is known as *yatamāna*, or the stage of attempt. It is to go on attempting not to engage the sense instruments, the eyes, ears, organs of speech and procreation, and so on, in their objects for sensual enjoyment. When one is successful to a certain extent in the *yatamāna* stage, one's attachment toward some objects of the senses is completely eliminated, and toward others, greatly weakened. In fact, many Hindus attempt this by means of vows *(vratas). Eka patnīvrata* (one person, one spouse), as opposed to promiscuity; abstinence for specific periods; control of one's diet by taking only *sattvic* food (conducive to *nivṛtti* thoughts) and rejecting the *rajasic* foods that make one highly aggressive and hyperactive, and *tamasic* substances like alcoholic beverages, which produce dullness and stupor, are examples of some of these vows. After this practice of self-control, there is a general disposition toward renunciation itself, arising out of mental clarity and a sense of well-being. Maintaining this level so that this partial self-control is firmly established is called the *vyatireka* stage. When this practice of abnegation is extended to all sense objects, and one loses completely all interest in pleasurable sensations so that only *citta*, the eleventh organ, or *antaḥkaraṇa*, retains the attachment in the form of old habits *(saṃskāra),* it is called *ekendriya*. Through further practice, when the mind by discrimination realizes the ephemeral character of itself, it is called *viveka* (discrimination), and one is said to have reached the fourth stage of *vairāgya*. There are many authorities on Indology who have concluded that the Hindu philosophies are dismal ones and are pessimistic. Anyone who reads the *vairāgya* portion contained in Yoga or Vedānta will naturally concur with this view. Sāṃkhya, the theoretical basis for Yoga, states that all of phenomenal existence is suffering of only three kinds. Furthermore, the other great philosophy, Buddhism, was born out of a great soul's intense feeling of despair on seeing the misery of all human beings. Hence, such people tend to become desireless and still reach the stage mentioned in Yoga. This is definitely a negative approach, in that those who are highly sensitive—as, let us say, is the eye when compared to the rest of the body—develop *vairāgya* naturally. But Patañjala yoga recognizes that this *vairāgya* is of an inferior nature. Such persons become merged in the feeling of existence stated above (*bhava,* existence, *pratyaya,* awareness) and subsequently get the power to concentrate completely and master the entire *prakṛti*, in its gross form, in its subtle form, or merged in the feeling of bliss or pure "I exist" feeling. It is also known as *samprajñāta samādhi,* or objective-knowledge-producing *samādhi.* On concentrating on the feeling of desirelessness *(vairāgya)* and by practice, they remain in that state.

The *apara vairāgya* of four states mentioned above may lead to a *citta* that becomes habitually nonresponsive to external stimuli. It does not lead, however, to self-establishment (or realization). To achieve an unbroken state of *nirodha*, for its permanent establishment in one's own true nature of total consciousness, knowledge of the principles mentioned earlier is necessary. Thus, after completely understanding the state of the observable *prakṛti,* one practices *vaśikāra vairāgya* and attains a state of *nirodha*. If, however, it is continued with the positive knowledge of the pure state of one's self, the *vairāgya* becomes strengthened. There is now a prop for the *citta* to remain quiet, as it knows that what is achieved is not merely due to a reaction from pain but is derived from the positive knowledge of the true nature of the Self. This is known as *paravairāgya,* or the highest *vairāgya.* The desirelessness *(vaitṛṣnya)* toward the ever-changing, qualitative, phenomenal, painful existence is fortified by the positive knowledge of one's own Self. It requires earnestness in the study of *nivṛtti* texts, enthusiasm to reach the goal, and constant deliberation in the mind, leading to total absorption *(samādhi)* of Self, resulting in perfect knowledge of the Self. This is the right royal path of yoga, according to Patañjali. It is thus the most optimistic philosophy, since it tells the aspirant about the highest goal of human existence and the definite means of achieving it.

Some more thoughts on *vairāgya* may be relevant. Sāṃkhyas point out that when the *citta*, or, more particularly, when the *buddhi* is *sattvic*, it can go in the direction of *dharma* (order), *jñāna* (incisive spiritual knowledge), *vairāgya* (dispassion), or *aiśvarya* (mastery of *prakṛti,* or nature). Except for those in the second *(jñāna)* group, the rest, without the correct perception and knowledge of the Self, tend to work toward achieving higher levels of happiness *(dharma and aiśvarya)* or avoiding unhappiness *(vairāgya).* The *dharmis* who faithfully follow the ritual worship and similar prescribed and optional *(kāmya)* procedures elucidated in the Vedas and subsidiary scriptures reach different heavenly abodes *(svarga)* and become gods and angels *(videha).* Then there are those that are pain-shy who withdraw into some aspect or other of *prakṛti,* say a *tanmātra* or *asmitā.* They are called *prakṛtilayas* (those that merge with an aspect of nature). This itself forms the foundation of *layayoga.* Sāṃkhyas say that from *vairāgya, laya* takes place *(vairāgyat prakṛti layaḥ).* Third are those who develop the capacity for contemplation *(samādhi),* master the entire universe, and attain supernatural powers *(aiśvarya)* called *siddhi* or *vibhūti,* and this is a yogi's approach, albeit of a lower order—lower with respect to the *nirodha* yogis. What is common in all three—the ritualists, the renunciates, and the *siddha* yogis—is that even as their *citta* is highly *sattvic,* because they lack the distinctive knowledge of the Self *(viveka),* they tend to have the attitude *(pratyaya)* of existence *(bhava).* The overriding concern of all three is that they must continue to exist forever *(bhava pratyaya)* with more happiness and less pain. Patañjali says those who have the I-should-exist-forever desire may follow any one of the three approaches and become *videhas* (gods or angels) or *prakṛtilayas* (*laya* yogis). On the other hand, a *viveka jñani,* one who has knowledge about the dichotomy between the entwined principles of *puruṣa* and *ahaṃkāra* (ego locus), is able to reach a state of *kaivalya* or permanent freedom. This *pratyaya*, or attitude, is dominated by—according to Patañjali—complete desirelessness (*virāma* = let there be an end to *saṃsāra*). And it is achieved by incessant practice (of the twenty-five principles) until the entire *citta* is transformed into one with the *saṃskāra* (habit) of not engaging in either *pravṛtti* or *nirodha*. The time it takes, which may be one or many births, will depend on the intensity of the practice. Those who practice yoga with great intensity *(tīvra)* get results quickly, and others are classified as either lethargic, moderate, or earnest in their practice and attain results in due time, even extending over several births.

It has been mentioned that *vairāgya* and *tattva abhyāsa* are the means of attaining the *nirodha* of *citta*. To the question of whether there is any other means of achieving the ultimate goal of a yogi, which is *kaivalya*, Patañjali suggests a second but equally important means known as Īśvarapraṇidhāna, which is a special devotion *(bhakti viśeṣa)* on the part of the devotee/yogi. It is a method of *prapatti*, mentioned earlier. Īśvara, or God, is a special *puruṣa*, but unlike individual souls, it is unaffected by afflictions *(kleśa)*, deeds (karma), the results of actions *(vipāka)*, or the desire for action and results *(āśaya)*. In Him are contained all knowledge in potential form, He being omniscient. He is the first preceptor, especially of spiritual knowledge, but transcends time and space. He responds and manifests to the devotee through repetition of the most sacred mantra, the *praṇava* (OM). *Praṇava* literally means "the highest praise," arising out of devotion. The repetition of OM, pronounced AUM, is known as *japa*, which is done while contemplating the secret meaning of the sacred syllable. Such deep meditations further help to remove all the obstacles confronting a yogi in his quest for self-realization. All deeds and results thereof are dedicated to Him in a spirit of loving and offering, with simultaneous total surrender. The obstacles that are overcome with Īśvarapraṇidhāna include distractions such as sickness and others such as attachment to yogic states and subsequent slipping to lower states. These are definite distractions a yogi should try to avoid. The symptoms of such distractions are a heavy heart resulting from sorrow, and also dejection, tremulous movements, and heavy breathing.

Patañjali's formulation of Īśvarapraṇidhāna, according to my teacher, is the more important or the only means available in this Kali Yuga. He would say that the word *vā* in the *Yogasūtras* should be construed as meaning "only" and not its usual meaning as "or." This corresponds to *bhaktiyoga* (devotional path) as distinct from the path of contemplation *(jñāna tattva abhyāsa)* propounded by the Sāṃkhyas and accepted in toto by Patañjali. The two approaches mentioned in the *Yogasūtras* have a parallel in the Vedānta *darśana*, especially in the Gītā school. Like the Sāṃkhyas' *tattvajñāna*, Vedāntins have developed the *jñāna mārga*, or path of vision (about the nature of Brahman), and *bhakti mārga*, or path of devotion to the Lord. There are lively discussions about the superiority or even the validity of either of these paths; suffice it to say that both have their adherents. A Purāṇic anecdote about the efficiency of each of the systems may be of interest.

Lord Śiva, with his consort Pārvatī, was in his abode Kailāsa. An old devotee offered him a delicious mango. Lord Śiva then turned to his two sons, Gajāmukha (the elephant-headed) and Ṣaṇmukha (the six-headed), and offered the mango to the one who could travel around the universe more quickly. Soon enough, Kārttikeya (or Ṣaṇmukha) mounted his peacock *vāhana* (vehicle) and in a flash started to fly around the universe. He knew that his obese and phlegmatic brother Vināyaka (Gajāmukha), using his *mūṣika vahana* (mouse vehicle), could never be a match for his speed. He was sure to win the contest and get the coveted sweet mango.

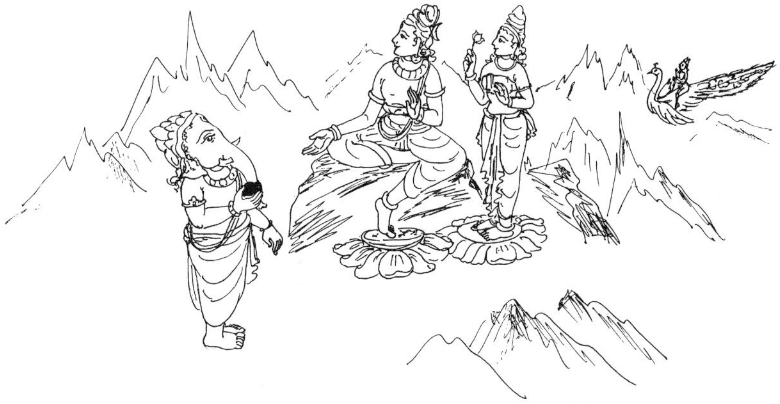

Vināyaka's prizewinning strategy

Vināyaka had his own strategy. He held his hands in *añjali* (salute) and went around his parents, Śiva and Pārvatī, with great reverence. After completing the *pradakṣina* (the going around), he told his parents that he had won the race and asked for the prized mango. He said to his quizzical parents, "You are the universe, my Lord. I have completed your task, and I deserve the fruit, and Kārttikeya is nowhere in sight." Sure enough, when Kārttikeya completed his round trip of the vast universe, he was flabbergasted to see Vināyaka feasting on the prized mango. That he become very angry and did not accept the verdict is another matter. He had lost the race. The moral of the story is that *bhakti* is easier to practice than *jñāna*. This is especially true in this Kali Yuga.

While on this subject of the *bhakti*, or devotion, of Vināyaka toward the universal parents *(Ādi bhagavan)*, it may be worth digressing a bit more to consider the peculiar deities worshiped in India. How do Hindus worship so many forms, some human and others human-animal hybrids? It is generally conceded by religions that God created man after Himself. That is to say, if God has a form, He would be like to a man (or human being). So several Hindu deities have a human form, except that they may have more arms to indicate several divine functions. But some deities have a human body but the head of a different species. God made man after Himself, but He also made several other species. So why should not God be considered to have both a human and an animal form? Then we have several possibilities for viewing the form of God. He can have a human trunk but with the head of the best of animals. If one considers the elephant to be the most majestic of animals, then

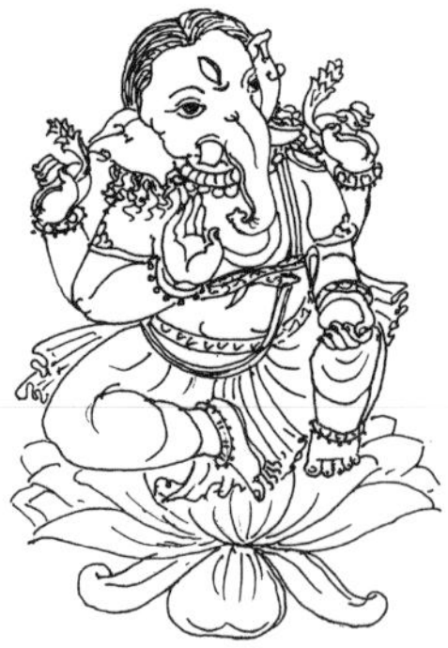

Vināyaka

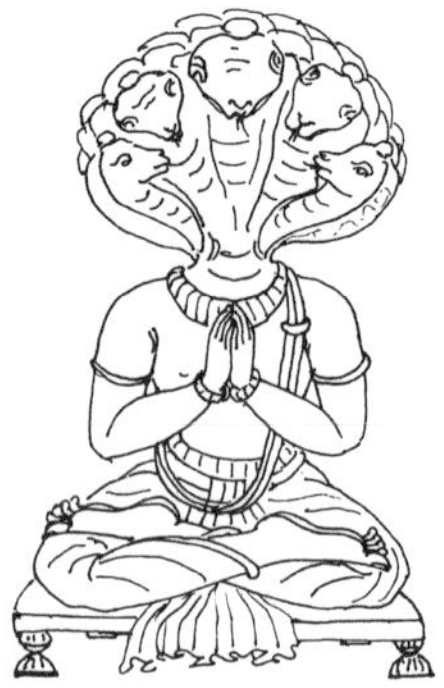

Ādiśeṣa

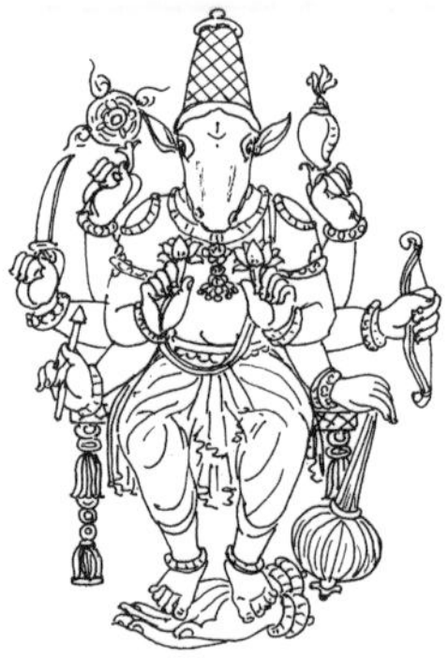

Hayagrīva

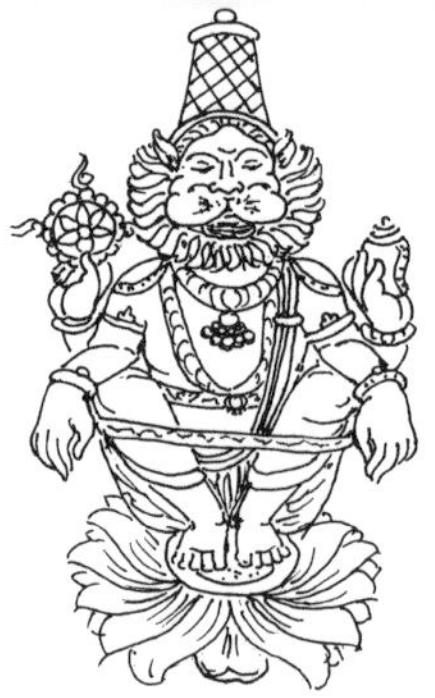

Narasimha

we have Vināyaka, the elephant-headed deity with a human body, who is the most beloved deity of all. The lion is the king of the forest, even though man rules his habitat. So we have Lord Narasimha, the man-lion incarnation of Lord Viṣṇu. The horse is one of the fastest animals, and it is a very lovable, intelligent animal that can be trained by a human. It is used in war and to travel long distances and proves its usefulness continually. Thus we have Lord Hayagrīva, considered the deity of knowledge, Vedic knowledge. He is said to save the Vedas, the repository of spiritual knowledge and *dharma*, at the end of each *yuga*. He has a human body and the head of a horse. There are several people who are fascinated by the reptile species. The cobra is the most venomous, but again highly respected and worshiped by different groups in India. Patañjali is an incarnation of the cobra Ādiśeṣa. Patañjali is depicted as having a human form but with a thousand cobra hoods.

Whenever a *samāhita citta* slips into a state of distraction, because of nonobservance of yogic practices, he could regain his original state of mind by *eka tattvābhyāsa* (meditation upon one principle). What is that one principle? It could be a reiteration of the Īśvarapraṇidhāna, to indicate that by surrendering to the one unique *tattva*, Īśvara, one could regain the *citta*'s *samāhita* state. According to some authors mentioned by my teacher, *ekatattva* refers only to Īśvara. It makes sense to take *ekatattva* as Īśvara, because Sāṃkhyas have mentioned the *pañca vimśati tattva* (twenty-five principles), the knowledge of which will lead to *kaivalya*, and, in contrast, Patañjali offers the alternative of knowing one principle alone. Referring back to the mango story, Vināyaka went after the one principle (Īśvara), and Kārttikeya, the twenty-four principles *(prakṛti)*. Patañjali also suggests the use of several other classical and traditional methods to regain mental equipoise whenever the mind deteriorates to a state of *vikṣepa* (distraction), manifested by the four symptoms mentioned earlier. These classical methods are discussed next.

Since the yogi is after self-realization, he or she needs to develop a *citta* that is not distracted by the attitudes of others toward him or her or toward others. Patañjali divides humanity into four attitudinal groups. It is said that the yogi should develop and practice a spirit of friendliness *(maitrī)* toward those that are contented and hence happy *(sukhī)*. Then there are those who suffer from the three types of mental afflictions *(duḥkhi)*; toward such unhappy mortals he should feel extreme compassion *(karuṇā)*. Those that tread the path of virtue *(puṇya)*, engaged in prescribed duties and working toward the welfare of society, evoke in the yogi a spirit of goodwill and appreciation *(mudita)*. But then to those who are influenced by *tamas*, who are steeped in indiscriminate actions and vice and cause suffering to others, he will be indifferent *(upekṣā)*. This attitudinal orientation of the *yogābhyāsī* gives rise to an untainted pure *citta (citta prasāda)*, and a purified mind regains one-pointedness and becomes serene. This particular method is prescribed in many religions and philosophical books in India. One of the mantras in the Lalitā Sasharanāma of the Brahmāṇḍa Purāṇa refers to this practice. The prayer is to the goddess Lalitā to give the devotee a boon to change his attitude so as to attain serenity and be able to meditate upon the mother *(maitryādi vāsāna labhyaḥ)*. I have seen some Buddhist treatises commend these attitudes as a part of the process for purification of the mind.

The second classical method of cleaning the *citta* is a special *prāṇāyāma*. Here the object of contemplation is *prāṇa* itself, with the emphasis being on "breath control," especially long exhalation *(pracchardhana)* and retention after exhalation *(vidhāraṇa)*. This practice, which can be done easily by many, requires some guidance. An awareness of *prāṇa* movement *(sancāra)* is necessary. It will have a better effect if it is done with mantras, which practice is known as *samantraka prāṇāyāma*. The use of mantras, however, requires proper initiation. Patañjali's *Sūtras* give the quintessence of *haṭhayoga: haṭhayoga* is *prāṇāyāma*, and in *prāṇāyāma* the essential element is *recaka*, or exhalation. My teacher used to say that all yoga accomplishments become possible with the efficiency of *recake bala* (the capacity for *recaka*, or long and complete exalation). *Pracchardhana* means to empty the lungs completely—as the stomach becomes empty when one vomits. After exhalation, one should develop the capacity to retain the breath out *(vidhāraṇa)*. During the period of *bāhya-kumbhaka* (external retention of the breath), the *bandhas* can be practiced, through which the union of *apāna* and *prāṇa* can take place. There are other schools that recommend the use of *prāṇāyāma* mantra after exhaling; normally, a mantra is recited mentally when the breath is held in. Therapeutically, this *vidhārana* has tremendous potential, as it becomes possible to access several internal organs *(kośas)* by means of the *bandhas*, including the heart *(hṛdaya kośa)*. There is yet another practice called *viṣayavatī pravṛtti*. It is common knowledge that objects are perceived through the sense organs—they are felt, smelled, seen, heard, or tasted. Without the objects, however, it has been found that yogis can get various sensations—of a higher order—by concentrating on specific centers or places in the body. From where the sensations arise, it is possible, under proper guidance, to focus attention on these specific centers to obtain mental fixity. The *nāsāgra* is the spot of higher smell perception that helps to fix the mind firmly, and, it is believed, helps remove doubts. Similarly one may direct attention to a spot between the eyebrows *(bhrūmadhya)*—the center of sight. That practice, called *rūpa pravṛtti,* is a necessary means for devotees to meditate on the form of the personal deity.

When such one-pointed attention leads to intense concentration, the sensations the yogi has are out of the ordinary. Several yogis have expressed reservations about this exercise, however, as it may take the yogi astray and lead him to increased involvement with objective pleasures and *siddhis.* My teacher used to say that according to his guru, a yogi can do without this particular practice of *viṣayavatī pravṛtti.* Yet another practice calls for attention on the principle of light *(jyoti),* the practice itself being known as *jyotiṣmatī vṛtti.* This is the realization that all higher and divine experiences take place in the region of the heart *(hṛdayakamala).* It is said that the heart lotus is normally closed and looks suspended. It is in the heart lotus that the various feelings associated with the ego *(ahantā and asmitā)*—the locus of self—are said to be established. It is thus the seat of the *jīva,* and many Upaniṣads and *upāsanā* portions of the Vedas commend this practice. Thus, by directing the attention to the heart region, and particularly the center, and by imaging the soul in the form of a bright light *(jyotiṣ),* one's mental energy becomes focused and the mind becomes free from sorrow *(viśoka).* This is a classical meditative *(upāsanā)* practice mentioned in the Vedas, and it is called *dahara vidyā* (the art of meditating within the heart). It is common knowledge that depression *(śoka)* is removed by light. In a state of depression, the cave of the heart *(dahara)* appears dark. But by positing the idea of light from the *puruṣa* remaining in the heart, this negative emotion can be eradicated. A passage in the Taittirīya Āraṇyaka that starts with *"Jyotiṣmatīm tvā sādhayāmi"* is a prayer to the soul to brighten the heart lotus. According to Bhatta, a well-known commentator, this prayer praises the light of the soul *(puruṣa)* in twelve epithets, although Sāyaṇa, another renowned commentator, relates these mantras to the consignment of the body to the fire. In the last chapter of the Yajur Veda, the idea of *viśoka,* a state free of depression, is attributed to the *puruṣa* (soul), which is described as being smaller than an atom *(aṇu)* and also greater than the greatest phenomenal principle (*mahat,* the first evolute according to the Sāṃkhyas). By meditating upon the light of *ātman (puruṣa),* the depression *(śoka)* goes away and the subject experiences immense bliss. The Mahānārāyaṇa Upaniṣad, in the passage praising the *sannyāsi* (renunciate), exquisitely describes the supreme soul inside the heart, which is seen directly by the *sannyāsi,* who then becomes free from *śoka (viśoka).* The classic Puruṣasūkta (prayer on the supreme indwelling *puruṣa*, or soul) describes the light as resembling lightning. The *trātaka* practice of *haṭhayoga* is in conformity with this Vedic practice. The Upaniṣad prayer *Tamaso mā jyotir, gamaya* is again a prayer for leading the yogi from *tamasic* darkness in the heart to the effulgence of the soul. Shedding the desire *(vīta rāga)* for external objects and sensations *(viṣaya)* by constant inquiry is another method, which is a very important practice to those who follow the *vairāgya* approach to *kaivalya*, or independence. It is also recommended that one repeatedly think of a person (saint) who is desireless. God, in His boundless compassion—as the people who follow the path of surrender proclaim—creates great spiritual souls for the benefit of every generation as objects for contemplation and subsequent emulation. Thus, many devotees of extraordinary spiritual personages do get mental peace by constantly thinking about their savior or guru. This is a very prevalent practice. Many people travel far and wide to see *(darśana)* great *sannyāsis*, such as the Paramācārya (since attained *samādhi*) of Kānci, and to experience immense peace. If one does not find such desireless people in the community, one may meditate upon such epic figures as Śuka, Sadāśiva Brahmendra, Śaṅkara, and others, and derive mental peace.

It is common experience that out of sound sleep, one gets a relaxed and clear mind. This sleep is known as *sattva nidrā*. In some Vedāntic literature it is said that in such *nidrā*, the *jīvātma* merges *(melana)* with the Universal Lord (Īśvara). By constantly remembering the pleasant, restful feeling of sleep, one can get a degree of mental peace. In addition, there are many pious people or devotees who once in their lifetime may get a divine dream *(divyam svapnam)* and experience a blissful feeling *(ānanda)* the like of which they or others may not have experienced in their normal waking state. By not ignoring it, but constantly drawing support from the divine vision, one can cultivate calmness of mind. Several religions accept dream experiences as valid, and some religious leaders discuss with their followers the experience and conversation they may have had with God in their dreams. A more involved explanation for the sūtra, *svapna nidrā jñāna ālambanam vā* ("by remembering dream and deep-sleep experiences"), can be found in Vedāntic literature. Study into the nature of sleep and dreams and comparing them with waking states has been the source of some great spiritual literature. Arguing that the dream experience and waking states are not materially different, Śaṅkara and other *māyāvadins* claim that the waking-state experience is, like the dream, only a virtual reality. Further, the absolute reality, the soul, undergoes no change whatsoever in any of the three stages of waking, dream, and deep sleep. The entire Māṇḍūkya Upaniṣad, along with the great commentary *(kārikā)* of Gaudapāda, have brought unique inspiration to the understanding of Advaita philosophy. The various religious rituals, *upāsanas* (devotional practices), are also intended for *ekāgra*, or mental fixity. The Hindu religion is often criticized for the multiplicity of deities (or different forms), even as the Vedas proclaim the one Īśvara. This multiplicity is mainly meant to take account of different inclinations among those who are religiously minded. Recognizing this, different methods or gods for worship *(mata)* have come into vogue. Śrī Ādi Śaṅkara, the founder of the present-day Advaita school of Vedānta, is credited with reestablishing six such major schools of worship, going back to the Vedic gods. These well-known schools of worship are still prevalent in many Hindu families, societies, and temples, with minor variations in the forms of worship. The six forms of worship are those of Gaṇapati, Śakti, Śiva, Subrahmaṇya (Kumāra), Viṣṇu, and Sūrya (sun). The religions are known as Gāṇapatya, Śākta, Śaiva, Kaumāra, Vaiṣṇava, and Saura, respectively. Patañjali's sūtra *yatābhimata dhyānāt* (1.39) is sometimes commented upon differently, in that the word *abhimata* can be taken to mean any object to which a particular practitioner finds his mind becoming attached. Such an explanation is erroneous, however, and is not according to the sanctions of the religion to which Yoga claims allegiance. In fact, going after an object to which the mind is naturally attracted, owing to sensuality, is the very tendency Yoga tries to correct, instead recommending that the focus of attention be on divinity. Thus the word *yatābhimata* should be taken to mean "according to one's religious practice."

The above practices can help one gain mental clarity and fixity of mind, once one has a balanced mind. When a yoga practitioner is able to achieve mental fixity easily, then other natural mental states *(citta vṛtti)* become reduced. Such a mind is compared to a high-quality transparent crystal, and it can grasp any idea or object presented to it, just as a spotless jewel takes on the hue of the objects near it. The yogi can fix his mind on any place inside or outside his body and its centers, from the most minute to the whole of creation (nature). When his contemplation matures so that the totality of mental energy merges, as it were, with the object of contemplation, this is known as *samāpatti* or *sabīja samādhi.* Such accomplishments lead to complete mastery, ultimate power, and supreme objective knowledge.

The awareness of such a yogi is different from the knowledge acquired by ordinary mortals whose mode of acquiring knowledge is sensory, mental (inferential), or secondhand and through authorities. And as this yoga *(samādhi)* method of understanding increases, it simultaneously destroys the normal habit *(saṃskāra)* of acquiring knowledge through the senses and through inference or acceptance of authority. The highest form of such a yogi's contemplation is the prevention of even the yogic knowledge-producing practices, in which case the mind develops the habit of becoming indifferent to both kinds of objective knowledge. The *citta* develops the habit of not entertaining any idea or thought. This is the highest evolution of the *citta*, as enunciated in the first chapter of Patañjali's *Sūtras.* A calm mind *(samāhita),* by the practice of *samādhi,* becomes a contemplative mind and becomes all-knowing *(dharma megha).* Then by further practice the yogi reduces it into the perfect equilibrium of the three basic constituent characteristics *(guṇas)*—called *sāmya avastā*—the closest palpable manifestation of *prakṛti.* In such a state, the Self—as pure consciousness—remains in its true nature, which is consciousness alone. This is the state of *kaivalya* for the self and of *nirodha* for the *citta.* That is yoga, Pātañjala yoga.

According to my guru, Patañjali had four students—Mastakāñjali, Kritāñjali, Baddhāñjali, and Pūrnāñjali—which implies four levels of yogic evolution. In the first chapter, for the yoga *ārūḍha,* the highest yogi, *nirodha* yoga is explained. Even here, one can find shades of difference in the studentship. The first sūtra is meant to eliminate all nonauthentic yoga practices. The second sūtra defines what yoga is, and the highest of the highest yogis requires no further elucidation. The next-level yogi is satisfied when he learns, in the third sūtra, of the state of the *puruṣa* at the time when *citta vṛtti nirodha* has taken place. Further explanations of the *vṛttis* and the many ways of achieving *nirodha* are meant for those *ārūḍhas* who need further answers. The alternative method is then detailed for the equally important, but temperamentally different, *bhakti* yogis.

At the end of the *samādhi pāda,* then, a vast number of yoga enthusiasts whose minds require more training even to become fit for *nirodha* yoga, whose minds are in state of disturbance *(vikṣepa)* and yet who are yoga *āruruksu* (desirous of treading the path of yoga), still need to be addressed. In the second chapter, called *sādhana pāda,* Patañjali thus starts from the fundamentals. This chapter is for the less accomplished.

# 5 Mantrayoga

*Since it's nature's law to change, constancy alone is strange.*

IN THE *SAMĀDHI PĀDA* CHAPTER of the *Sūtras,* two types of *samādhi*—objective and objectless *(nirbīja)*—are discussed, with *nirbīja samādhi* of *citta* being the ultimate stage for the *citta* to remain in a state of *kaivalya.* To achieve this, the highest form of dispassion *(paravairāgya)* was mentioned as the primary means. This is possible for perhaps very few in the great sea of mankind, those whose mental evolution is so high that *vairāgya* comes to them easily and naturally. The whole chapter is on the final stage of spiritual evolution and gives the practices appropriate to that style. But what of those who yearn for liberation but whose minds are in a state of perpetual distraction? For them, Patañjali starts from the root causes of distractions and pain and recommends *sādhana,* or more mundane practice.

According to my *ācārya,* yogis are divided into three classes in Pātañjala yoga. The highest or most evolved is the one who starts with a balanced, steady *citta (samāhita),* but the generally distracted aspirants *(vyuthita)* could be further classified into middle-order *(madhyama)* and lower-order *(manda)* aspirants. Both classes are dealt with in chapter 2 and in part of chapter 3 of the *Yogasūtras.* For the *manda* the yoga of activity *(kriyāyoga)* is recommended. Many people, because of their obligations to society and family, and also because of their own low level of (spiritual) evolution, keep their desire for spiritual progress in a dormant level for a long time, until they are free from many of life's obligations. This aspect is acknowledged in the well-known Hindu approach to the different stages of life, or *āśrama,* which consist of first, the stage of a student *(brahmacāri);* second, the family man *(grahasta);* third, the retiree *(vānaprastha);* and finally the recluse *(sannyāsin).* The latter necessarily have to start their yogic disciplines rather late in life, and Patañjali, out of great compassion, recommended *kriyāyoga* for them.

What is *kriyāyoga? Kriyā eva yoga,* where action alone is the predominant factor, is *kriyāyoga.* It is basically a purification process of the aspects of action, of body *(kāyika),* speech *(vācika),* and mind *(mānasika).* The three parts of this yoga are *tapas, svādhyāya,* and Īśvarapraṇidhāna. The word *tapas,* like *dharma,* is very widely used and encompasses different shades of meaning. It is a Vedic word, and those who are adept in *tapas* are called *tapasvins,* many of whom are subjects of adulation in the Purāṇas. Without *tapas,* no yoga is possible: *Na atapasvino yogaḥ. Tapas* means "to heat up intensely" *(tapa dāhe).* Just as intense heat is used to burn away dross in a nugget of gold, *tapas* is a well-planned regimen of purification. It may be noted that *tapas,* or austerity, should be such that it does not affect the humors of the body; one does not want to throw out the baby with the bathwater. Several yoga texts warn against some practices of extreme penance, like fasting for several days, or repeatedly doing *sūryanamaskāra,* a strenuous form of exercise. Brahmānanda, a commentator on the *Haṭhayogapradīpikā,* several times warns against doing *sūryanamaskāra* (sun salute)—as is vigorously advocated these days by many yoga exponents *(bahu sūryanamaskāram vrajet).* Fasting on *ekādasī* (the eleventh day after a full or new moon) is acceptable. But a practice such as fasting for forty days, for example, followed by some adherents of different religions, is not acceptable to a *yogābhyāsī.*

Moderation in food and diet is also *tapas.* Sadāśiva Brahmendra, a commentator on the *Yogasūtras,* says, *"hita, mita, medha āśanam tapaḥ." Tapas* is partaking of food that is *hita* or nourishing, easily digestible, and basically *sattvic.* What are *sattvic* foods? Several texts catalog them. Some, like the *Haṭhayogapradīpikā,* would ask the practitioner not to eat food that is not helpful to yoga, such as *rajasic* and *tamasic* foods and those that are sour, pungent, hot, or spicy. Mustard, a very common item in Indian food, is to be avoided. So should the yogi avoid *tamasic* alcohol and *rajasic* meat, fish, and so on. Yogurt, especially at night, should be avoided, as should jujube fruit, oil cakes, some hard peas, asafoetida—a favorite spice in south Indian food—and also garlic and onion. Why garlic and onion? Even though they are supposed to have health benefits, they are to be avoided by a yogi, as both are supposed to be non-*sattvic* foods. Why so? A Purāṇic story may not be out of place here.

The *devas* (good angels) were repeatedly defeated by the *asuras* (demons). As is their wont, the *devas* approached the Lord and pleaded that since good has to overcome evil in the scheme of things, they should be able to defeat the *asuras* and remain immortal. Immortality can be achieved, so the myth goes, by the *devas* being able to obtain nectar and drink it. But it could be obtained only by churning the milky ocean with the help of huge Mount Mandara as the axis of the churn, the serpent Vāsuki as the rope, and the *devas* and *asuras* holding Vāsuki at either end. The *devas* could not accomplish this stupendous task by themselves, and the only way they could get additional help was by roping in the *asuras*. So they agreed to share the nectar with the *asuras* after it was churned out of the milky ocean. The *devas* never had any intention of keeping their word, and besides, the Lord would help them for the sake of good triumphing over evil! After considerable effort, the nectar was churned out and contained in a pot. The *devas* and *asuras* sat in separate rows awaiting the distribution of the nectar. Now the problem was how to deny the demons their share of the precious nectar. If they also tasted it, parity would prevail, and the whole exercise would end in futility. It could even be worse: If the *asuras* became immortal, they would forever defeat the *devas* and dominate the universe, with evil *(adhama)* ruling always. Hence the Lord took the form of a bewitching damsel, named Mohinī (one who bewitches others with *moha*, or a spell), and went about distributing nectar to the *devas* first, instead of alternately distributing it between the two rows (slightly different versions of this story appear, but what is important is that the *asuras* were cheated). The *asuras* looked at Mohinī as if spellbound, without noticing that they were being deprived of their share right under their noses. Toward the end, however, two of the *asuras*, realizing what was happening, crossed over to the other side and managed to get just a drop of the nectar, the last drops from the vessel. Except for Rāhu and Ketu, none of the *asuras* got to taste the fruits of their hard labor. Sūrya and Candra (sun and moon), members of the *deva* clan, realizing that two of the *asuras* had tasted the nectar, beat them up (or the Lord beat them up with the ladle, aided by the two *devas*). The two hurt *asuras* spat blood and phlegm, but did not die, since they had taken the nectar, albeit a small portion.

What is the relevance of the story? From the blood and phlegm that fell on the ground sprouted two species of plants—onion and garlic. These two have medicinal values because they have traces of nectar in them. But since they were from the excretions of *asuras*, who are basically non-*sattvic*, people who eat them tend to develop *rajasic* and *tamasic* or *asuric* characteristics that are antagonistic to the *sattvic* quality the yogi wants to strengthen in himself. Hence, these are taboo for a *yogābhyāsī*. Reheated food is also to be avoided. Cooked food kept for more than three hours is not fit for consumption, according to the Gītā. In this microwave age, freshly cooked food is a rarity. Foods with an excessive amount of salt and that are acidic (such as the tamarind dishes of south India) are also to be avoided. Food that is hard to digest, such as those made of ulud, a high-protein lentil (and compared to meat by conventionalists), are likewise to be avoided. Other practices such as using a heater (with naked flames) in cold season (rather than blankets), long travel, and hard labor that requires spending a large amount of calories (some yoga classes are good examples) should be avoided as well.

Which food items are agreeable to a yogic way of life? Wheat and wheat products, rice, cow's milk, ghee (melted butter), rock salt (small amounts), honey, ginger—preferably in a dried form—vegetables—especially those that are grown locally—cucumber, fresh water, and fruits are good, and the food is to be offered to a favorite deity before eating. It is customary in many households in India religiously to offer cooked food to the deity after daily *pūjā* and before having lunch. Such food offered to the deity and then eaten, called *prasāda,* is said to increase *medhas* (offerings to God). The Upaniṣads stress the need for taking *sattvic* food. The Chāndogya Upaniṣad proclaims, *"āhāra śuddhou, sattva śuddhiḥ"* (with the intake of pure *sattvic* food, the *citta* becomes pure and *sattvic*). Of course, the term *āhāra* is given a wider connotation by such stalwarts as Śaṅkara to include all that is taken into the system—what one hears, smells, touches, sees—apart from food. *Mitāhāra* or *mitāśana* (moderation in food) is also part of *tapas.* Several yoga texts point out that obesity can be prevented with control over the diet. As a matter of guidance, it is said that one should fill the stomach with two parts food and one part water (liquids), and the fourth part should be kept empty, for digestion and to avoid gastric problems. One should stop eating when one feels that an extra helping can be had. In short, *tapas* in relation to food is taking *sattvic* food *(hita)* in moderation *(mita)* and after offering it *(medha)* to God.

Another aspect of *tapas* is with respect to speech and communication. It is the considered view of many yogis, including my teacher, that one who exercises no control over his speech has lost control of his mind. When one tends to talk aimlessly—such as with gossip and backbiting—the mind tends to get disturbed. My teacher used to say moderation in speech and food, *mitāśana* and *mitabhāṣaṇa,* is *tapas.* Here again there are extremes—some people resort to total silence during different parts of the day or for long periods of time. One should speak purposefully and in such a way that others will eagerly want to hear one. Śaṅkara and Āñjaneya of the Rāmāyaṇa are said to be perfect examplars of good communication skills. *Mouna,* or complete silence, is again divided into *kāṣta mouna* and *ākāra mouna.* When one does not speak at all, this is called *ākāra mouna*, but if one refrains from communicating, even through gestures, this is called *kāṣta mouna.* Let me be brief at least with this aspect of *tapas.*

*Tapasvins* are those who do *tapas* and are eulogized in the Purāṇas, or myths. In them, *tapas* refers to an extraordinary intensity of purpose that overcomes all difficulties and obstacles. Both the gods and the demons have resorted to *tapas* for achieving their ends—some *sattvic* (generally good), some *rajasic* (selfish ends), and some without any motive except the intense desire to have a vision of their god.

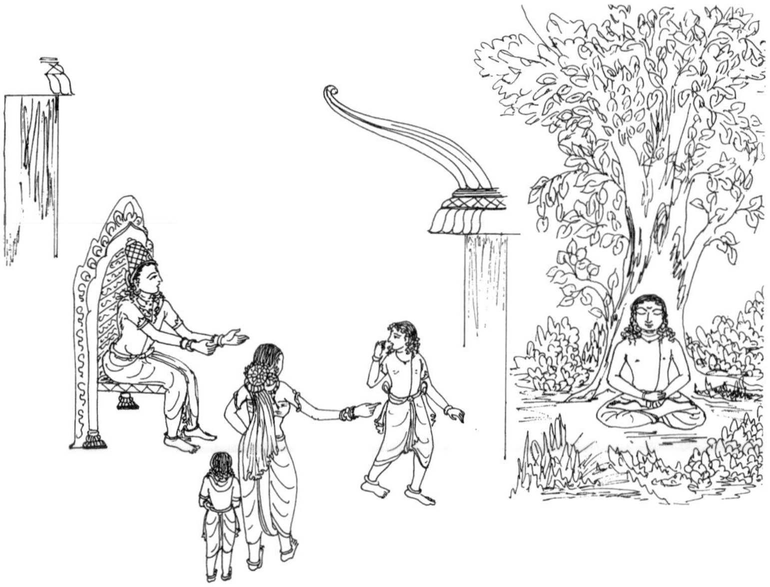
A distraught Dhruva leaving the palace and then attaining peace through *tapas* on the Lord

Here is a story from the Purāṇas. Dhruva, the young crown prince, upon seeing his younger half brother sitting there, wanted to sit on the lap of his father-king, who himself was occupying the throne. His stepmother, Suruci, would not allow it, and his henpecked father would not intervene. Dhruva's abandoned mother could do nothing except to suggest that he pray to the Almighty Lord, Viṣṇu (Nārāyaṇa). Determined to have a meeting with the Lord, the young prince, who was on his way to the forest, was met by Nārada. The little prince, not even ten, performed enormous *tapas,* or penance, in the forest, alone, in the cold, in the rain, and in the summer heat, all with single-minded devotion. At long last, the Lord answered his prayers and gave even more than had been asked. His father accepted him and he was made king later on. In addition, the Lord gave him a unique place in heaven, a fixed and permanent place, even as the other celestial beings have only tenured positions. Dhruva (meaning "steadfast") was made the Pole Star.

In yet another story, Prahlāda (great bliss) was the son of the *asura* Hiraṇyakaśipu. He had such great love and devotion for Lord Nārāyaṇa that the father, desiring everyone to accept him as a god, subjected him to all kinds of tortures, including drowning him, throwing him into an inferno, and so on. The son's love for the Lord never diminished, and he was always doing *tapas* of the Lord. He saw the Lord everywhere. The story ends with the Lord taking the form of a lion-man to destroy the demon king and finally absorb Prahlāda into Himself *(sāyujya).* Prahlāda exemplifies unadulterated *bhakti,* as does Bhagīrata, who did *tapas* standing on one leg (see *bhagīratāsana*) in order to appease Lord Śiva to let the river Gaṅgā flow down to earth from the Himālayas and thus get salvation for his dead forefathers, over whose remains the Gaṅgā's waters then flowed. The intensity of purpose, called *tapas,* is also evident in the Upaniṣadic episode of Bhṛgu, who attained Brahmanhood by intense *tapas* on Brahman. Bhṛgu asked his father,

Varuṇa, to teach him the nature of Brahman as described in the Vedas. The father, rather than giving a direct definition, gave him the direction or way to attain Brahman *(taṭasta lakṣana).* "Know that from which all these elements are created and sustained and into which everything merges, as Brahman." Bhṛgu intensively thought (did *tapas*) and found that matter was the source of everything and asked his father if this were so. Varuṇa, finding that his answer was only partial, asked him to go back and do more *tapas* (think deeply). In stages, Bhṛgu realized that the life force *(prāṇa),* mind *(manas),* intellect *(buddhi),* and happiness *(ānanda)* were all aspects of Brahman and the consciousness beyond all these manifestation was Brahman, the absolute. This intense pursuit of the knowledge of the ultimate is *tapas.* The Yajur Veda says several of the Vedic disciplines come under the rubric of *tapas.* They are: speaking the truth; speaking the essential; Vedic chanting; mental equanimity; control of the senses; calmness; charity; performing Vedic rites and doing prescribed duties; and worshiping the Lord.

In my experience of my teacher's method, *svādhyāya* is perhaps the most important aspect of yoga practice apart from *āsanas* and *prāṇāyāma.* Svādhyāya, according to my guru, is the study of the scriptures, here the Vedas. It is *sva-śakhā-adhyāyana,* or studying that branch of the Vedas with which one is traditionally affiliated. The Vedas are countless *(anantā vai Vedāḥ).* Hence each family used to study first the branch of the Veda corresponding to its family tradition. Presently in south India most people study the Taittirīya Śākha (Taittirīya branch) of the Yajur Veda. In the olden days, Vedic study included the memorization of the Veda as the first step. Since in the Vedic days the various scripts (written characters) were not developed, the Vedas were intently listened to and memorized and thus were known as *śruti,* or "that which is heard." If one wants to know about the other Vedas, one should master one's own Vedic branch before going to different teachers to study the others. In the olden days, those who went beyond their assigned Vedas were known as *dvivedi, trivedi,* or even *caturvedi,* depending on whether two, three, or all four Vedic renditions were studied. A *caturvedi* of present day may have no faith in the Vedas, but he carries a surname one of his forefathers may have earned.

Once the Vedas were got by heart, then, according to several Vedic commentators such as Sāyaṇa and Bhattabhāskara, one has to learn the meaning. Only then is such study known as a *vedādhyayana* or *svādhyāya.* To know any subject, one should study and understand the meaning of the texts. With the Vedas being the source of knowledge, *svādhyāya* became the main method of learning in the olden days. Since the development of the various scripts, most Vedas are now available in several different versions, like *nāgari* and *grantha,* or *telugu* and *kannada.* The mere memorization of the Taittirīya Śākha takes about seven years of continuous study and is taught in special full-time schools called *pāṭhaśālas.* To maintain the purity of the recitation, the entire text has fixed notes and methods derived to check and preserve the purity of the rendition. The number of words, paragraphs, and sections have all been calculated. There are a few experts who perform the recitation in several different ways such as *pada, krama, jhathā,* and *ghana.* When the text is recited continually as it is, this is called a *saṃhitā* recitation. This is the basic textual recitation. It is said that if one recites the Vedas regularly, one attains heaven. Furthermore, the gods, pleased with the prayers contained in the Vedas *(yenam triptaḥ),* bless the devotee with long life and make him a leader among men, glowing with glory, and bestow upon him popularity, scholarship, and wealth—according to the Vedic sayings. At the end of this life, the devotee merges with Brahman *(sāyujya).* When the sentences of the Vedic texts (mantras) are divided or split into individual words and recited one word after the other without *sandhi* (conjunction), this order of recitation is known as *pada pāṭha* (*pada,* "word," *pāṭha,* "reading"), or reading word by word. It is said that the benefit that accrues to the one who recites a text is twice as much as it is for one who merely reads it.

Yet another method of recitation is to take two words of the text, read them together, and then immediately recite them, as in the *pada* method. This method is called *krama,* and it is said to give the chanter four times the benefit of just reading the text. *Jhatha* recitation is like the strands of a braid: The first word is recited once, followed by the second word twice, then the first word twice, followed by the second word once, as in the *krama* method. For example, taking the three-word Śiva Pañcaksari mantra from the Yajur Veda, *namah śivaya ca,* and chanting it according to the *jhatha* method would yield: *namas śivaya śivaya/namo namas śivaya/śivaya ca ca/śivaya śivaya ca* (the first word once and second word twice; the first word twice and second word once; the second word once and third word twice; the second word twice and third word once). The benefit of more complicated recitations such as this increases exponentially! It is said that the *jhatha* method of recitation will bring one thousand times the benefit of the *saṃhitā* recitation. It is customary that this kind of *krama pāṭha* of Vedic chanting is arranged by experts for the benefit of devotees. If the procedure followed is done without splitting the words, but as a block of mantras following the rules of conjunction *(sandhi),* then it is called the *ghana* (heavy) method of recitation. Those who are able to do this kind of recitation from memory are called *ghanapāṭhi* (one who recites the Vedas using the *ghana* method). It is said that one's memory increases enormously by the use of this method.

*Ghanapāṭhis* are few and are a highly respected lot. Normally people with excellent memory and a booming voice attempt to be *ghanapāṭhis.* They were the preservers of the Vedas in the olden days when writing was not prevalent, and the purity of Vedas was well maintained generation after generation. In the Kṛṣṇa Yajur Veda, there are forty-four chapters of Saṃhitā that make up the mantra portion, apart from thirty-eight chapters in the Brāhmaṇa (ritualistic, forest, and Upaniṣad portions included). There are places where the recitation of the Saṃhitā portions is carried out continuously by one method after another. Those who chant, those who listen, and those who organize such chanting programs all derive benefit. Veda *pārāyaṇa* (chanting) occurs in many public places, like temples, so that everyone can benefit from listening to it. In the olden days it used to be presented for the public good as a charitable endeavor. Vedic chanting produces *sattvic* vibrations, and the *sattvic* quality in the environment is churned out, and everyone attains merger with Brahman in due course. My teacher and I belong to the Yajur Veda school of the Taittirīya section; in fact, this is the *śākha* to which most in south India belong. Śrī Kriṣṇamācārya taught us several of the important chapters in the Yajur Veda that are recited regularly. They should be chanted with *svara* and proper pronunciation.

Perhaps the most commonly recited chapter is the first chapter in the Āraṇyaka (forest) portion. The Yajur Veda (Taittirīya) consists of eighty-two chapters, forty-four of Saṃhitā, twenty-five of Brāhmaṇa, three of Kāthaka, and ten of Āraṇyaka the last four of which are the Upaniṣads. The first chapter, called Aruṇa Prapāṭhaka, or the chapter on Aruṇa, is also known as the Sūryanamaskāra, or sun salutation. It consists of thirty-two sections *(anuvāka)* subdivided into 132 paragraphs. Its recitation, if done unhurriedly, takes about an hour, and it is customary to chant it early on Sunday morning. This particular *prapāṭhaka* was chanted by my teacher and many of his students, times without number. The sun is worshiped for general health, longevity, and good eyesight *(arogyam bhāskarāt iccheth).* In the olden days it is said that sick and even terminally ill patients would be brought to the temple hall, where the recitation of this particular chapter would be done and the patients would listen to the chanting. My teacher once said that he, along with a few other Vedic scholars, would do Aruṇa *pārāyaṇa* aloud, even as they walked along the streets of Mysore. He was the *yogācārya* at the Mahārājah's *yogāśalā,* and the point of the walking chant was so that very ill people who were bedridden and unable to come out of their homes would hear at least a few mantras of this potent chanting. There are also a few devotees who do *saṣṭāṅga namaskāra* while facing east at the end of chanting each of the thirty-two *anuvākas* of Aruṇam. There are some yogis who do thirty-two *namaskāra* using *vinyāsakrama.* Thus it may be possible to combine the physical *namaskāra* with the Vedic mantras. Another method still used in south India is to do the Aruṇa *pūjā* to a *kalaśa* (vessel) containing pure water and complete the Aruṇam recitation after doing Varuṇa *pūjā* to the *kalaśa.* At the end of the recitation the holy water is sprinkled on the devotees, who chant or listen to the recitation and do *namaskāra.* The water may also be taken (in a spoon) as *ācamana.* There is also a practice by which a *sūrya yantra* and *pūjā* are done with the Aruṇa mantra with flowers and *akṣata* (rice). Of course, a regular *yajña* (fire sacrifice) also used to be performed that made use of the mantra. Several translations in English and other languages are available for those who want to know the meaning of these mantras. With 132 paragraphs, this is the longest chapter in the Yajur Veda. It would be beneficial if yoga schools could organize on Sundays and have Aruṇa recited by those who can do such recitation. Students who can do *sūryanamaskāra* can do the same at the end of each *anuvāka,* and others who have faith in Vedic mantras can sit down and listen to the chanting.

The second chapter in the Taittirīya Āraṇyaka is on *svādhyāya* or Vedic chanting itself. It stresses the importance of the regular practice of Vedic chanting and knowing the meaning of the mantras. If one chants the mantras with total concentration and dedication and also knows their meaning, this is as good as performing the various religious rites such as the *yajñyas* associated with the mantras *(yam yam kratum adhīte, tena tena api iṣtam bhavati).* Based on this, Patañjali (2.44), while explaining the benefits of Vedic recitation *(svādhyāya),* says that by *svādhyāya* one gets to communicate with the deity of the mantras and obtain all possible benefits *(svādhyāyād iṣṭa devatā saṃprayogaḥ).* This particular chapter narrates the glory of the famous *gāyatrī* mantra and how through its recitation during daily oblations *(sandhyā vandana)* the demonic characteristics of the mind are cleared. The chapter is an important one containing mantras for the repentance *(prāyascitta)* of the sins one tends to commit repeatedly, such as those committed with our minds, words, hands, and feet, the eating of unwholesome food, secretive indiscretions, and so on. The sins committed through words include, for instance, lies, backbiting, and rumormongering *(samkusuka, vikusuka, nirṛta).* It is said that if a person feels he has committed deeds that are *adhārmic* (not *dharma* or correct), then he should chant this chapter. It is also used to perform a *homa* (minor fire rite) called *kūśmāṇḍa homa.* This also contains the prayer to the *devas* of the four quarters, which is normally recited at the beginning of a gathering of scholars who came together from different directions. It is also recited before undertaking any major auspicious activity, such as the construction of a house, a wedding, a Vedic initiation *(upanayana),* or as a process to clear up mental cobwebs. The third chapter, called "Caturhotṛ Citi," contains the Puruṣasūkta (the prayer to the Lord in human form). Some of the mantras in this chapter are also related to last rites and to meditation on the soul as a form of light. The fourth and fifth chapters of the Taittirīya Āraṇyaka are recited early in the morning, and this recitation is again supposed to remove the ill effects of any *adhārmic* acts. The fifth *prapataka,* called Pravargya Brāhmaṇa, consists of 108 *anuvākas* or sections. The Pravargya is the only chapter that has a peace invocation at the beginning as well as at the end. These *anuvākas* are also recited before a wedding, before beginning study of the Vedas by initiates, and also at the end of these studies. It is a very important part of the famous fire sacrifice of the Vedic god Soma (Soma *yajña*). Basically this particular rite involves the use of mantras to boil cow's milk. The milk, when boiled to the accompaniment of the chanting of these mantras, becomes nectar. Those who perform this rite, or those who only chant these mantras, develop sharp intellect, a luster arising out of spiritual knowledge, energy, and power. The milk turns into nectar and is said to give one a very long, disease-free life. The Pravargya mantras have a number of beneficial effects. For example, they are efficacious in begetting adorable children. If one circles the *aśvattha* tree 108 times while chanting each of the 108 *anuvākas* of the Brāhmaṇa, it is believed that this will eradicate infertility in women; this is still a common practice in rural India. If one has dull children, then if one fills a pot *(kumbha)* with water, invokes the sun lord in the waters of the *kumbha,* does a recitation of the Pravargya mantras, and then bathes *(abhiseka)* the children, their minds will become sharp. During the afflictive periods of the Sun and Venus, those who suffer the ill effects, as well as those who desire the removal of the ill effects, of Rāhu and Śani (Saturn), can recitate the Pravargya mantra, do the mantra *japa* for *navagraha* (the nine planets), and make appropriate charitable offerings to reduce the ill effects. When one is unable to get cured from using medicines, or when one is unable to diagnose the cause of an ailment, one may listen to the chanting of these two chapters of majestic mantras to get relief. Sudden mental stress can be overcome by chanting these chapters in the shrine of Lord Śiva or of his other (formless) form, Dakṣiṇāmūrti. These mantras can also be used when one becomes weak or when one is involved in litigations. It is also said that those who suffer from terminal ailments may listen to these mantras and achieve a peaceful death without suffering *(anāyāsa maranam).* The second through fifth chapters are recited in public on the eighth day of the new or full moon *(aṣtamī),* or any other festive days when the village or town's temple deity is taken around the streets. This is said to ensure general prosperity to the region. Wherever one wants to do Veda *pārāyaṇa* (Vedic recitation) but cannot do the chanting himself, he should intently listen to its recitation by others. The mantras have the power, it is said, to create the right vibrations, both in the outer environs and in the *cakras.* I have always felt extremely good and peaceful at the end of an hour's chanting, especially of the Pravargya.

Another section that is recited regularly is the one containing the mantras used in the *aśvamedha,* or horse sacrifice. Among all the Vedic rites, these are supposed to be the most elaborate and efficacious. Later on, the horse sacrifice became a very important religious rite performed by kings who would establish their suzerainty over the neighboring kingdoms. Lord Rāma is said to have performed this *yajña.* In the rite itself, a thoroughbred horse, having been subject to the necessary preparations through the chanting of various Vedic mantras, would be let loose, followed by the king's army. The horse would wander around to the different kingdoms, and anyone who dared to stop and take possession of the horse would be fought tooth and nail by the king's army. The horse would be repossessed after the victory, and the hostile enemy would be taken prisoner. As prescribed by the scriptures, after the successful completion of the rite by the victorious king, the king would become an emperor, and if he completed one hundred such *yajñas*, he would, after death, take over as Indra, the head of the *devas* or celestial beings. Since this particular *yajña* required enormous resources and manpower, only kings used to perform the *yajña*, with the priests and scholars helping in the performance of the rite.

According to Vedic traditions, however, sincere recitation of the rite with an understanding of the meaning would itself produce the same results as performing the *yajña* with material objects *(yam yam kratum adhīta, tena tena api iṣṭam bhavati)*, and it has been the practice to recite this portion in its entirety. It is normally recited on the eleventh day *(ekādaśi)* after either the full or new moon. The *ekādaśi vrata* (vow) includes fasting, and in the afternoon the whole of the three central chapters (Acchidra and Aśvamedha) is chanted, which takes about three hours to complete. Aśvamedha is supposed to remove the disastrous consequences of committing such a heinous crime as killing a Vedic scholar as well as other despicable acts. It also includes mantras to the sun deity that help cure some terminal ailments such as a heart ailment *(hṛd rogam mama sūrya harimaṇam ca nāśaya)*. In India, there are several societies that arrange for scholars to come and recite these mantras on *ekādaśi* day, with several others joining in to listen to the three-hour recitation, even while fasting completely for the day. The fourth chapter in the same third section of the Taittirīya Brāhmaṇa is also recited with Aśvamedha. This fourth chapter is called the "Puruṣamedha." On the following day, *dvādaśi* (the twelfth day after the new and full moon), the last four chapters of the Yajur Veda, called the Upaniṣads, are chanted. Vyāsa, who wrote a commentary on the *yogusūtras*, comments that study of the scriptures leading to *mokṣa* (or release) will also come under *svādhyāya*. While Vedānta represented by the Upaniṣads is termed a *mokṣa śāstra*, other *nivṛtti* approaches like Sāṃkhya and Yoga will also qualify as *mokṣa śāstra*. Thus, study of these three subjects, namely Sāṃkhya, Yoga, and Vedānta, are part of *svādhyāya*. Without theoretical study (for a beginning practitioner), how can one know about spiritual matters? Sooner than later, people who practice yoga should study the texts supporting the yoga systems.

The last four chapters of the Yajur Veda are called Upaniṣads. According to the *dharma śāstra* (the treatises on *dharma*), the Upaniṣads are to be recited and studied daily. The Taittirīya Upaniṣad consists of three chapters (the seventh, eighth, and ninth of Taittirīya Āraṇyaka). This Upaniṣad is the one most often recited, and it is one of the ten major Upaniṣads that form the basis of the Vedānta system of defining the nature *(svarūpa)* of and means *(tatasṭha)* for experiencing the ultimate Vedānta truth. This Upaniṣad, even though it can be recited daily, is especially chanted on the twelfth day *(dvādaśi)*, immediately after the *ekādaśi vrata*. These three chapters describe the nature of the study of the Vedas *(śikṣā)*, the nature of Brahman *(ānanda)*, which is unalloyed bliss, and the step-by-step approach to realizing Brahman—which was explained above (in discussing *tapas*). The last chapter of the Yajur Veda is known as the Mahānārāyaṇa Upaniṣad and contains several of the Vedic mantras used in the daily religious oblations and in *upāsāna*, as well as various Vedic prayers *(sūktas)* to Sūrya and Durgā, and the Aghamarṣana, the prayer addressed to Varuṇa, lord of the element water, recited when one bathes. In addition, mantras used in daily *sandhyā* and *prāṇāyāma;* mantras to improve memory and for proper attention in class; the famous mantras used for meditation in the heart *(dahara vidyā);* mantras used before taking food; Śiva mantras; and the *trayambaka* mantra for longevity—all can be found there. Taittirīya Kāṭhaka, a distinct section between the Brāhmaṇa and the Āraṇyaka portions, is the source of the Kaṭha Upaniṣad, which itself in the inspirational basis for the Bhagavad Gītā. Of these three chapters, the first deals with the glory of Sāvitrī (the sun's luster); the second deals with story of Naciketas and is the basis for the Kaṭha Upaniṣad; and the third contains religious rites and mantras, like *caturhotriya.* All three chapters together take about two hours to recite. Some adherents recite *Kāṭhaka* again on *dvādaśi* day. Other important recitations include the famous Puruṣasūkta, and the Rudram and Camakam, from the Saṃhitā portion.

Since many will not be able to recite these Vedic passages, Vācaspatimiśra, the commentator on Vyāsa's *Yogabhāṣya,* includes those prayers consistent with the Vedic gods and philosophies as an acceptable form of *svādhyāya* for the *kriyāyogi* and *aṣṭāñgayogi,* grouped together as yoga *sādhakas.* His selections are taken from the two epics and the scores of Purāṇas, Upapurāṇas, and mythologies based on the Vedic revelations and Vedic gods.

Of all the Purāṇas, those on Viṣṇu are many and are perhaps the most widely read, and several portions are recited as prayers. One of the better-known prayers is the Viṣṇu Sahasranāma (Thousand Names of Viṣṇu) from the Mahābhārata. It is recited daily by thousands in houses and temples. The benefits accruing to one who recites or who hears the recitation is given in the *phalaśruti* following the *sahasranāma.* It is customary for all prayers to contain what is known as *phalaśruti,* or statement of benefits. It may be worthwhile cataloging the benefits mentioned by Vyāsa. Nothing inauspicious or unwholesome will ever come to pass to one who listens to or recites the Viṣṇu Sahasranāma daily. All four castes will get their due. A *brāhmana* gets the knowledge of the Veda and Vedānta; a *kṣatriya* conquers all his enemies; a *vaiśya* acquires immense wealth; and others will experience great happiness *(sukha).* A person wanting to lead a meritorious life will do so. One desiring wealth, on reciting the one thousand mantras of Viṣṇu, will acquire riches, and the sick will get well again. Those who want progeny get children. One who chants the *sahasranāma* of Viṣṇu becomes famous, a leader in his community, and acquires undiminished wealth and prosperity. He never falls sick and acquires a luster. He will become strong with noble qualities. If he suffers from any disease, he will be rid of it. If he is in bondage to another, he gets released. A habitually timid person becomes brave, and those with innumerable difficulties overcome them. The one who chants finally attains *mokṣa,* or total release, which is the main goal of human life. The chanting is done both in the morning and in the evening. Several commentaries including that by Ādi Śaṅkara are available explaining each and every mantra in the Viṣṇu Saharasnāma.

There is a convention by which the Viṣṇu Saharasnāma is recited along with the Indrākṣi and the Śivakavacam, two minor works on Śakti and Śiva, for protection from evil forces and cure of diseases, especially fevers. The other well-known work *(mūla grantha)* from the *itihāsas* that is routinely recited is the Rāmāyaṇa, especially the Sundarakānda, the part in which the monkey god, Āñjaneya, finds Sita and paves the way for her being rescued by Lord Rāma. This portion, consisting of over 2,800 stanzas, can be recited in about ten hours, and it is customary to do it over a period of seven days *(saptāha).* Girls aspiring to get married to pious men, when they are confronted with insurmountable legal or financial difficulties and no hope, are advised to recite or listen to the recitation of the Sundarakānda. Those who want to perform an extraordinary feat will get inspiration from the exploits of Āñjaneya narrated in this work. Another important work that is recited is the Devī Māhātmya or Candi, also known as the Durgā Saptaśatī, from the Mārkaṇḍeya Purāṇa, which consists of seven hundred stanzas. It is recited during the month of *purattasi* (September 15–October 15) for nine days following the new moon day. Several other works are recited regularly, such as the Lalitā Sahasranāma, already mentioned, and short prayers, such as the Āditya Hṛdayam.

The *mokṣa sādhana,* or philosophical works, are mainly the Sāṃkhya and Yoga philosophies and, directly from the Vedas, the Upaniṣads, ten of which are the most important and for which great Vedānta exponents have written lucid commentaries. The other works that follow the Upaniṣads are found in the Brahma Sūtras and the famous Bhagavad Gītā. These are not only chanted, but also studied in great depth by spiritual aspirants. *Svādhyāya* is not mere recitation, but also knowing the meaning and meditating upon the import of the mantras. The recitation of the Vedas and related scriptures is *svādhyāya.* It is always stressed that society should encourage the study of original works *(mūla pārāyaṇa).*

In his commentary Vyāsa includes the chanting of mantras from the Vedas and related scriptures as *svādhyāya* (for example, the *praṇava* and *mantra japa*). Patañjali introduced the *japa* of *praṇava* in the *samādhi pāda. Japa* is the chant of a mantra, aloud or silently with the lips barely moving, or else mentally, depending on the level of mental relaxation and concentration. Immediately after chanting the mantra, the *yogābhyāsī* has to meditate on the meaning of the mantra *(tat japaḥ tadartha bhāvanam).* Mechanical repetition of the mantra with a wandering mind is not *japa*. There are several mantras that are suitable for *japa*. According to old commentators like Mādhavācārya, mantras are of two kinds, Tantric and Vedic. Tantric mantras are basically *kāmya mantras*, and a very large body of knowledge is available explaining the various Tantric mantras and their elaborate rituals *(japa vidhāna).* They are highly potent, but beyond the scope of this discussion on *svādhyāya*, which is a Vedic word. The well-known Vedic and Purāṇic mantras that are chanted are quite numerous. The mantras can be one syllable, a word, a line, or a few lines. These are repeated a fixed number of times—10 times, 108 times ($1^1 \times 2^2 \times 3^3$), or 1,008 times, or several thousand times, even up to one crore (10 million), this last being done in a common place by several people over several days for the common good. Perhaps the most well-known Vedic mantra is the *praṇava*, or OM, and this mantra is the most fundamental and potent of Vedic mantras. The *praṇava* is extensively dealt with by philosophers, including Patañjali in his *Yogasūtras*. The *praṇava* is chanted alone or in combination with several other mantras, both Vedic and Purāṇic. It is customary to chant any mantra with the *praṇava*, with the latter usually as prefix. The other well-known Vedic mantra is the famous *gāyatrī* mantra of twenty-four syllables. The mantra is used to help the mind be rid of the dross of *tamas* and glow with enlightenment. The deity invoked is the effulgent sun, and the *ṛṣi* or sage who discovered this potent mantra is Viśvatmitra; the meter is called *gāyatrī*. It is customary among many devout Hindus to do *gāyatrī japa* thrice daily. On special occasions, one may chant it 1,008 times. There are a few who take the vow to chant it 1,000 times daily for several years. If one does this for about thirty years, one will have done this *japa* 10 million times, by which time one becomes a *siddha* of the particular mantra.

There are similar mantras for other deities in the *gāyatrī* meter and they are known by their respective deities, for example, Nṛsiṁhagāyatrī, Agnigāyatrī, Durgāgāyatrī, Śivagāyatrī, Viṣṇugāyatrī, and so on. Single-word Vedic and Purāṇic mantras are also popular among many devotees. The Śiva *pañcākṣarī*, the five-syllable Śiva mantra *(namaśśivaya);* the eight-syllable mantra on Lord Nārāyaṇa *(Om namonārāyaṇāya);* and the twelve-syllable Vāsudeva mantra *(Om namo bhagavate vāsudevāya)* are also popular among many *āstikas* for *japa*. Like the *gāyatrī*, there are a few other Vedic mantra passages that are also repeatedly chanted. The Mṛtyumjaya mantra is chanted to overcome the fear of death and attain *mokṣa*. It is a prayer to Śiva to save the devotee from the pain of death (physical and mental) and make him immortal: "I pray *(yejāmahe)* to the three-eyed Śiva, who emanates a pleasant smell (as against the stench of disease and death) and gives nourishment to all. May He release me from the clasps of death like a cucumber separates, imperceptibly, from the creeper." This highly poetic but poignant wish of the devotee for a painless release is a favorite mantra as one gets older.

My mother was very ill and the doctors attending her said that they might not be able to be of much help any longer. It was about 9 P.M., and when we asked her if she would like to be taken home, she agreed to go immediately. She was brought home in an ambulance. My wife arranged for drip-feeding for her, and the house was full of relatives. At about 3 A.M., she called me and asked me to fetch our family astrologer-priest after dawn. "Why?" I asked her. She would only say that she was ready to go, but wanted to talk to him. I managed to fetch him at about 11 A.M. on the following day. He immediately sent for a few Vedic *paṇḍits*, who were asked (all three of them) to chant the Mṛtyumjaya mantra 1,008 times. After the preliminaries, they started the chant of the mantra: *Trayambakam yejamahe sugandhim puṣtivardhanam. Urvārukamiva bandhanāt mṛtyor mukṣīya māmṛtāt.* After the initial *saṅkalpa* to state that the *japa* was being done for the benefit of my mother, the *japa* went on for about forty-five minutes. Before it started I asked my mother if this is what she wanted done, and she immediately said yes. The framed picture of her favorite deity *(iṣṭa devatā),* Mother Karumari, was hanging in the wall in front of her. After doing about six hundred or so *japa,* my mother, who was lying down, was put into the reclining position. She slowly closed her eyes, and her lids appeared heavy. After about one hundred chants, when I asked her if she could hear me, she nodded her head. I then asked her if she could hear the chanting, and with eyes still closed, she nodded with a relaxed smile.

After about three minutes, my wife said that her pulse appeared to start threading. My mother turned her head a couple of times, then opened her eyes and gazed at the picture of her favorite deity. She died with her gaze fixed on the divine picture. She was gone, separated from life—like a cucumber separates from the vine. It is customary among Śaivites to mutter "Śiva, Śiva" in the ears of a dying person. In my mother's case, Śiva's favorite mantra, the Mṛtyumjaya mantra, was repeated several times as she passed away from life to the eternal.

There are other Vedic passages that are chanted to improve memory, concentration, health, longevity, wealth, progeny and so on. Among the mantras from the Purāṇas that are popularly chanted are Rāma, Kṛṣṇa, Govinda, Śiva, Ambā (mother), and Añjaneya. *Tapas* and *svādhyāya* are very well ingrained in the ancient religious ethos. The Rāmāyaṇa starts with the words *tapas, svādhyāya nirataḥ,* "the sage well established in *tapas* (austerity) and *svādhyāya* (spiritual studies)."

The next aspect of Patañjali's *kriyāyoga* is Īśvarapraṇidhāna, a term used to describe an alternate method for attaining *kaivalya* in the *samādhi pāda*, intended for the highest-level yogi. It should be understood that Īśvarapraṇidhāna is a complete spiritual practice whose range includes practices appropriate to the three levels of yoga. It is included as a *niyama* (prescribed duty) for the midlevel *aṣṭāṅga* yogi. In the context of *kriyāyoga* it would refer to Īśvarapūjana, or worship of the Lord, as ordained in the various *śāstras.* The Gītā talks about the Lord becoming pleased with any offering from the devotee, whether a *tulasī* leaf, a fruit, a flower, or a spoonful of water for *ācamana.* Īśvara *pūjā* as an aspect of *praṇidhana* is a well-established religious practice. There are several *pūjā* methods in vogue—some are very elaborate and some brief, and several methods based on Vedic tradition are quite comprehensive. Temple worship will fall under Īśvara *pūjā,* which varies from tradition among families.

*Nitya* (daily) *pūjā* of the Lord is considered a daily routine in orthodox families. Of the several methods, the *pūjā* of Īśvara in the form of Śiva, or Śiva *pūjā,* is well known. A Śiva *liṅgam* is used for the *pūjā,* or worship. Even though I am tempted to describe this *pūjā krama* (method of doing *pūjā*) in detail, it is beyond the scope of this book. Other well-known *pūjā kramas* include, among Vaisnavites especially, the *saligrām pūjā.* The Śiva *pañcāyatan pūjā* (worship of five deities at once) is also popular among *smartas,* with a Śiva *liṅga* in the middle, Ganapati in the form of a small lump of turmeric or a red icon in the southwest, Mother Śakti in silver in the northwest, Viṣṇu in the form of *saligrama* in the northeast, and Sūrya (the sun) in the form of a crystal *(sphaṭika).* There are other methods by which one's favorite deity, for example, Viṣṇu, can take center stage. There are some who would add a small spear representing Lord Subrahmaṇya, the sixth deity of the orthodox system of *ṣaṇmata* (six forms of religious worship). It should be noted that *kriyāyoga* is the essence of Hindu religious practice, embodying austerities, the study of scriptures, and devotion to the Lord.

Patañjali (2.43) indicates the manifold benefits of *kriyāyoga.* It stops depression and unhappiness and prepares the *citta* for *samādhi,* which itself is the prerequisite to attaining *citta-vṛtti-nirodha.* Doing *tapas* purifies the body and especially the senses *(kāyendriya siddhir aśudhi kṣyāt tapasaḥ). Svādhyāya* gives one a first glimpse into the nature of self, and the mind gets the desire to experience *puruṣa.* Thus the individual gets a measure of control over the senses and *citta,* and, rather than being engrossed completely in worldly *vṛittis,* starts contemplating spiritual pursuits. Īśvarapraṇidhāna helps the *citta* to develop the capacity for *samādhi,* a necessary condition for bringing about direct perception of *puruṣa.* It should be noted that Patañjali, even as he advocates the procedure for inquiry, gives equal importance to the yoga of devotion by including Īśvarapraṇidhāna for all three levels of yoga, in *kriyāyoga,* in *aṣṭāṅgayoga,* and in yoga. Īśvarapraṇidhāna is a comprehensive devotional path for reaching *kaivalya.* At the level of *kriyāyoga,* the first-stage aspirant is required to make use of the well-developed system of *pūjā* to the Lord. Through its rather elaborate ritual, it helps the *yogābhyāsī* achieve *ekāgratā,* or one-pointedness. For the middle-level yogi, as an aspect of *niyama,* it requires surrendering the fruits of all action to the Lord and a sense of total submission. For the *kriyā* yogi, Īśvarapraṇidhāna helps to prepare the mind for *samādhi (samādhi bhāvana).* For the more advanced *aṣṭāṅga* yogi, Īśvarapraṇidhāna facilitates the attainment of *samādhi* itself *(samādhi siddhi),* along with the other *aṅgas.* The born yogi with a natural ability to go into *samādhi* is able to achieve the ultimate goal of *kaivalya* with Īśvarapraṇidhāna or meditation on Īśvara as mentioned in the *samādhi pāda.*

What are the *kleśas,* or causes of pain, that *kriyāyoga* is able to reduce significantly? The worst *kleśa (kliśnāti iti kleśaḥ)* is misconception about the nature of the self. *Avidyā,* or nescience, produces impressions that are not consistent with reality. The goal described in the first chapter of Pātañjala yoga is to make all five *kleśas* of the *citta* cease. The objective is to attenuate the five causes of pain, the five *kleśas.* Misconception, mistake, and misunderstanding are the cause of all pain, whether in worldly or spiritual matters. *Sāmyak darśana,* correct perception, is what is to be obtained. Now, what is *avidyā?* It is the general term used to denote misconceptions about permanence, wholesomeness, happiness, and the Self. When what is not is taken to be what is, this is *avidyā.* The results of this generalized *avidyā* are manifold. The most fundamental misconception is about the Self. When one wakes up from deep sleep, the waking takes place while the feeling of "I am," or "I exist," arises. The *vṛtti* that one experiences as one wakes up is called *asmitā (aham asmi iti bhāvana asmitā).* Since it is a *vṛtti* that is experienced, the "I exist" feeling is not the Self, the experiencer, say all philosophers including Patañjali. The thought of "I," with its firm locus in the *citta,* becomes more and more established from childhood to adulthood. It divides all other external objects into those that are favorable and those that are not, even though none is favorable or unfavorable to the nonchanging, overseeing Self. Then *citta,* without knowing the real nature of the Self, develops an affinity for objects that are favorable (because they produce happiness to *citta*) and a dislike for objects that are unfavorable. It culminates in the final *kleśa,* or affliction, called *abhiniveśa,* or fear of losing what is favorable and being harmed by what is unfavorable. Hence the fountainhead of all these afflictive causes is *avidyā,* or the misconception about one's own Self.

The *cit* or consciousness is the seer—the one that constantly oversees whatever happens in the *citta,* in which the locus of the "I" feeling resides. When the *citta* does not distinguish the difference between the seer and the "I exist" feeling, or self-locus, which itself is a thought, or a *citta vṛtti,* that is experienced, this affliction or misconception is *asmitā.* The *citta,* when it develops a desire for objects that appear to create happiness—even as no object really affects the Self one way or the other—is called *rāga,* and the other side of the coin is *dveṣa* (dislike). Fear is *abhiniveśa,* and the greatest of the *abhiniveśa kleśa vṛtti* is the fear of death, the fear of losing everything, including the pseudo-self. This phenomenal fear is in all of us, even the best of scholars who have studied the nature of the self. *Kriyāyoga* helps to reduce these five afflictions. They have to be reduced because in the *udāra avastā*, the highest afflictive stages, they become an obsession—an obsession about one's own interests to the detriment of all others, of getting what one wants and destroying what one hates, and the great fear of disease and death. These *kleśas* seldom go away, but instead remain dormant. Patañjali exhorts the first-level *yogābhyāsī* that these *kleśas* have to be rolled back, and *kriyāyoga* helps greatly to reduce the *kleśas*.

But then the *kleśas*, the harmful *vṛttīs*, have to be completely rooted out, and one has to look beyond *kriyāyoga* for guidance. Patañjali then addresses the second-level *yogābhyāsī* in suggesting that these *kleśas* can be rooted out by *dhyāna*, a representative term used by him to indicate the yogic practices called *antaraṅga sādhana*, part of the eight-limbed yoga (*aṣṭāṅgayoga*) that he later discusses. If the seer or the Self is always free and only oversees the functions of the *citta*, what causes these apparent endless misconceptions and their cyclic effects? The next important concept regarding action and results, called the karma hypothesis, the cornerstone of Vedic philosophy, is taken up and succinctly explained by Patañjali.

The *kleśas* are the roots *(kleśamūla)* or causes of the actions' fructifying and producing results, in the here and the hereafter. The corollary to this is that actions not actuated by *kleśas* will not result in experiences. Individuals act desiring what they think is favorable to them, and what they think is favorable is governed by desire *(kāma)* and greed *(lobha)*. They also act in anger *(krodha)* to avoid or destroy what is unfavorable. *Moha* (infatuation or confusion) also governs our actions. The acts themselves can be classified into those that are uplifting, *dhārmic* or *puṇya*, and those that are despicable *(adhārmic* or *pāpa)* or mixed *(puṇyāpuṇya)*. Thus what is desired can be achieved by actions that are *dhārmic* and on other occasions *adhārmic*. It becomes an issue of means and ends. The three, *kāma, lobha,* and *moha,* are degrees of *rāga,* and *krodha* is intense *dveṣa.*

Having their roots in the five *kleśas*, arising basically out of spiritual misapprehension, individuals tend to act. Actions sometimes produce results immediately or later on in life, or in a life beyond. But since the residual action bundle (actions that are yet to give rise to results) produce a specific birth, life span, and incidental experiences (happiness and misery), the roots of them all, the *kleśas*, have to be removed. Once the *kleśas* are removed, like removing the chaff from the grain, they lose the capacity to produce results. Paddy (rice with husk), when planted, grows, but not rice. The residual karmas are called *karmāśaya*, inasmuch as they remain within all beings who go from birth to birth; and they are *dharma* and *adharma,* those that sustain *(dharma)* and those that let one down *(adharma)*. Hence *dharma* and *adharma* are what are said to be right and wrong actions. The motives are there and they propel individuals to act to get the benefits in the future, even as they experience the results of past karmas. If there is a desire (motive) to obtain a place in heaven, for example, one tends to do all the actions mentioned in the scriptures, such as *aśvamedha* and *jyotiṣṭoma,* rites that are said to take the individuals so motivated to the heavenly abodes at the end of this life. These acts are called *iṣtis.* One may also do other socially relevant and charitable acts (called *pūrta*), such as feeding the poor, creating public parks, the construction of temples and roads, planting trees, and others. Here the motive is desire, and the actions are righteous *(dharma).* But one may have the desire for good things, especially worldly pleasures, and one may achieve wealth, but instead of taking the right means *(nijakarma),* one may use prohibited means such as stealing, cheating, and so on.

By doing such *adhārmic* or prohibited actions *(niṣiddha* or *pāpa),* even though one may get what one wants, one will simultaneously acquire *adharma* or *pāpa,* which will produce its own ill effects in due course, whether here or hereafter. One may, due to infatuation, or *moha,* indulge in cruelty to scholars or those who are weak and cannot defend themselves. One may indulge in actions prohibited in scriptures, though consistent with the laws of the land, and still acquire *adharma.*

*Dharma* and *adharma* that are yet to give results are *karmāśaya,* and remain as *saṃskāras.* The *karmāśaya* are divided into *dṛṣṭajanma vedanīya* and its opposite. All actions done with the present life (body) are *dṛṣṭajanma* and those results that are experienced in this *janma* are called *dṛṣṭajanma vedanīya.* Thus life runs on parallel lines: On one side one keeps on acting, and on the other one continues to experience the results of past karma. All experiences that would take place in the next life for actions due in previous lives are all *adṛṣṭajanma vedanīya.* Of all the pious *(puṇya)* actions, those done with extreme intensity with the help of mantras, *tapas,* and *samādhi* or by propitiating gods (deities), great sages, and so on may give rise to effects even in the same life. An example found in the Purāṇa is that of Nandikeśvara, who because of his intense devotion to God acquired enormous *puṇya* and in the same life attained the state of a *deva* (angel). On the other hand, one who commits atrocities on those that are helpless, sick, or trusting, or who are great personages *(mahātmas), tapasvins,* and similar precious beings, suffers the consequences in the same life. The Mahābhārata narrates the example of Nahuṣa. He was a king of the lunar race *(candra vamśa),* and was the son of Ayus, grandson of Purūravas, and father of Yayāti. He was a very wise and powerful king. Indra, the king of *devas,* had killed a demon called Vṛtra, making use of the backbone of the seer Dadhīci (who is believed to have performed penance in *vajrāsana,* also known as *dadhīcyāsana*). His backbone was hard *(vajra)* and was used by Indra as a weapon (thunderbolt). Vṛtrāsura had to be destroyed because he had all *devas* in captivity owing to his enormous *tapas,* which strength he wrongfully used to confine the *devas.* But since Vṛtra, even though he was a demon *(asura),* was also a *brahman* scholar, and killing a scholar *(brahmahatti)* was considered a *doṣa* (sin). In order that he may expiate the sin *(pāpa),* Indra lay concealed under the deep sea for a considerable length of time. There are some versions that say he hid himself in the tip of a grain, through *layayoga*. The *devas* were looking for a temporary leader, and imposed on Nahuṣa to occupy the exalted position of leader of the angels. This great advancement happened because of the *dhārmic* activities he had performed as a king. After a while, Nahuṣa, becoming conceited and thinking of his position as permanent, wanted all the perquisites of Indra, including the hand of Indrāṇī, the celestial consort of Indra. He became so conceited and cruel that he even went to the extent of forcing the seven highly respected and genial sages *(sapta ṛṣayaḥ)* to be his palanquin bearers. Sitting smugly in the palanquin, he directed the sages to carry him to the abode of Indrāṇī. One of the sages—believed to be Agastya (rhymes with Augustus, though some say it was Aṣṭavakra)—was short and had a limp and hence could not keep pace with the other sages. And every time Agastya planted his shortened leg, jerking was felt by Nahuṣa. Irritated at the slow pace of the palanquin and the bumpy journey, and unable to control his *adhārmic* lust, he shouted at the deformed sage to speed up by saying *"Sarpa, sarpa,"* meaning "move fast" or "run." Agastya, who had the *tapas* to bestow boon *(anugraha)* or administer a curse *(śāpa)*, cursed Nahuṣa by saying *"Sarpo bhava"* ("Become a snake"; *sarpa* means "snake" as well). The weight of his sins was so much that with the curse of the *ṛṣi*, the *adhārmic* activities of the once-upon-a-time *dharmi* instantly produced their effect. Nahuṣa fell immediately from the exalted position of Indra to that of a snake and remained in that pitiable state—to be stoned by urchins passing by. He was later resurrected by Yudhiṣṭhira, a great *dhārmic* soul.

It follows that since the *kleśas* are the roots that produce the effects to the karmas one has performed but which have not yet produced results, if the *kleśas* can be removed, then the *karmāśayas* will not produce a different future life, with the attendant life span and its related experiences. Therefore, by the fire of the knowledge of the Self, one will be able to "burn away," as it were, the potency of the past karmas to produce a future birth. Each birth produces an inexplicable variety of experiences. It could, therefore, be hypothesized that at the time of death, several of the actions, some *dharmic* and some *adharmic,* that can produce experiences with a particular kind of birth (a bird, a reptile, a human being) combine to produce a future birth. Thus, as is mentioned by Lord Kṛṣṇa in the Gītā, it is difficult to pinpoint the course of karmic effects, or to pinpoint which karmas will produce effects when, even though one can state that karmas produce results. It is the considered view of the *śāstras* such as Yoga that several actions combine together to produce a new birth.

Some actions performed during a given life span will produce effects in that same life span. But other karmas may not be able to produce their effects because that particular birth and its life span do not allow for the results of those karmas to take effect. For instance, if a human being performs meritorious acts whose beneficial effects go beyond the limitations of the human form and—shall we say—can only be experienced by celestial beings, those karmas thus created by the performance of the meritorious acts will remain dormant as *karmāśayas* all through that life span. In addition, karmas acquired during past births that did not come to fruition in those previous births or in the present birth will also carry forward as *karmāśayas.* Then, from among all the *karmāśayas* of previous births and the present birth, one powerful karma becomes the major karma. Several other karmas out of the *karmāśaya* bundle, which are consistent with or in league with the main karma, join it as subordinate karmas. They start acting at the time of death to produce one life. These karmas, working in unison, will determine the type, span, and experiences of the next immediate life. More specifically, one main karma *(pradhāna)* determines the particular form of that life (man or lion, for instance), and all the subsidiary karmas whose effects can be experienced in that particular form will produce their effects during that life span. All other karmas not taking part in that birth remain dormant as *karmāśayas.*

The idea is that only those experiences that a human being can have will come to fruition during a human life, its effects produced by a *pradhāna* (main) karma that has the potential to give a human life. But the experiences and the life span will vary depending upon the subordinate karmas that may produce effects, constantly modified of course by karmas that can produce effects even in the same birth *(dṛṣṭajanma).* To reiterate, if the main *(pradhāna)* karma gives rise to the birth of a bird or a *deva*, only those that can give rise to the experience of a bird or *deva,* as the case may be, become the subordinate karmas. The *karmāśaya* that are inconsistent with the present *janma* will have to wait for a long time to be operative, but at the appropriate time will give the experiences. How does it happen that one who was a human being is able to get the instincts to behave like a bird in a future birth? The answer is that since this stream of birth and death *(pravāha)* has no beginning and is believed to go on forever, each individual contains the karma *vāsana* (the memory or innate nature) of all species within itself. At the time of death, owing to the variety of karmas, the *vāsana* of the imminent birth comes up only along with *pradhāna* karma. Therefore, the *vāsanas* in our *citta* have accumulated over countless births and, like the knots in a fishnet, are bewildering. Several acts done in the same life produce effects in that same life. Those that can take effect only in a future birth or those that can produce effects in the future of the same life are the *karmāśayas* that can be modified, for better or worse, as in the case of Nandikeśvara and Nahuṣa. These *karmāśayas* are called *aniyata,* or "subject to change," and are uncertain to produce a particular effect, as they may be modified, or even made ineffective, before they can bear fruit.

The *karmāśayas* that are yet to produce results can be grouped into three classes: (1) those that can be destroyed before they become ready to come to fruition; (2) those that can produce effects only in conjunction with a main karma; and (3) those that are waiting for their time, but are prevented from coming to fruition for the duration of the present birth (main karma), and will therefore have to wait for a future birth. All three are called *aniyata* karmas. Now, the next question to be addressed is, how can any karma in the form of *karmāśaya* be destroyed before it can produce an effect? Is this not inconsistent with the general belief that the effects of karma or fate cannot be changed? It is said that *dharma* can nullify the effects of *adharma (puṇyena pāpam apanudati).* The *śāstras* contain several *parihāra a prayascitta* karmas, or rites, that have the potential fully or partially to nullify the effects of *adhārmic* karmas that are yet to come to fruition. The daily *sandhyā (nityakarma),* specific religious rites and *vratas,* and the accepted charitable acts are believed to have such a potential. The second situation is when one does a main karma, which may be a pious act, like *jyotiṣṭoma, paśumedha,* or *aśvamedha,* that also involves harming animals such as cows or horses. Hence one has to suffer the consequences of the *pāpa* of harming the animals, since this violates the dictum *"Na himsyāt bhūtāni,"* even as one reaps the benefits of a *puṇyakarma.* Thus the *pāpakarma* has to wait until the main karma starts producing effects. And then there are karmas that may not be able to be part of the experiences of the next birth and will have to wait until the appropriate birth *(janma)* comes to pass. It is almost impossible to exactly predict, therefore, if a particular karma will produce effects at a definite time, place, and life from out of the myriad karmas done in this life or one before. But it is certain that *puṇyakarma* will give rise to happy experiences *(hlāda phala)* and that *pāpakarmas* will give rise to tortuous experiences. Patañjali puts it succinctly, *"Te hlāda paritāpa phalāḥ, puṇyāpuṇya hetutvāt."*

Now, the *śāstras,* especially the *nivṛtti śāstras,* make a case for getting out of this beginningless cycle of life after life. Yogis, like Sāṃkhyas and Vedāntins, argue that the whole continuous and endless existence from birth to birth is only misery. All objects tend to change *(pariṇāma).* Objects that give happiness at a particular time undergo change over time and can become a source of misery, as, for instance, our own bodies, which were a source of great happiness in youth but become a burden of misery and sorrow as we age. Then there is always a tinge of unhappiness in all of us. We are never completely, thoroughly happy for any length of time because of *tāpa. Tāpa* is of two kinds, not getting what one wants and being unable to distance oneself from what one does not want. When one finds another having more success than oneself, a tinge of jealousy or unhappiness creeps in. It is common to find people, in spite of their fairly comfortable position in life, comparing themselves with those who are more successful and lamenting in frustration, "What have I not done to get that kind of success" *(Kim aham sādhu na akaravam).* By thus comparing, people become miserable *(tāpa).* Then, on the other hand, when one suffers, say, from a terminal ailment or from a great personal loss of wealth or prestige, one tends to lament what *pāpa* or misdeeds has one committed to suffer so *(kim aham pāpam akaravam iti).*

A third point to be noted is that *karmāśayas* or *saṃskāras* produce habits. People who are used to *pāpakarma*, such as lying, harming others, and so on, have difficulty changing the bad habit *(saṃskāra).* How difficult it is to stop smoking or drinking even when the first bad health symptoms appear? Then there are those habits that pertain to one's own *citta.* The *citta* is made of three *guṇas, sattva* (order), *rajas* (energy), and *tamas* (disorder). The *citta* keeps changing in its *vṛttis* of *sattva, rajas,* or *tamas.* When the *citta* is *sattvic,* one tends to be righteous, but when it becomes *tamasic* or *rajasic,* the same person acts differently. This change in moods and the resultant actions produce their own *pāpa* and *puṇya* results. So the entire future is strewn with dangerous uncertainties and the possibility of experiencing sorrow has a high probability. But one may say, "You are looking only at the thorns and not at the roses that come along in life." Vyāsa here compares a *viveki* (a discriminating person) to the eye, which is extremely sensitive when compared to other parts of the body. The eye reacts and instantly suffers even when a spider's web brushes against it, for example, whereas the rest of the body will barely feel it. So is the sensitivity of the *viveki* who feels that everything in life is only misery, and to him the following is addressed. Having realized that the beginningless, endless, and aimless journey from birth to birth gives rise to misery alone, Patañjali advises the sensitive yogi to find ways and means to end this misery once and for all *(heyam dūḥkham aṅagatam).*

If we have to eradicate an ailment, we have to know its cause. If the *kleśa* of *avidyā* is to be destroyed and not merely weakened, as *kriyāyoga* can help facilitate, one has to know the nature of *avidyā.* It has already been said that *avidyā* is a *kleśa.* If one is to completely eradicate transmigratory existence, the fundamental confusion *(avidyā)* about the nature of the Self has to be removed. The true Self and the ego appear to be one and the same—they appear so completely intermingled *(samyoga)* that one does not see that they are absolutely different from each other. This *samyoga,* or apparent identity or sameness of the two distinctly different principles, in the ordinary, nondiscriminating mind, is the cause of all *kleśas.* The self-locus or ego is something that is experienced. When one is awake or in a dream state, one experiences the separate identity of the individual. Since it is experienced, it is called *dṛśya*—that which is seen. Anything that is seen is not the seer. If the *citta* can realize that the seer *(draṣṭṛ)* is different from the seen, including the ego or self-locus, half the battle is won. To reinforce the understanding of the dichotomy between these two subtle principles, Patañjali explains that what is seen *(prakṛti)* is composed of three *guṇas* and consists of twenty-four *tattvas,* evolving in four stages, the stages being the unmanifest *(aliṅga),* the manifest *(liṅga),* the subtle *(aviśeṣa)*, and the gross *(viśeṣa)*. What is seen gives experiences and, in the case of a *yogābhyāsī*, triggers involution *(apavarga)* of the *citta* to its basic constituents so as to attain a balance of the *guṇas (sāmyāvastā)* through *sāmyak-darśana*, or correct perception of the self. The twenty-fifth principle, *puruṣa*, the seer, which only sees (without likes or dislikes, unlike the ego), has none of the changing qualities of the *citta*. Even so, the *puruṣa* is constrained to oversee all the *vṛttis* of the *citta* all the time. Thus, while the true Self is pure consciousness, the ego is subject to likes and dislikes, as part of the observed *prakṛti*. And the *prakṛti* or *citta* has no function except to act for the assumed benefit of the seer. The Sāṃkhyas use an example to explain this concept. Take the case of a sincere performing artist, a *nartaki* (dancer). She is a very skilled performer and her only aim is to satisfy her patron, who is sitting in front of the stage and watching her perform. The *nartaki* exhibits all her skills to humor the patron, but has no way of knowing what will please him or if he is satisfied with her performance. She makes her own judgments and keeps changing her strategem, until after dancing a long time, she wonders if her patron/observer is really interested in her performance. Slowly she realizes that the observer has no particular interest in her skillful performance, that he is self-contained. Once she realizes that her patron is totally uninterested in her performance, she will cease to dance. Likewise, when the *citta* realizes that the real Self is self-contained and is totally unaffected one way or the other by the various *vṛttis* aimed at satisfying the Self (after all, the mind always endeavors to satisfy the Self), it will cease to function. That is the *nirodha avasthā* for the *citta* and *kaivalya* (freedom) for the *puruṣa*. This takes place owing to the correct perception by the *citta* of the nature of the Self. So the yogi will keep the *sāmyak-darśana*, or perfect vision, without any intrusion by an imperfect impression of the Self that results from *avidyā*.

When once a yogi is able to maintain this correct perception of the true nature of *puruṣa* without any slide back to *avidyā*, or confusion, he crosses, according to Patañjali, seven mental levels *(citta bhūmis)*. For the yogi who has acquired the sharpness of a *viveki* (discrimination), the seven lower levels of *citta* in which the vast majority of humanity functions will have been transcended. These levels are easily recognizable. The first is called *jijñāsā*, or the general desire to know. All of us have an insatiable desire to know about several things. The person who has not acquired the correct picture will continue to have the desire to know. The *viveki-yogi*, however, having known the nature of the Self, concludes that his search for knowledge has come to an end and no other aspect of this world or other worlds interests him any longer. He transcends *jijñāsā*, the desire to know. The second level common to all *aviveki* beings is to get rid of anything that is considered undesirable. Having known that "I" should really refer to the nonchanging pure Self, the yogi has nothing to get rid of, since the Self is not affected by anything at all. If I am not affected, what should I get rid of? Hence, he transcends the desire to get rid of undesirable pain *(jihāsā).* The third level that he has crossed is the desire for achievements *(prepsā).* By the *sādhana* of yoga, he has obtained the state of *kaivalya,* or freedom, and he has nothing more to achieve. His *citta* stabilizes at the thought that he has nothing higher to achieve, having achieved the highest, his own Self, the precious treasure. The next level that he would have transcended is the desire for action *(cikīrṣā).* He has practiced yoga *sādhana* so that his *citta* is absolutely purified and brought up to the level of *nirodhaḥ samādhi,* and he has nothing else to perform. Because of the changing qualities of the three *guṇas*, there are three more conditions of the *citta* that are also transcended. One is *śoka,* or depression. The yogi overcomes *śoka* as the mind attains absolute peace, having completed all activities with respect to the Self. He has no reservations or fear that the *citta* will again degenerate into nonyogic states and get into the mire of *saṃsāra.* Thus he is not afraid *(bhaya)* anymore. Last, there is absolutely no reason for the *citta* to deviate from the state of *samāhita citta* to that of other *vṛttis (vikalpa).* Thus the yogi's *citta,* after the practice *(sādhana)* of *aṣṭāṅgayoga,* will be beyond the stages of *jijñāsā, jihāsā, prepsā, cikīrṣa, śoka, bhaya,* and *vikalpa.*

What is the difference between *kriyāyoga* and *aṣṭāṅgayoga*? It is in the degree of the cleansing of the *kleśas.* An empty earthen pot that previously contained a highly pungent liquid, even if cleaned with water several times, will still contain the pungent material (like kerosene) in its pores. Likewise *kriyāyoga*, even as it cleans the *citta* of the *kleśas,* to a great extent cannot completely eradicate them. When the pot is heated, the pores are also cleaned, and the pot does not smell of the pungent substance anymore. In the same way, *aṣṭāṅgayoga* completely purifies the *citta* of the *kleśas.* It is done in stages. *Aṣṭāṅgayoga* is a step-by-step, deeper, and subtler cleaning process of the body, senses, mind, and intellect.

# 6 The Eight-Part Yoga and Its Ten Commandments

PATAÑJALI STATES THAT THE PRACTICE of *kriyāyoga*, which helps to reduce mental *kleśas*, is for the old and the weak, whereas the practice of the more elaborate *aṣṭāṅgayoga* is recommended for the middle-order yoga aspirants. *Aṣṭāṅgayoga* effects a deeper and subtler cleansing process of the body, the senses, the mind, and the intellect, weakening, in the process, one's attachments and also aversions to material objects and desires, such as reaching heavenly consciousness and avoiding hell. One's mental clarity is phenomenally enhanced by *aṣṭāṅgayoga*, and the limit is perfect objective knowledge—up to achieving the distinctive knowledge *(viveka kyāti)* of the *puruṣa* (seer) and the observable *prakṛti*. *Aṣṭāṅgayoga*, which comprises eight different types of activities, is, however, divided into external and internal processes *(bahiraṅga* and *antaraṅga sādhana)*. Of these, the first two *aṅgas*, *yama* and *niyama*, the self-controls and restraints (dos and don'ts), are the preparatory steps. The first *aṅga*, called *yama*, means control. It consists of an attitudinal practice of the yogi toward objects that are external to him. This helps the *yogābhyāsī* to reduce significantly the distraction caused by the external world. In fact, the *niyamas* and *yamas* taken together form ten commandments (*mahāvratas*, "great vows") that the *aṣṭāṅga* yogi has to follow. The don'ts *(yamas)* are don't harm *(ahiṃsā)*, don't lie *(satya)*, don't steal *(asteya)*, don't philander *(brahmacarya)*, and don't accumulate (wealth) *(aparigraha)*. The dos *(niyamas)* are keep clean *(śauca)*, develop contentment *(saṃtoṣa)*, practice austerity *(tapas)*, study the scriptures *(svādhyāya)*, and surrender to the Lord (Īśvarapraṇidhāna). These two, *yama* and *niyama*, are the first steps the yogi has to be firmly established in before the other steps like postures and yogic breathing can be effective. Since these "commandments" are not stressed sufficiently in modern days, I shall expand upon them here.

*Ahiṃsā hi paramo dharmaḥ: ahiṃsā,* or nonviolence (not harming), is the greatest piety. Not harming any being, whether by mind, words, or physically, is *ahiṃsā*. Among all the *yamas, ahiṃsā* is the most important. All other aspects of *yama* are there so that the yogi will be a harmless person. The definition of a Hindu is *hiṃsāt dūyata iti hinduḥ,* "one who refrains from harming anyone."

Not lying, or always speaking the truth, is the next aspect of *yama*, but it should be consistent with the earlier injunction "Don't harm." A sage, dedicated to the law of always speaking the truth, was walking along the bank of a river. There were a few urchins stoning a turtle that had climbed up the bank from the river. It had managed to save itself with its hard back and by its instinct, drawing in all its limbs and its head. The urchins asked the pious sage how they could kill the turtle. Being given to speaking the truth always *(satya vrata),* he said what was obvious to everyone except the children. Thereupon the urchins turned the turtle over and attacked its soft belly, whereupon it died. The sage had to bear the karmic effects of killing a helpless animal in his next life. Even as he spoke the truth, the more important Vedic and yogic injunction of not harming any being *(na hiṃsyāt sarva bhūtani)* was transgressed. It is therefore said that one has to make sure that what one does, does not violate this injunction. In situations where speaking the truth will be harmful, the yogi is advised to keep mum *(mouna).* According to Manu, *Satyam bhrūyāt priyam bhrūyāt, na brūyāt satyamapriyam. Priyañca na anṛtam bhrūyāt, yeṣa dharmo sanātanaḥ,* "One's communication is to be guided by *ahiṃsā* and *satya.*" The *sanātana,* or perpetual *dharma,* is that one should speak what is true and what will result in good. Furthermore, one should not speak untruth even if it is good. In the above case, the sage could have kept quiet, as his telling the truth was not going to create any good but, rather, would only harm a helpless animal. Both *satya* and *ahiṃsā* are Vedic injunctions. The Taittirīya Upaniṣad advises Vedic students to speak the truth and never deviate from the path of *satya (satyam vada, satyāt na pramaditavyam).* It also says that compassion for all beings is a law *(bhūtyai na pramaditavyam).*

Anything that is taken unlawfully, or anything that is taken by any mode not approved by the *śāstras,* is *steya,* or stealing. Not taking anything that is not the result of one's own honest work is *asteya. Steya* includes crimes of all colors. To collect money by coercion or deceit is *steya.* There is a story in the Mahābhārata that may be of interest. Two brothers, Śaṅkara and Likhita, were great *tapasvins* (sages). They had set up two hermitages *(āśrama),* each one on the banks of the river Bahudā. The banks had plenty of trees bearing fruits and plentiful flowers. One day Likhita went to his elder brother Śaṅkara's hermitage. Śaṅkara was not in at that time. As he was waiting, Likhita saw a tree in the *āśrama* with fully ripe fruits hanging from it. Without hesitation, and since he was hungry, he plucked a couple of them and started eating. Śaṅkara returned presently and, seeing his little brother eating the fruits, asked him whence he got them. Knowing that Likhita had taken the fruits without his permission, Śaṅkara angrily told Likhita that this was tantamount to stealing, and as a *tapasvin,* he should not let this sin of stealing remain in a dormant state. He directed him, therefore, to go to the king, confess his theft, and receive due punishment. The king, knowing the greatness of the sage Likhita, said he would use his discretionary powers and let him go. But the sage insisted that he be given the punishment, so that he would be rid of the sin of stealing. The king reluctantly awarded the punishment and the hands of the sage were duly severed. Glad that as a yogi and *tapasvin* his crime sheet was clean, Likhita returned to his brother and told him about his encounter with the king. Śaṅkara, glad for his brother, asked him to bathe in the river and offer oblations to the sun and the *devas (arghya* and *tarpaṇa).* How was that possible for a person who had both hands severed? As he bathed and attempted to do *ācamana* with his hand, both the hands grew back, so the story goes. The happy Likhita narrated the incident to his brother, who said that since he had received the punishment for his crime, he was free of all defilement, and his own *tapas* had the capacity to restore his arms, so that he could continue with his spiritual journey.

Since anything that is unlawfully taken is a theft, those who practice yoga should eradicate from their minds the evil desire to covet. *Brahmacarya,* here, refers to self-control and scrupulously respecting the institution of marriage. *Parigraha* is the desire to accumulate material things and wealth, and *aparigraha* is the conscious effort to overcome this desire for material objects. As one develops this controlled attitude toward other beings and objects, the mental tribulations arising out of transactions with others and objects in the world around one are reduced.

Once the *yogābhyāsī* develops *yama*, then he is less likely to be disturbed by external things. He can then examine his own personal habits and make necessary changes so that his bad habits *(saṃskāras)* are not a hindrance to *samādhi.* The first *niyama* is called *śauca,* or cleanliness. It is again divided into *bāhya* and *antaḥ*, or external and internal. The *Haṭhayogapradīpikā* gives a fairly comprehensive list of requirements and methods for *śauca*. External *śauca* refers to keeping the body clean by having regular baths in pure water. References are also made to bathing with mud. In fact there is a Vedic mantra that is spoken while taking a bath using certain kinds of mud. The prayer to the *devatā* is to give health and remove all diseases through the pores of one's skin. Internal cleanliness generally refers to keeping the mind free of haughtiness, jealousy, or being unduly touchy. There are a few religious *kriyās* for cleaning the internal organs, which will also come under *antaḥśauca*. *Ācamana*, which is drinking three spoonfuls *(uddharanī)* of water held in the cupped right palm, one after the other, is an internal cleansing procedure. The mantras *acyutāya namaḥ, anantāya namaḥ,* and *govindāya namaḥ* purify the internal organs and the mind as well. Acyuta is the Lord who never falls down from the highest pedestal, Ananta is the one who pervades the universe and is unbounded, and Govinda is another name of Kṛṣṇa and means a cowherd. God is considered the superintending force over all beings. As the cowherd gathers the cows and protects them, so Govinda protects all beings. Similar metaphors, such as the shepherd, are found in other religions. *Ācamana* as a cleansing process is well known. All the Hindu rites or *pūjās* start with *ācamana.* In the Āditya Hṛdayam from the Vālmīki Rāmāyaṇa, Rāma is described as being purified by *ācamana* before his final encounter with Rāvana: *trirācamya śucir bhūtva* ("having done *ācamana* and becoming clean").

The next *niyama* is *saṃtoṣa,* or contentment. It is the way to reduce the two types of *tāpa* mentioned in chapter 5. A yogi or a *yogābhyāsī* has to be content with his present position and not hanker after anything that is worldly, as that will only take him in the direction opposite to the the yogic goal. The other three *niyamas,* namely, *tāpas, svādhyāya,* and Īśvarapraṇidhāna, have been discussed already. Īśvarapraṇidhāna here would refer to surrendering the results of all pious activities done by the *abhyāsī* with love and devotion to Īśvara. One stops accumulating *puṇya* by such an offering.

It is said that no person, not even a dimwit, will commence an arduous undertaking without knowing of its benefits. Some of the benefits of *yama* and *niyama,* or the ten yogic commandments, should be described. These two preliminary *aṅgas,* by their own strength, impart their own benefits, even if one is not able to achieve the ultimate goal of yoga in this lifetime. If one becomes, by diligence, firmly established in *ahiṃsā,* friendliness will be reciprocated. One will encounter no enemies, and hence will be free from being harmed by secret or openly inimical activities. One can progress, therefore, without hindrance in one's chosen ambition of self-realization. One's nonviolence should be total—of thought, word, and deed. It should be noted that many religious rites in the Vedas and other scriptures permit harming other beings as part of the rituals. But the performers of the rites not only get the benefits of the religious rites but also have to bear the cross, as it were, for causing pain to other beings. A yogi is advised to observe nonviolence without any exception—not only because he is convinced about the uplifting effect of nonviolence but also because he is not interested in heaven and the higher worlds mentioned in the *śāstras.* So his nonviolence is total. If the *yogābhyāsī* is well established in truthfulness, his actions will always produce the right results. The Purāṇas talk about those sages who stick to truthfulness getting the power for *śāpa* (curse) and *anugraha* (conferring a boon). When one is established in nonstealing, or develops a trusteeship approach toward wealth and earns money only from honest *(nijarkama)* and prescribed *(svadharma)* duties, he paradoxically comes to possess and manage wealth. Nonpossession, or *aparigraha*, frees the mind from worries and activities about protecting one's wealth and helps one continue on the path of self-realization.

Some reflections on the dos and don'ts *(yamaniyamas)* for an *aṣṭāṅga* yogi are in order. Certain practices and attitudinal changes are necessary and sufficient prerequisites before the practices pertaining to one's own body and senses can be taken up, which practices require a mind free from internal and external distractions. What is called for is a deliberate attempt to practice these dos and don'ts so that the earlier habitual and slavish tendencies of the mind to follow the dictates of the senses and their objects are minimized. This is, however, easier said than done. Patañjali recognizes that the difficulty is mainly the result of our childhood habits and conditioning, as well as the latent tendencies acquired through many previous births. To help the earnest *yogābhyāsī*, he suggests keeping in the back of one's mind the thought that one has taken up yoga after having been convinced that it is the only and last resort to attain peace of mind. The *yogābhyāsī* should think repeatedly that the motivations behind all actions inconsistent with the commandments are greed, enmity, and infatuation, and these will only and invariably lead to endless misery and confusion. All yoga practice, whether *āsana, prāṇāyāma,* or *antaraṅga sādhanas* (internal or mental exercises), will be of little use, and the benefits, if any, will be only temporary if done without the preparatory *aṅgas*. Practice of mere *āsanas* without change in diet and other attitudinal changes is perhaps the cause of much disappointment among *yogābhyāsīs*.

Patañjali, in his great compassion for the struggling *yogābhyāsī*, has thus indicated the benefits that accrue even from preliminary practices. In the Gītā, Kṛṣṇa encourages Arjuna and other devotees to take to the spiritual path through the practice of classical yoga. He cautions them that they may not be able to achieve the end result of yoga, whether it be self-realization or God-realization. But their *saṃskāras* will lead them (through the grace of God) to be born into a family of yogis or to be born into a well-to-do family. Then they can pursue the practice of yoga without the compelling need to spend all their time and energy earning a livelihood or without spending a lifetime in search of a yogi or guru.

PART TWO

# *Yoga Sādhana,* or Practice

# 7 Standing Postures

*There are sixty-four arts. Yoga is one of them.*

HAVING WITHDRAWN THE MIND FROM THE EXTERNAL environment by *yamaniyamas,* the next set of distractions, which arise from one's own body, need to be addressed, and thus Patañjali mentions *āsanas* as the third *aṅga* of *aṣṭāṅgayoga.* He does not, however, describe the techniques or the variety of *āsanas* that are possible, nor their specific benefits. But following the dictum *anuktam, anyato grahyam* ("what is not mentioned in a text has to be acquired from other texts"), one needs to study other relevant texts on yoga to get a detailed understanding of *āsanas* and their benefits. Since *āsanas* are an *aṅga* of purification, Patañjali has only to state that perfection of the body accrues to one who has mastered this aspect of yoga. Mastery in this case would mean being able to stay in an *āsana* comfortably and steadily, which requires the good circulation, respiration, muscle tone, and nerve strength that *āsanas* help one to achieve. Since *āsanas* are an important and perhaps the most widely known aspect of yoga, it is necessary to dwell on this part of yoga practice. Mine is a humble attempt to explain the techniques and benefits of the practice of *āsanas,* given my limited capacity to appreciate the nuances of the *vinyāsa* system of my teacher.

It is said that the total number of *āsanas* is uncountable: *Āsananica tāvanti, yāvanto jīvaraśayaḥ.* Yoga texts mention that there are as many *āsanas* as there are species of animals. Even so, about eighty *āsanas* are currently believed to be in vogue. In the olden days, it is said, people prevented and even eradicated diseases by means of *prāṇāyāma* and *āsanas* (breathing exercises and postures). According to some Āyurvedic books, ailments that are chronic and those that are not curable by medical science *(vaidya śāstra)* and drugs can be cured by *āsanas* and *prāṇāyāma.* Since Āyurveda and Yoga derive inspiration from Sāṃkhya philosophy, it may be worthwhile for Āyurvedic practitioners to make use of yogic methods of treatment along with Āyurvedic applications. Because yoga is a proactive method of treatment requiring the involvement of the patient, the patient's confidence level rises when the cure is brought about with the help of yogic breathing, *āsanas,* and meditative methods. Unfortunately, during the dark centuries of the past, many of our ancient scriptures on yoga therapy have been lost.

The practice of *āsanas* has become popular again after a lapse of a number of years. It is suggested that the daily practice of yoga should start with a prayer to one's *iṣṭa devatā* (favorite deity) and also to Ananta, or Nāgaraja, or Patañjali. A mechanical approach to the practice of *āsanas*—merely achieving a posture somehow—may not give the anticipated results; a certain degree of preparation is necessary. The chanting of the Vedas, for example, should be done with *udātta, anudātta,* and *svarita* (three notes); this *sasvara* (with notes) chanting has been going on since time immemorial. There are also specific rules for composing traditional music and poems. Finally, if one offers *pūjā* to a deity *(pūjā vidhāna),* there are various requirements that need to be observed for fruition of the *pūjā.* The practice of yoga, especially *āsana* and *prāṇāyāma,* will not deliver its full benefits without similar kinds of preparations and variations *(vinyāsas)* in the various postures. Without these *vinyāsas, āsana* practice is only as good as any other physical exercise. It is of little use if one learns a dozen well-known *āsanas* and practices them without the *vinyāsas.* It was my *ācārya's* contention that the disillusionment of many *yogābhyāsīs* with yoga results from their practicing *āsanas* without the *yama-niyamas, vinyāsas, pratikriyās,* synchronous breathing, and work with the *bandhas* and instead with a nervous urgency to achieve quick results.

Yet another important factor in *āsana* practice is the use of breath while doing the *vinyāsas* and *āsanas.* Here also, many schools teach yoga without any reference to breathing in *āsana* practice, and some actually discourage the use of the breath, on the plea that the practice of breathing is a separate "limb" of *aṣṭāṅgayoga, prāṇāyāma.* Actual practice shows, however, that deliberate synchronous breathing with *vinyāsas* is necessary in *āsana* practice to attain the results mentioned in various texts. In the *Yogasūtras* (2.46), Patañjali mentions making use of the breath to achieve perfection in posture, which entails steadiness and comfort *(sthira* and *sukha).* In the sūtra immediately after defining *āsana,* Patañjali suggests the means of attaining perfection in postures when he says (2.47), *prayatna śaitilya ananta samāpattibhyām.* The word *prayatna* is normally taken to mean "effort." While this is generally correct, the word should be construed as a technical one, and its appropriate meaning investigated. Several authors and commentators have taken the word to mean "general effort," which translates into asking students not to force themselves into a posture but, rather, to ease into it. Nyāya, a sister philosophy, splits *prayatna* into three groups. These are *pravṛtti, nivṛtti,* and *jīvana prayatna. Pravṛtti* and *nivṛtti* are the *citta vṛttis* (discussed earlier) and their corresponding physical actions, such as moving forward to meet and greet a friend or taking evasive action from being hit by a speeding car. *Jīvana prayatna,* however, refers to the efforts made by the individual to maintain life and, more especially, breathing. This is the *sāmānya vṛtti* referred to in chapter 4. Hence the word *prayatna* should be taken to mean "the effort of breathing." And it should be made smooth (*śithila,* from which comes *śaithilya,* "relaxation"). Thus, during the practice of *āsanas,* the breath should be smooth, and in my teacher's system it is therefore mandatory to stop one's practice and to rest when the breath is not smooth. Shortness of breath is associated with a fragmented mind *(śvāsa praśvāsaḥ, vikṣepa saha bhuvaḥ)* and thus synchronized, smooth, long breathing (both inhalation and exhalation) becomes the sine qua non for *āsana* practice in *vinyāsakrama.*

Patañjali's sūtra also mentions *samāpatti,* or "fixing the mind." It is common to find people's minds wandering as they practice *āsanas,* especially when they get used to them. One's effort becomes mechanical, a habit, like driving a car, when one is not completely focused. So what should the mind focus on? The answer is also in the sūtra, in short, on *ananta (ananta samāpattibhyām),* which word literally means "unbounded" or "infinity" *(an + anta = ananta);* certain schools suggest that one should concentrate on infinity while practicing *āsanas.* This is difficult—almost impossible—for the beginning practitioner even to attempt. Ananta, however, is the name of Nāgaraja or Ādiśeṣa, whose *avatāra* Patañjali was. One should therefore—some yoga traditions require it—contemplate the figure of Nāgaraja or Patañjali, whose icons and idols are available in certain temples, and in yoga schools that have installed the *vigraha* (icon) of Patañjali. The *dhyāna sloka* (invocation prayer) of Patañjali describes his form *(ākāra)* and his greatness *(prabhāva),* and as Ananta, he is the premier proponent and guru of yoga.

The word *ananta* also means "breath," which meaning is most appropriate here. *Ana* is breath *(ana śvāse),* as in the word *prāṇa (pra + ana).* Thus it is correct to say that one should mentally follow the breath while doing the movements in the *āsanas.* Close attention to the breath, which should synchronize with one's movements, is *samāpatti,* and breath is the connecting link between mind and body. Thus it may be concluded that while practicing *āsanas,* done with purposeful breathing and fixity of mind, one achieves steadiness and relaxation, which is *āsana siddhi* (accomplishment in *āsana*). Then, one is not affected by pairs of opposites such as fever and hypothermia and other opposing conditions, whether physical or mental. The *āsanābhyāsī* develops a tolerance for pain deriving from opposites *(dvanda)* such as heat and cold, ridicule and praise, success and failure; his endurance is greatly improved.

There are four factors in yogic breathing. The first is *pūraka,* or inhalation. The second, holding in the breath after inhalation, is called *antaḥ-kumbhaka.* The third is *recaka,* or controlled exhalation. The fourth, holding the breath out—as it were—is called *bāhya-kumbhaka.* All yoga movements are done deliberately and with a specific type of breathing. There are some movements that should always be done while inhaling, and there are others that should be done while exhaling. Then one could stay in a posture while holding the breath in or holding the breath out, or one could do a controlled cycle of yogic breathing while remaining in the posture. But there are some movements that can be done during either breathing in or breathing out, depending upon the condition of the practitioner and the results desired from the practice. Moving during inhalation and holding the breath in is *brahmana kriyā,* and moving while breathing out and holding the breath out is *langhana kriyā.* In Āyurveda, or the science of medicine (or life), *brahmana kriyā* refers to nourishment and *langhana kriyā* to fasting, but these words mean something different in *yogābhyāsa.* The *kriyās* in *sattvic* yoga practice are the use of natural air in cleaning the *nāḍīs* and not the use of cloth or other external aids. Thus the use of breath in *āsanas* helps one to relax and attain the desired posture. The breath helps one to reach and work on the deeper muscles and organs inside the body, which may not be possible otherwise. In addition, it has been found that with deliberate breathing, one's mind is not allowed to wander, but is committed to following the breath. Yoga practice becomes much more purposeful. Yogi Nāthamuni, believed to be the author of *Yoga Rahasya,* calls each of the sixteen chapters of his treatise a *kalā,* a word that means "art." As in music or any other art form, one has to develop sensitivity and skill with deliberate practice and intense concentration.

Like medicines, *yogāsanas* have good effects but may also have some minor side effects, which are essentially physical. To counteract them, every involved posture has a counterpose or a sequence of countermovements that help to preserve the effects of the main *āsana* and counteract any undesirable aspects. For instance, *śīrṣāsana* has positive effects on the system. But it has to be followed by *sarvāṅgāsana.* If *sarvāṅgāsana* is done as the main posture (say, for ten minutes or so), it has to be followed up with a mild back-bending and neck-stretching exercise, like *bhujaṅgāsana* or *śalabhāsana,* and followed by the sitting posture *padmāsana.* In fact, some of the counterpostures, or *pratikriyās,* help to retain the benefits of the main posture. The *śīrṣāsana-sarvāṅgāsana* combination of main posture and counterposture is but an example. One has to see the effect of doing *āsanas* and their counterposes diligently to feel the difference between an organized regimen or planned sequence of doing *āsanas* and *vinyāsa* and practicing *āsanas* at random. Apart from the emphasis on conscious breathing in *āsanas,* as one makes progress in one's practice, the use of *bandhas*, which involves the contraction of specific groups of muscles, is recommended for gaining more benefits from *āsana* practice. Of the many such *bandhas*, three are very important. The *mūla bandha* requires the drawing in of the rectum, the pelvic diaphragm, and the lower abdomen as if to touch the backbone (to reach perfection). This is done after exhalation. It should be noted that, at least in the initial stages, one has to practice *brahmacarya* (abstinence) to attain a mastery of *mūla bandha*. The *uddīyāna bandha* is the in-drawing of the navel region, again as if to touch the back bone, and the raising of the diaphragm so that the abdominal region becomes scaphoid, or boat-shaped. It is obvious that people who are obese will not be able to do *uddīyāna bandha* satisfactorily, and hence the need for dietary control, or *tapas*, in *āsana* practice to bring the body back to its proper shape. The *jālandhara bandha* involves stretching the back of the neck and pressing the chin against the breastbone, about three inches below the neck. This effectively controls the air passage during breathing, and it is a great aid for both *prāṇāyāma* and controlling one's breathing in the practice of *āsana vinyāsas*. These three *bandhas (bandha traya)* are important in the practice of *āsanas*. It may not be possible for beginners to practice these at the outset of their yoga practice, but they will have to do so as they progress. It should be noted, however, that work with the *bandhas* should not be attempted without the guidance of a competent teacher who himself has practiced and mastered them. (For more on the *bandhas*, see chapter 8.)

The author of the *Haṭhayogapradīpikā* mentions that, irrespective of age and physical condition, anyone can start the practice of *yogāsanas*, but that it is regular and involved practice that brings results *(siddhi): Yuva vṛddho ati vṛddho vyadhito durabalopi vā. Abhyāsāt siddhim āpnoti, sarvayogeṣu atandritaḥ.*

It should be mentioned that yoga is useful to children and women as well. Traditionally, in ancient India, among Hindus, children at the age of seven used to be initiated into Vedic *karma* (activities mentioned in the Vedas and complementary scriptures) after their *upanayanam* (initiation). *Sandhyā*, or the daily oblations done at dawn, dusk, and midday, includes *āsanas* like *utkaṭāsana, uttānāsana, padmāsana*, among others, and *prāṇāyāma*, or breath control, with mantra followed by *japa* (repetitive chanting and meditation) of the sacred *gāyatrī* mantra. It is apparent that children were practicing yoga in ancient India, and they may do so as well in the present day, even though such practices are not as commonplace now.

With regard to the controversy about whether women are fit for integral yoga, there is ample evidence to show that interested women were initiated into yoga. The *Yoga Yājñavalkya* and the Śiva Saṃhitā, two authentic texts on yoga, are actually the teachings of Mahāṛṣi Yājñavalkya to his highly talented wife Maitrayi, and of Lord Śiva, known as Lord of Yoga *(Yogeśvara)* to the goddess Pārvatī, respectively. In the *Yoga Rahasya*, Nathamuni specifies *āsanas* such as *pañca konāsanas* (five *kona* postures) as aiding the development of the fetus, and certain others, such as *pāśāsana,* are said to prevent conception *(garbha nirodha).* Furthermore, there are a number of *āsanas* and *prāṇāyāma* that are useful in the correction of such gynecological conditions as prolapse of the uterus, postnatal disorders, menstrual disorders, and so on. It should be noted that *yogāsanas* should be practiced according to *sampradāya* (tradition) to attain the benefits mentioned in the texts. The *paddhati* (system) of our *ācārya* based on the *śāstras* is that one should practice *āsanas* with the necessary constraints *(yamaniyamas)* or prerequisites. Any practice should be done with preparation, progression, and variation of postures *(vinyāsa),* as well as corresponding synchronous, conscious, and modulated breathing, the whole interspersed with stipulated counterposes and countermovements *(pratikriyās)* that employ the *bandhas* and *mudrās* at the appropriate stages.

## *Tāḍāsana,* or *Samasthiti,* and Its Variations *(Vinyāsas)*

*Āsana* practice directly helps to improve one's health and flexibility *(arogyam aṅgalāghavam ca). Āsanas* can be broadly classified into standing, sitting, supine, prone, balancing, and inverted *(viparīta karaṇī)* postures. In this chapter the important standing *āsanas* and their useful *vinyāsas* will be discussed. *Samasthiti,* or *tāḍāsana,* is the starting and ending position in the practice of *āsanas.* It involves standing erect, with one's feet together and fully resting on the floor. It is better for the standing postures to stand on a hard floor rather than on one heavily carpeted, because one's feet will sink into the pile of the carpet and balance will be more difficult to maintain. The ankles should be kept together, and those who can should also try to keep the knees and thighs close together. Be sure that the knees are not flexed. The chest should be kept erect and the shoulders slightly thrown back, so that the shoulder blades are drawn closer to each other, forming a canal along the spinal column in the back. This *samasthiti* is the first standing posture in the *vinyāsakrama* of the *tāḍāsana* (mountain or tree posture) group.

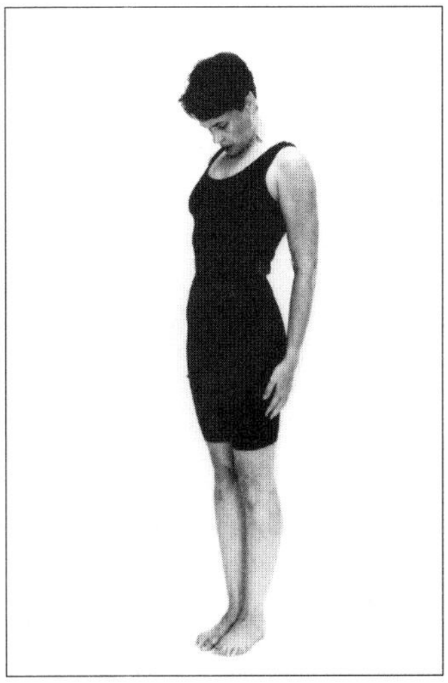

*Samasthiti* with *jālandhara bandha*

Since this group of *āsanas* and *vinyāsas* involves doing movements while standing, a good sense of balance is necessary and desirable. Thus you should check how good your balance is. In *samasthiti,* keep your head down, close your eyes, and observe closely how well you balance on both feet. There will be some swaying felt, but if you feel that you sway too much, and this swaying is accompanied by rapid breathing, this indicates that you are not in a fit condition to do yoga, at least for the time being. This could be the result of temporary illness, lack of sleep and rest, or a distracted or disturbed mind. If you otherwise feel fine, start slowly following the body's balancing act as it sways from side to side. Stay in this position for at least two minutes, and slowly the amplitude of the sway is reduced, and you will feel that you are in a better condition to proceed with the practice. Then check your breathing by directing your attention to your breath, to the air going in and going out. Or better still, focus your attention on the point from where the chest starts expanding and toward which it appears to contract. If your breathing appears heavy and fast, you may not be able to do *āsanas,* because long and smooth breathing is necessary. As you watch the breath, the whole movement will slow down, and after watching the breath closely, you will be in a position to start the *vinyāsas* and *āsanas* in this group. Breath and balance are the first things checked by the *yogābhyāsī* before proceeding further.

The variations, or *vinyāsas,* of *tāḍāsana* now follow. In each of the following *vinyāsas,* except in cases where the head is turned to the side or the neck is bent back, after complete exhalation lock your chin against the top of your chest (against the breastbone); this is the *jālandhara bandha,* or chin lock, mentioned earlier. For *vinyāsa* 1, slowly and deeply inhale with a rubbing sensation in the throat and raise both arms straight overhead, interlocking your fingers and turning your hands outward. The movement of the arms is made alongside the body, slowly stretching the knees, hips, sides of the chest, shoulders, elbows, wrists, and neck. The inhalation and the completion of the movement should synchronize. One should adjust the pace of the movement to the breath, the slower the better. Breathing should be done with a hissing sound in the throat—the sound created by the partial closing of the glottis, which is aided by the chin lock. After a momentary pause, slowly exhale with a hissing sound in the throat and again lower your arms along the sides of your body, synchronizing your arms' movement with the outflow of the breath.

The next *vinyāsa* (2) involves raising your arms overhead, but moving them in front of the body as you inhale while pressing your feet, especially the big toes, into the floor. This helps to stretch the front of the body *(pūrva bhāga),* especially the shins, knees, thighs, pelvis, abdomen, chest, and arms. Your fingers should be kept straight (not interlocked as in the previous *vinyāsa*). Exhale slowly while lowering your arms, in the reverse route taken to raise them up. For the third *vinyāsa,* cross your hands and put them on the opposite thighs. As you inhale, sweep your arms (slowly, please) and bring them up to the level of the shoulders so that they are fully extended sideways. Exhale slowly and lower your arms to the sides. This helps to open the chest. While completing the inhalation, gently push your chest slightly forward so that your shoulder blades touch each other.

For a third *vinyāsa* in *tāḍāsana,* start from *samasthiti;* as in the inhalation part of the first *vinyāsa,* raise your arms overhead, interlock your fingers, and turn your hands outward. As you exhale, bend your elbows, keeping your chest pushed forward, and while bending your elbows, lower your forearms (with fingers interlocked) to the farthest extent possible, keeping your hands behind your neck. Your hands, with fingers interlocked, should continue to be turned upward. Then, while inhaling, raise your arms overhead, stretching your body along the sides in the process. Then exhale and return to *samasthiti.*

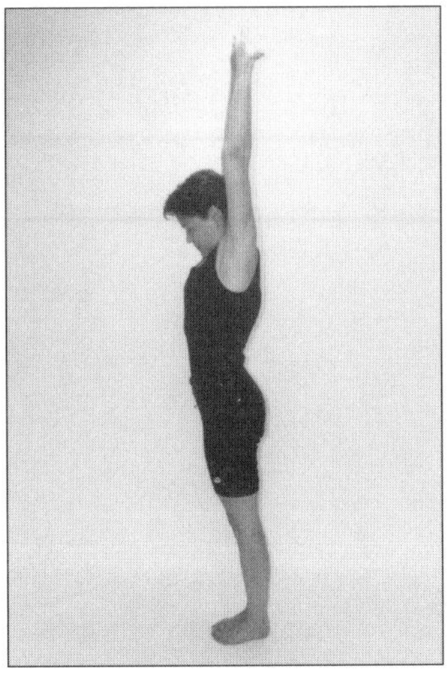

Tāḍāsana (*vinyāsa* 1)

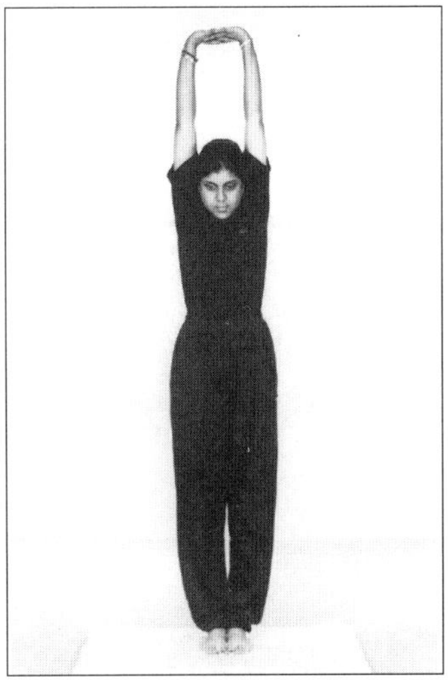

Tāḍāsana (*vinyāsa* 1) (front view)

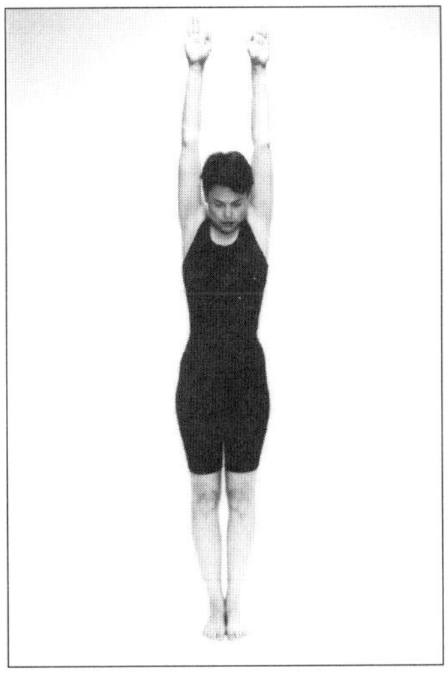

Tāḍāsana (*vinyāsa* 2)

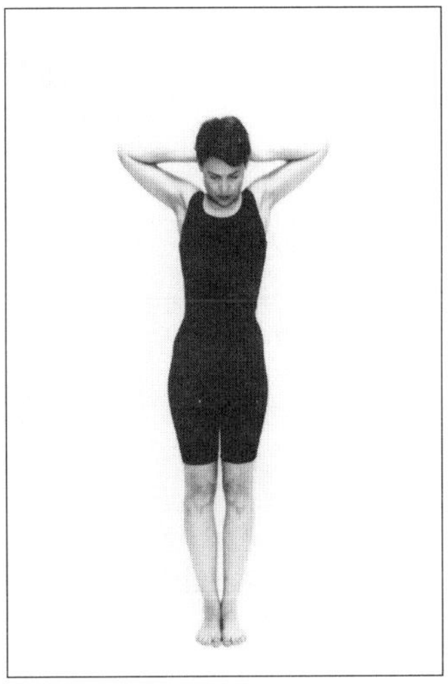

Tāḍāsana (*vinyāsa* 3)

The fourth *vinyāsa* begins with the same initial movement as the first *vinyāsa*—that is, raising the arms while keeping the fingers interlocked and turned outward. Then, separate your hands and keep them facing front. As you exhale, bend your elbows and place your palms on your shoulder blades, with your elbows pointing up, keeping the chest slightly pushed forward. Then inhale, raise your arms overhead, exhale, and lower your arms.

For the fifth *vinyāsa,* the initial movement is again the same as for the first *vinyāsa*, in which the arms are raised with the fingers interlocked and turned outward. In this sequence, as you exhale (as in the fourth *vinyāsa*), bend your elbows but place your palms on opposite shoulder blades, crossing your hands behind your

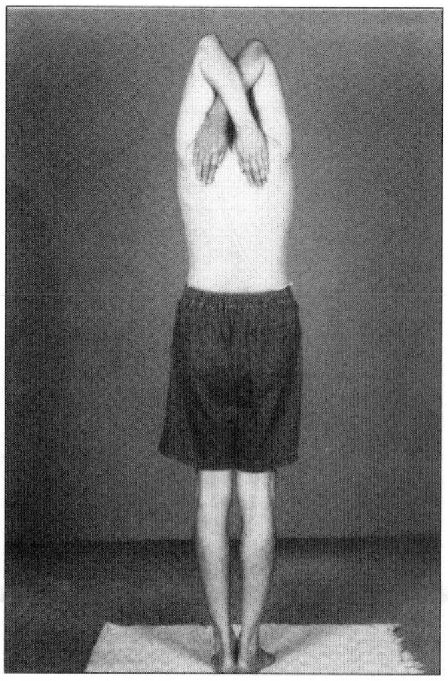

*Tāḍāsana vinyāsa* 5

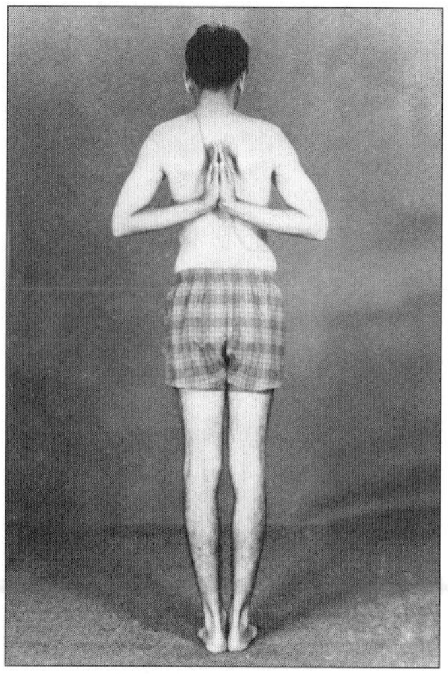

*Tāḍāsana-hasta vinyāsa* 6, (variation of hand position; *pṛṣṭāñjali*)

neck so that your elbows are pointing up again. Your chest should be pushed forward. Then, as you breathe in, raise your arms overhead, interlock your fingers and turn them outwards. Exhale, lowering your arms back to *samasthiti.*

For the sixth *vinyāsa*, as you can probably predict, begin by raising your arms overhead as in the first one. While exhaling, bring your arms all the way down and bring your hands behind your back, joining the palms. Now turn your joined hands with fingers pointing up and touch your back near the bottom of your spine. As you continue the exhalation, gently slide your hands upward, all along the spine, until the joined hands (palms against each other) are between your shoulder blades. The hands' position is known as *añjali,* and because it is on the back, it is called *pṛṣṭāñjali.* Those who have stiff necks and shoulders should not force themselves to do this particular *vinyāsa.* Inhale slowly, lower your arms, and then raise them upward, interlocking the fingers. Exhaling, return to *samasthiti.*

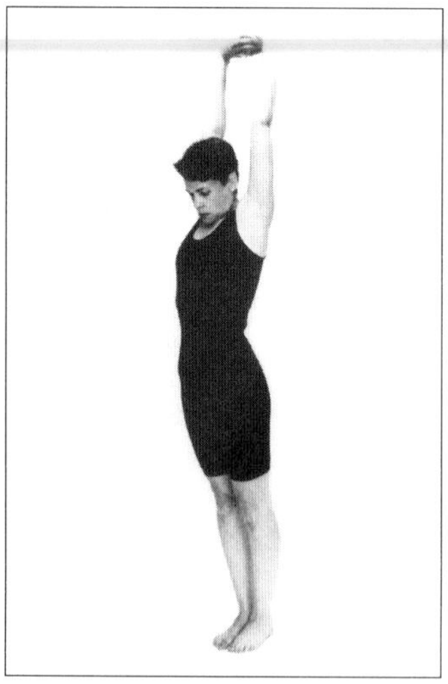

*Tāḍāsana* (preparation for shoulder movements)

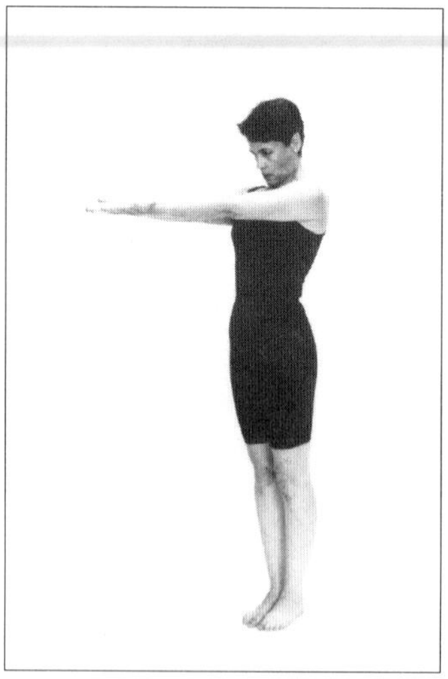

*Tāḍāsana* (shoulder movement)

For yet another variation, inhale and raise both arms overhead, interlocking your fingers and turning the hands outward. Release the interlock, and, as you exhale, slightly bend back, rotating your shoulders with the outward movement of your arms at shoulder level, then bring your arms forward so they are straight in front. This provides a good rotating movement to the ball-and-socket joints of the shoulders. Then as you inhale, retrace the path and end with your arms up with fingers interlocked and turned outward. Then as you exhale, release your hands, lower your arms in front of you up to shoulder level (your palms facing downward), and continue the movement of pushing or sweeping your arms back at the level of the shoulders. The movement of the arms is done at shoulder level, until the shoulder blades touch each other and the chest is pushed forward. Inhale and return. This *vinyāsa* is a good and complete exercise for the shoulders. Together these will be a fairly exhaustive set of *vinyāsas* for the arms.

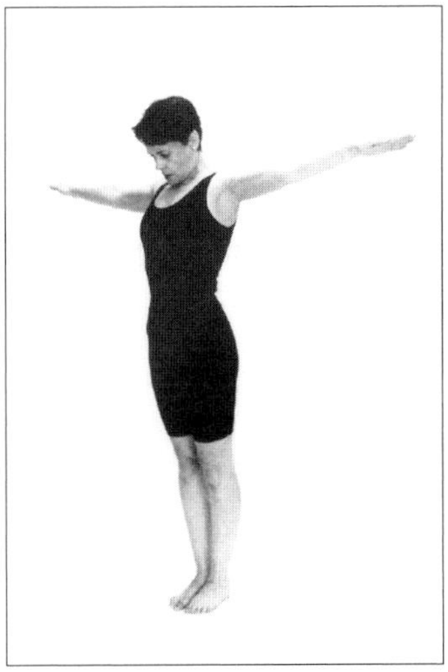

*Tāḍāsana* (shoulder movement)

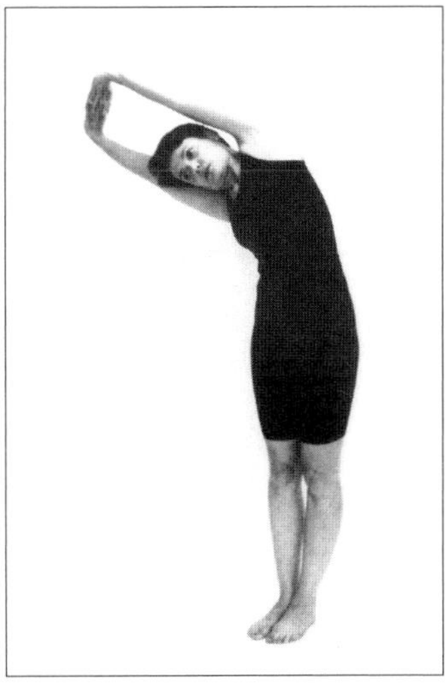

*Tāḍāsana pārśva-bhaṅgi*

Still another *vinyāsa* is called *pārśva-bhaṅgi,* or side posture. Raise your arms while inhaling, as in the initial *vinyāsa.* As you exhale, press your feet into the floor, push your left hip out slightly, and bend to the right side, stretching the left side of your body, especially the side ribs. The posture resembles a small, supple tree swaying in a heavy north wind. The upper body should neither stoop forward nor be pushed backward. The whole movement should be done in the vertical plane. Inhaling, return to the starting position. The same movement is repeated in the opposite direction as well, so the movements act as *pratikriyās* (countermovements) to each other. It is good to keep feet and knees together (without bending) all through the process.

The next *vinyāsa,* "the torso twist," is a variation of *pārśva-bhaṅgi* and will again require the same initial movement as the first. Then while exhaling,

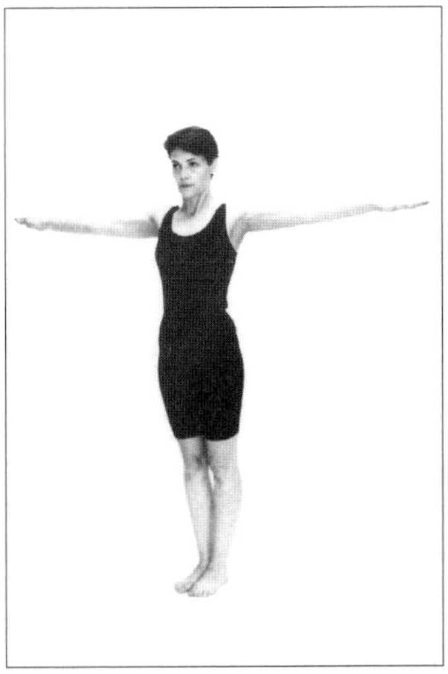

*Tāḍāsana pārśva-bhaṅgi,*
torso twist (preparation)

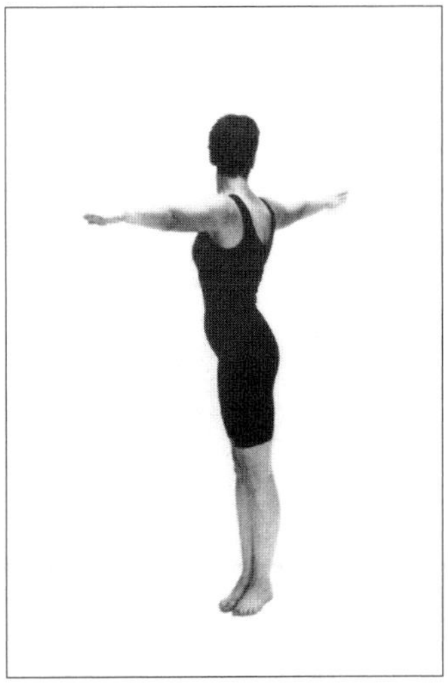

*Tāḍāsana pārśva-bhaṅgi,*
torso twist

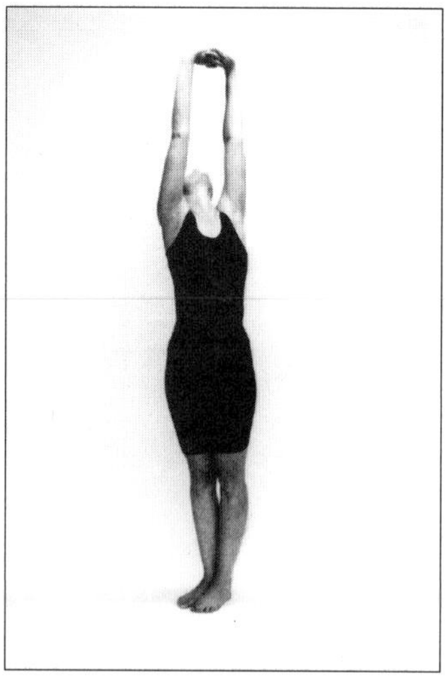

*Tāḍāsana pārśva-bhaṅgi*
(*vinyāsa*)

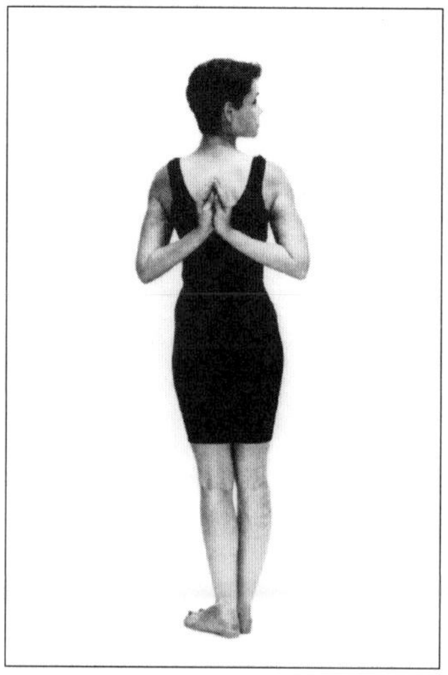

*Tāḍāsana pārśva-bhaṅgi*
(with *pṛṣṭāñjali*)

twist your upper body to the right side to the farthest extent possible, stretching your neck, and look up. The position of your feet is not altered, and your knees should be kept together without buckling. Then inhale and return to the standing position. You should then do the same movement on the left side. The same twisting movement can be done with different positions for the arms. The easier *vinyāsa* involves raising your arms to the sides up to shoulder level on inhalation. Then as you exhale, turn to the right side, pressing your feet into the floor and not moving them. As you turn, your head is also turned and looks over your right shoulder. The spine is given a good twist (like a half turn, or less, of a screw); the entire spine participates in the whole movement. Inhale, return, and repeat the movement on the other side. A more difficult hand position involves doing *pṛṣṭāñjali* for the hands, as mentioned earlier. Then, after inhalation, exhale, and, with your hands completely locked behind your back, slowly turn to the right side and also turn your head to look over your right shoulder. Since the arms are locked, it will be rather difficult to maintain your balance and also do the turning movement in the *vinyāsa* satisfactorily. Inhale, return to the starting position, and repeat the movement on the other side as well.

It should be noted that the above set of *vinyāsas* in *tāḍāsana* helps to exercise the chest muscles and all the auxiliary muscles used in breathing. Since the whole set is done with deep and full breathing, the chest muscles are also exercised from within. The thorax and the spine—which is not free, being attached to the ribs—are also exercised in a unique way, due not only to the extensive stretching of the arms and the chest muscles but also to the extension provided by slow and deep inhalation, which acts as a more complete and natural traction on the spinal column. Since the muscles associated with breathing are completed exercised, this set of *vinyāsas* will prove beneficial to people who suffer from periodic asthma attacks. These *vinyāsas* should not be done during such attacks; but the muscle spasms in people who have breathing problems can to a very great extent be corrected by this set of *vinyāsas* for the arms and the torso, done in *tāḍāsana*. Purely for therapy, if the patient cannot stand and do the *vinyāsas*, he or she may be permitted to sit or even lie down and helped to do some of the simpler *vinyāsas*. Which *vinyāsas* are to be done and in what sequence can be determined by the therapist upon seeing the patient, as most asthmatics have poor chest-muscle tone. And for those who tend to have neck spasms or a narrowing of the vertebrae, the combination of movements and breathing will form a good traction exercise. The above group of *vinyāsas* based in *tāḍāsana* are useful for slowly and deliberately working on the joints, hands, elbows, shoulders, neck, spine, and torso in general. Next in the sequence will be *āsanas* and *vinyāsas* for the backbone, hips, knees, and ankles.

The next *vinyāsa* is again done by raising the arms overhead while inhaling and keeping the fingers interlocked, turning them outward at the end of the movement and the inhale. Then, as you exhale, push your hips back and bend forward, keeping your back straight and horizontal. Your knees should not be bent. Inhaling, return to the original position, slightly arching your back as you come up. This posture is called *ardha-uttānāsana,* or half-stretching posture. Then, after coming into the posture, inhale and bring the arms, stretched outward, to shoulder level and exhale. Then, as you inhale stretch the arms overhead even as you stay bending forward, pushing the hip and stretching the leg muscles and back. After exhaling in the posture, inhale and return to the starting position. Exhale and lower the arms. Another variation of the arms' position will be to do the same movement with the hands in back salute *(pṛṣṭāñjali).*

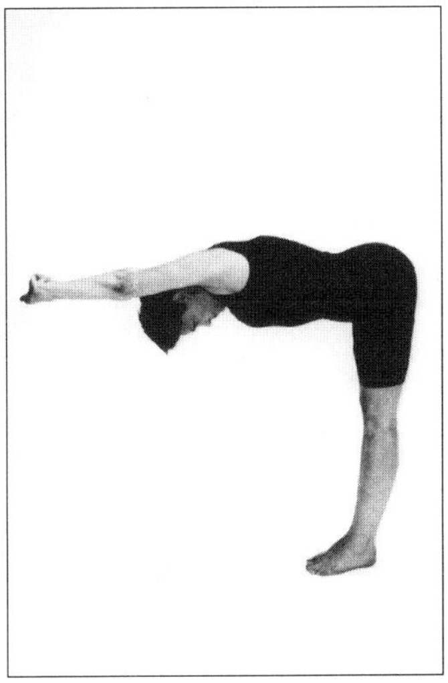

*Ardha-uttānāsana*

The next *āsana* in the group is *pūrṇa-uttānāsana.* Inhale once again and raise your arms overhead, keeping them in front. As you bring your arms up, bend back a little bit, looking up. As you breathe out, press your feet and, without bending your knees, slowly bend forward and place your palms by the sides of your feet, on the floor. For those who have stiff posterior muscles, it may not be possible to go down all the way; in this case you may touch the ground with your fingertips, or hold your ankles and shins. Then as you inhale, pressing your palms against the floor, raise your head, stretching your neck in the process. As you exhale, try to touch your knees with your forehead; then inhale as you return to the original position. *Pūrṇa-uttānāsana,* or full-stretching pose, involves the posterior parts of the legs, back, neck, and shoulders. If you hold your big toes with your thumb and fingers, the pose is known as *pādāṅguṣṭhāsana.* There are a number of variations or *vinyāsas* on this *āsana* pertaining to the position of the hands and palms. One important variation will be to interlock your fingers with your hands

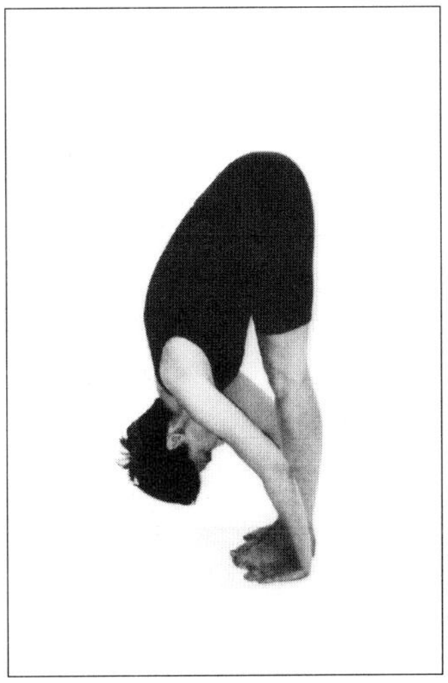

*Pūrṇa-uttānāsana*

behind your back. On the next exhalation, bend forward and touch your knees with your forehead, simultaneously stretching your arms behind your back, stretched almost to behind the back of your head. Keeping your palms on your back in *pṛṣṭāñjali*, or keeping your arms stretched at shoulder level and completing the posture, are some of the variations for the position of the arms in this posture. *Pārśva-uttānāsana* (see p.109) is yet another variation on the *uttānāsana* posture.

The next group of movements involves the knees. In *samasthiti*, inhale and raise your arms in front to the level of the shoulders. As you exhale, still keeping your feet on the floor, bend your knees and squat halfway, with your thighs parallel to the floor. You should keep your chin locked. This posture is called *ardha-utkaṭāsana*, or half-squat posture. There are many *vinyāsas* for this posture depending upon the position of the arms. From *samasthiti*, move your arms to the different positions as mentioned in the beginning of the *tāḍāsana* practice; for example, your arms can be kept stretched out to the sides at shoulder level, or kept overhead, or kept behind the back with the hands in the position of *pṛṣṭāñjali*, or your palms can be kept on the back of their respective shoulder blades, or on the opposite shoulder blades.

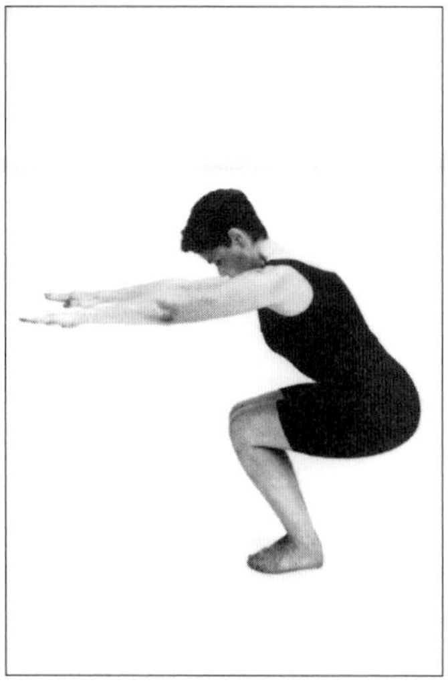

*Ardha-utkaṭāsana* (*vinyāsa* 1)

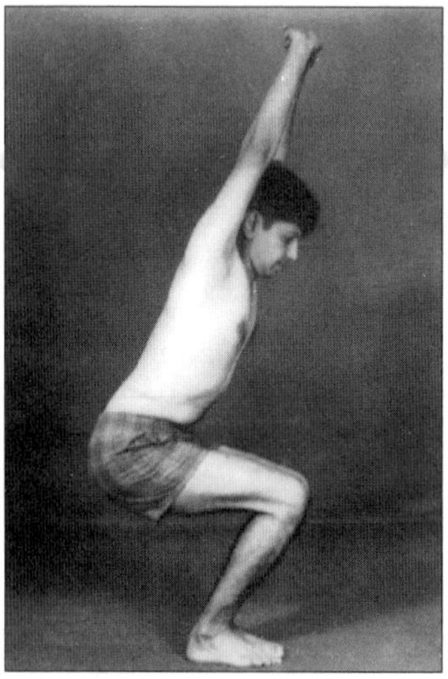

*Ardha-utkaṭāsana* (*vinyāsa* 2)

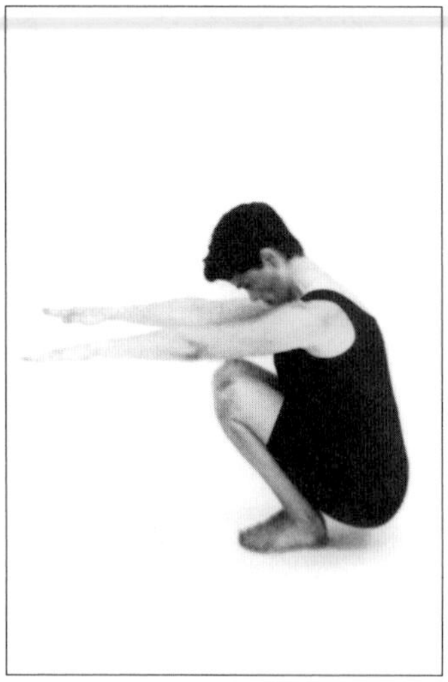

*Utkaṭāsana* (*vinyāsa* 1)

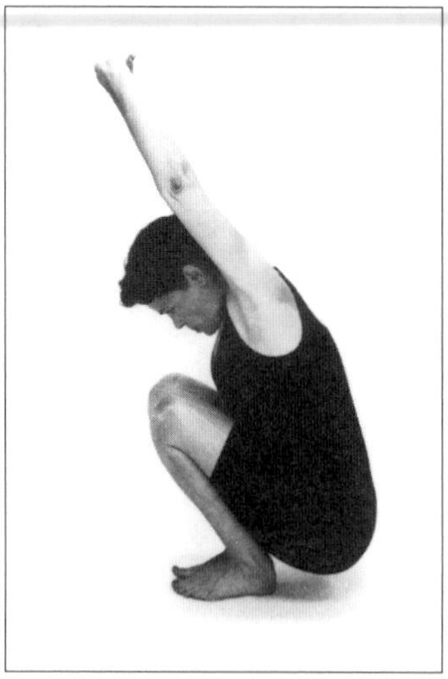

*Utkaṭāsana* (*vinyāsa* 2)

The next *āsana* in this sequence is *utkaṭāsana*, or sitting on one's haunches (without sitting on the floor). Begin as you would for *ardha-utkaṭāsana*. Inhale and raise your arms in front to shoulder level. Then as you exhale, keeping your ankles together and without spreading your legs, bend your knees all

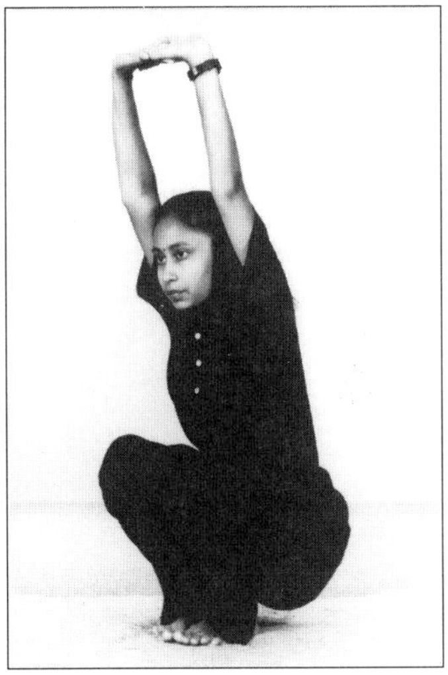

*Utkaṭāsana* (*vinyāsa* 2)
(front view)

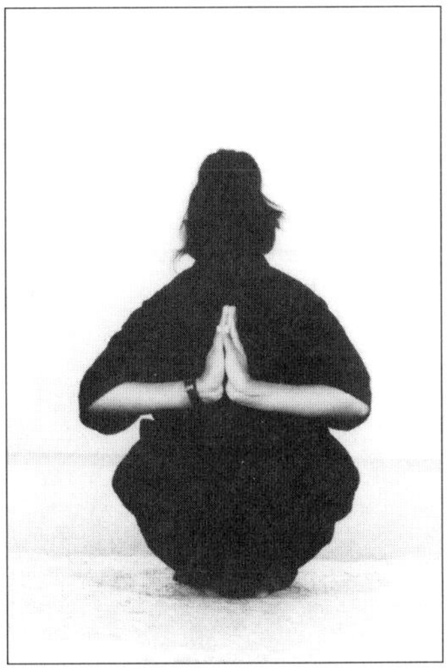

*Utkaṭāsana pṛṣṭāñjali* (*vinyāsa* 3)

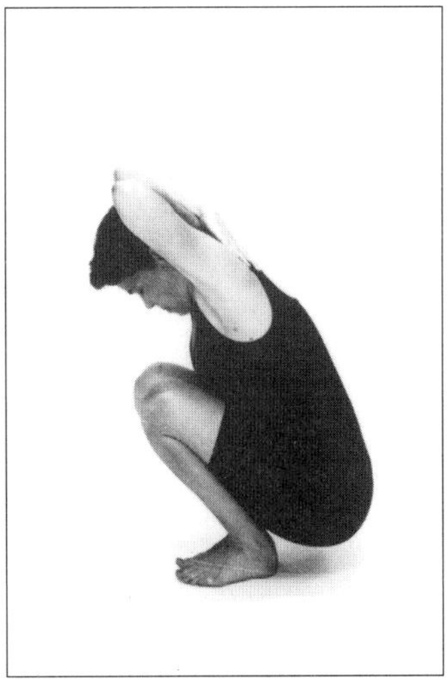

*Utkaṭāsana* (*vinyāsa* 4)

the way until your thighs touch your calf muscles and your knees are fully bent. Your outstretched arms in front will help you maintain balance. You should be sure that your heels are not raised in this posture. Indeed, in all the *āsanas* and *vinyāsas* that have been described so far, your feet should be kept together. As you inhale, rise to *tāḍāsana,* pressing your heels and stretching your ankles, back, shoulders, and neck. As in *ardha-utkaṭāsana*, the same hand positions *(hasta vinyāsas)* can be tried while moving into the posture, for example, arms overhead; hands on the back in *pṛṣṭāñjali* (*vinyāsa* 3)*;* arms at shoulder level; or palms on the shoulder blades or on opposite shoulder blades (*vinyāsa* 4). Of course, one should follow the breathing pattern mentioned while moving the arms to the different *vinyāsa* positions.

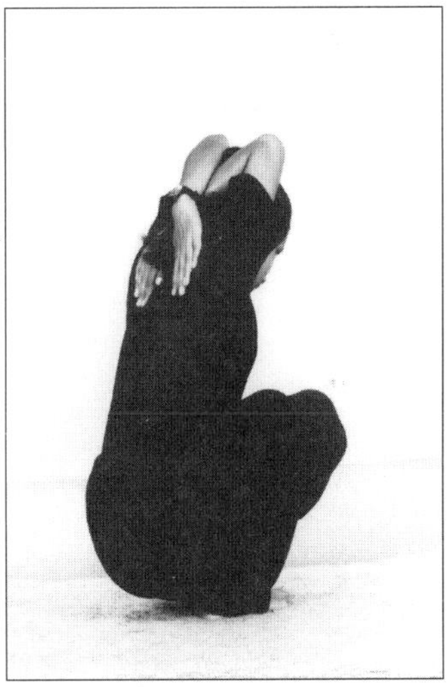

*Utkaṭāsana* (*vinyāsa* 4)
(back view)

Yet another *āsana,* a bit more difficult for beginners and older people, requires being in *utkaṭāsana* and then spreading the knees and thighs while still keeping the feet together. As you exhale, bend forward between the legs, bring your arms back and around your legs, and hold your heels from behind. You may bend forward and touch the floor with the top of your head, forehead, nose, or chin, each of which is progressively more difficult. This is called *malāsana*, or garland posture. Instead of holding your heels, you may bring your arms back around your legs and hold hands behind your back. This is called *kāñcyāsana,* or belt posture. Inhale to get back to *utkaṭāsana,* exhale, and then return to *samasthiti* while inhaling.

Another important posture that requires keeping the feet together is *pāśāsana,*

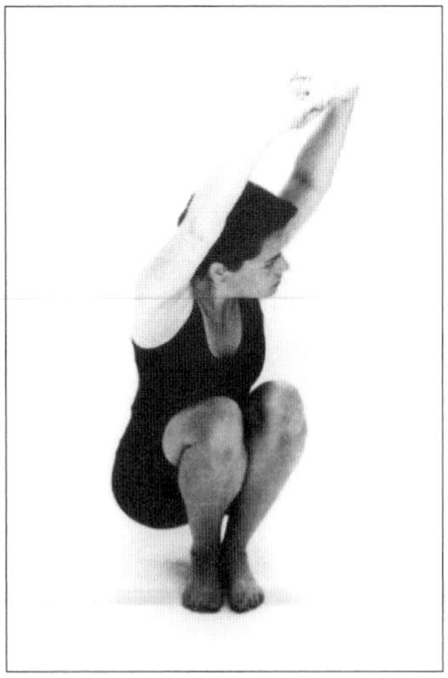

*Utkaṭāsana* (preparation for

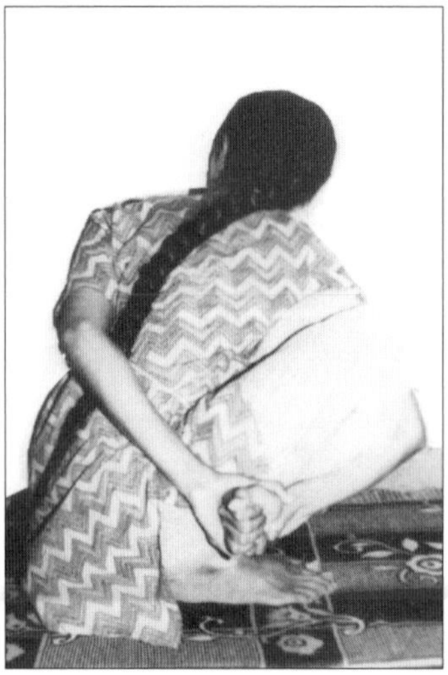

*Pāśāsana* (rear view)

or noose posture. It requires starting from *samasthiti.* Inhale, raise both arms overhead, interlock the fingers, and turn the hands outward. As you exhale, turn to the right side, pressing your feet. As you exhale again, sit on your haunches as in *utkaṭāsana*, except that your upper body is now turned to the right. On the next exhalation, sweep your left arm around the knees and hold it with your right hand, which has been swept around from behind on the right side. Having a good hold of your hands and pressing your feet, turn to the right side as much as possible as you exhale. Inhale, relax the grip, bring your arms overhead, and return to *samasthiti.* Exhale and lower your arms. *Pāśāsana* is a very good posture to tone up the entire backbone; it also helps tone the lower abdominal muscles. Digestion improves and relief from constipation can be obtained with this posture.

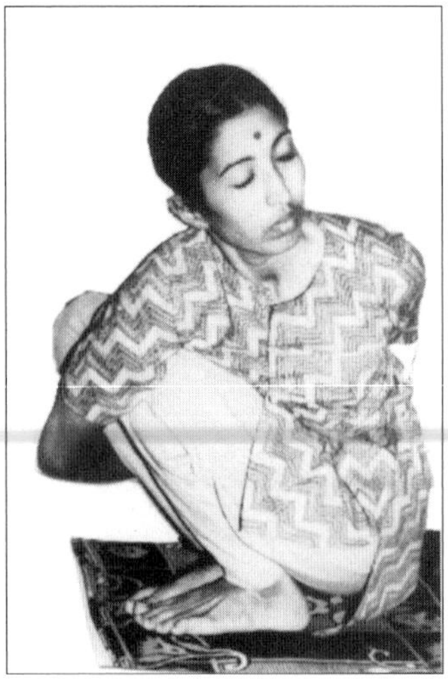

Pāśāsana

Yet another *āsana* that can be done while in *utkaṭāsana* involves exhaling while lowering the arms and placing them by the sides of the feet. Inhale, exhale, and then hold the breath out *(bāhya-kumbhaka),* press your palms, and raise your trunk, even while staying in *utkaṭāsana.* Your feet are now off the ground, and you should maintain the posture of *utkaṭāsana* and balance on both hands. After a few seconds, lower the body and plant the feet on the ground. This method of raising the trunk, pressing the palms, and balancing in a posture is called *utpluti.* It provides a very good sense of balance and strengthens the arms, and perfection in the posture is achieved. Children and more flexible adults love to do these balancing *āsanas.* In fact, all sitting postures such as *padmāsana, vajrāsana, daṇḍāsana,* and so on, lend themselves to this balancing act that is called *utpluti* (raising up).

Another dynamic sequence of *vinyāsas* involves doing *utkaṭāsana* and *ardha-uttānāsana.* From *tāḍāsana*, inhale, raise your arms overhead, and interlock your fingers. As you exhale, push your hips back and bend forward, making your upper body parallel to the floor. This is *ardha-uttānāsana.* Then inhale and bring your arms to shoulder level, stretched out to the sides. After the next exhalation, hold your breath out and, slightly bending your knees, gently jump forward a couple of feet, land softly, and squat on your haunches in a *vinyāsa* of *utkaṭāsana.* Your arms should be kept outstretched. Then as you inhale, come up to *ardha-uttānāsana,* still keeping your arms outstretched at the shoulder level. Inhale, hold your breath, and jump back about two feet, land gently, and sit on your haunches in *utkaṭāsana vinyāsa* once again. Inhale, come back to *ardha-uttānāsana*, inhale and stretch your arms overhead, then inhale again to get back to *tāḍāsana*, and finally return to *samasthiti* while exhaling. This set of *vinyāsas* is called *khagāsana, khaga* meaning "bird." Just as a bird with its wings spread out lands on the ground, this set of movements resemble the bird's movement. Children love these additional *vinyāsas.*

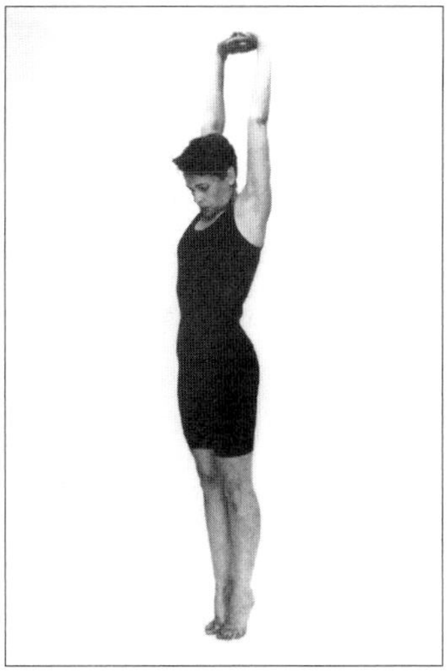

*Tāḍāsana*

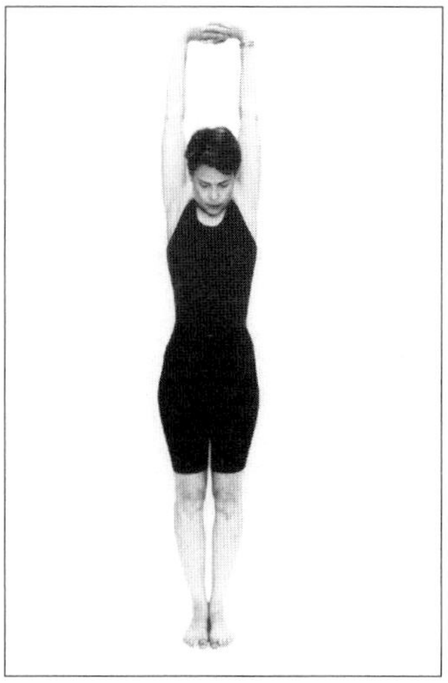

Preparation for *pārśva-uttānāsana*

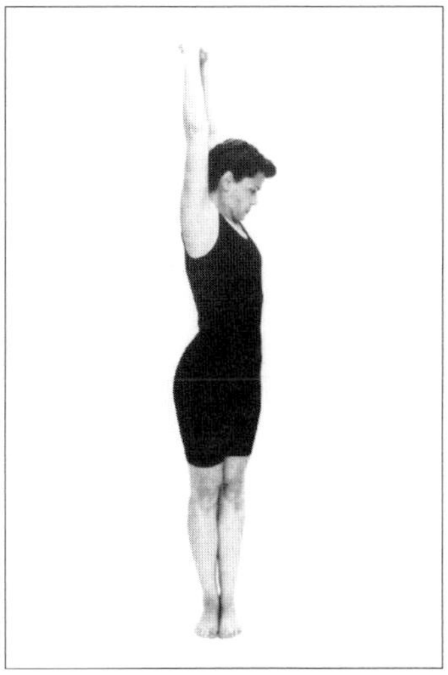

Preparation for *pārśva-uttānāsana*

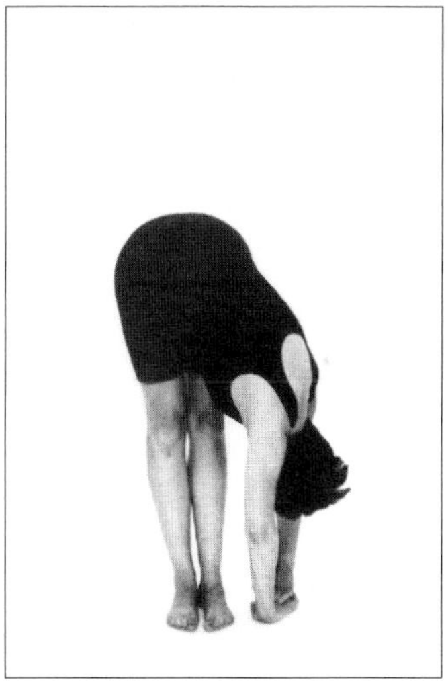

*Pārśva-uttānāsana*

Finally, from *tāḍāsana*, inhale, raise your arms overhead, interlock your fingers, and turn your hands outward. Exhaling and pressing the balls of your feet close together, raise your heels as high a possible, stretching your body, especially your ankles and calf muscles, in the process. Then while exhaling, bring your heels down slowly and deliberately, again synchronizing the movement with your breathing. In the beginning you may have difficulty maintaining balance or keeping your ankles and knees together or stretching your ankles, but if you proceed step by step, a few millimeters at a time, you can reach the full stretch of the posture comfortably. This is a good stretching movement, especially if done in the morning, and it has a tonic effect on the muscles and joints *(sandhis).* Growing children should practice this stretch to aid in increasing their height. It helps to align all the *cakras* and consequently all the *kośas* (five sheaths of the body). The *tāḍāsana* group could also be considered a good beginning set of exercises for limbering up the joints and toning the muscles. It should be noted that it may not be possible to reach the final position itself in the beginning. For some, owing to their physical condition (*śarīra sthiti*), age, and constitution, it may not be possible to do the stretch even after considerable practice. But the benefits start accruing when one does it consciously and with the correct breathing, and when one feels the stretching.

A word of caution against overdoing is warranted here. The built-in control against overdoing it, which is to be avoided, is the breath itself. When it tends to become short, it is an indication to the practitioner to rest. One may rest by returning to *samasthiti* and breathing normally with the mind closely following the breath without interfering with it. This built-in check is an additional advantage in our *ācārya's paddhati.* Unless otherwise noted, breathing should be done with the throat constriction mentioned in the beginning. This group of *āsanas*, especially *utkaṭāsana,* helps tone up the digestive system. After some practice, when one is steady in the posture, *mūla bandha* and *uddīyāna bandha* can be attempted after exhalation (have your teacher by your side when you start to learn this practice). After some experience has been gained, one may stay in a *vinyāsa* or *āsana* for a specified time, doing long smooth inhalations and exhalations. These *vinyāsas* are especially good for women, since they work on the pelvic muscles and are useful against certain cases of menstrual disorder and dysmenorrhea. They also improve the tone of the pelvic muscles that are used during labor and help reduce postnatal complications such as prolapse of the uterus. The *mūla bandha, uddīyāna bandha,* and *vinyāsas* involving *utkaṭāsana* are contraindicated during pregnancy. Practice of *āsanas* should be avoided during menstruation; that is the tradition. There are cases in which some of the more involved *āsanas* (such as *utkaṭāsana* and the lower *bandhas*) could lead to menorrhagia. Simple and long inhalations and exhalations are good during menstruation.

For all aspiring yogis, the morning, either at or before sunrise, is ideally suited for practice. *Abhyāsa* in the evening, however, is better than skipping the practice for the day. One should not practice until three hours after a solid meal and at least a half hour after the intake of fluids.

## More-Difficult *Vinyāsas* in *Tāḍāsana*

The above group of *vinyāsas* is fairly comprehensive, though there are many more-difficult ones that are not included. Some *vinyāsas* require changing the position of one leg while keeping the other leg firmly planted on the floor. These *ekapādāsanas* (one-legged *āsanas*) are usually associated with severe *tapas,* or penance, and some are named after sages who are believed to have attained various *siddhis* in these positions, which require an excellent sense of balance and an enormous capacity for endurance.

The simplest of these *vinyāsas* requires starting again from *samasthiti.* Keeping your head down and back straight, inhale, bend your right knee, raise your leg, and hold the big toe of your right leg with the fingers of your right hand, keeping your left hand on your hip. Inhale and stretch your right leg straight out, holding your big toe. Inhale and, holding your right big toe in position, rotate or swing your right leg to the right side, maintaining balance. This posture is called *ekapādāṅguṣṭāsana;* with the leg to the side, it is *pārṣva-ekapādāṅguṣṭāsana;* squatting, it is called *utkata-ekapādāṅguṣṭāsana.* There is still another variation. Exhale and bring your leg to the starting position in front of you. Then lean forward slightly and, while inhaling, hold your right foot with your right hand and then with both hands, and inhale. During the next exhalation, bend forward and touch your right knee with your forehead without changing the position of your leg or bending either of your knees. Inhale, raise your trunk, and lower your right leg. You may repeat this *vinyāsa* on the other side as well.

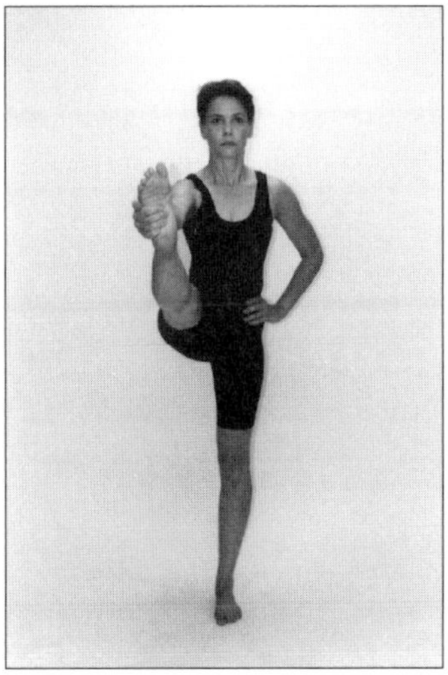

*Ekapādāṅguṣṭāsana*

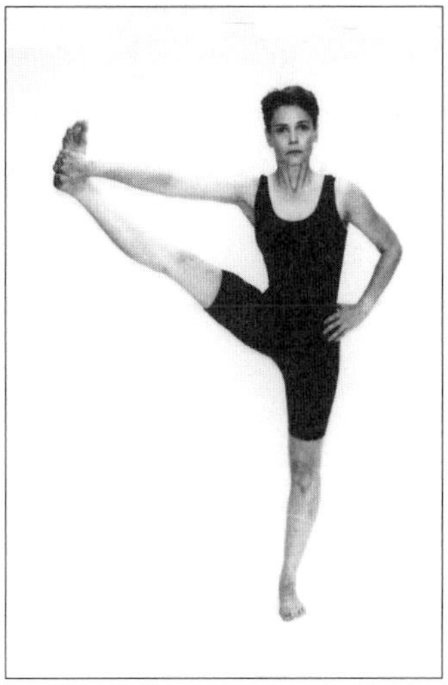

*Pārśva-ekapādāṅguṣṭāsana*

The next *vinyāsa* will require you to bend your right knee and place it on the top of your left thigh, with the heel touching or close to the left groin. This is the half-lotus position, and the movement is done on the exhalation. Inhale, raise both arms overhead, interlock your fingers, and turn your hands outward. On the next exhalation, keeping your left arm overhead, bring your right arm around your back and hold the big toe of your right leg with the fingers of your right hand. During the next exhalation, you may lower your left hand as well and place it on top of your right hand. You may try to stay in this position for a while, watching your balance and doing normal inhalation and exhalation. Your head should be kept down, since this will better facilitate maintaining your balance. This

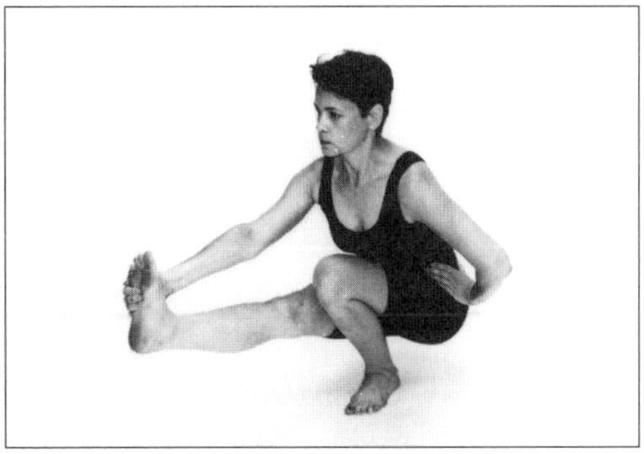

*Utkaṭa-ekapādāṅguṣṭāsana*

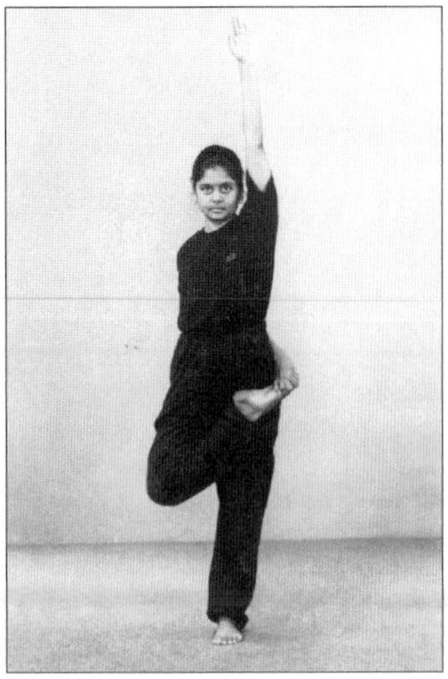

*Vṛkṣāsana*

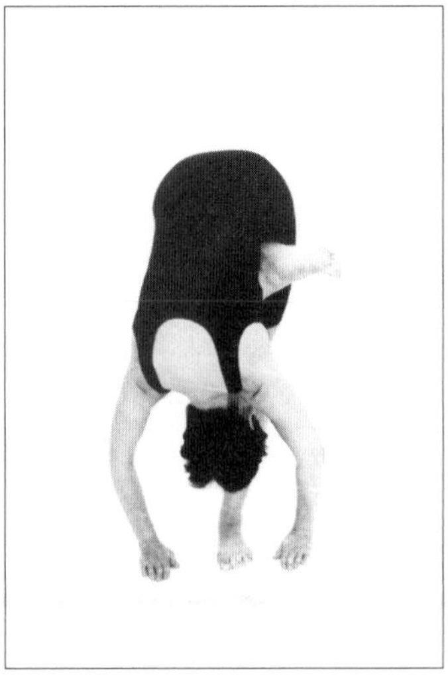

*Uttānavṛkṣāsana*

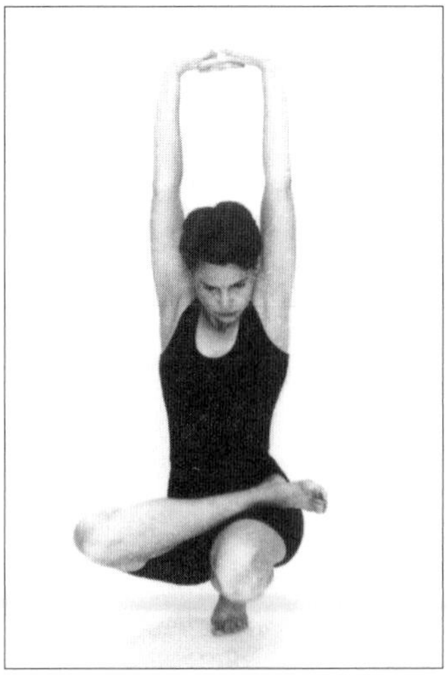

*Utkaṭavṛkṣāsana*

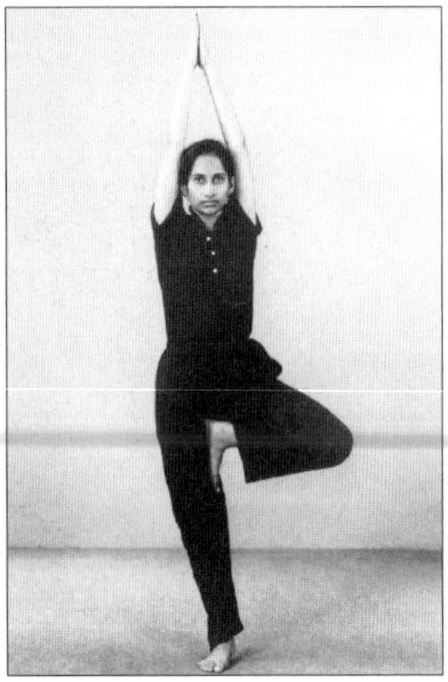

*Bhagīratāsana*

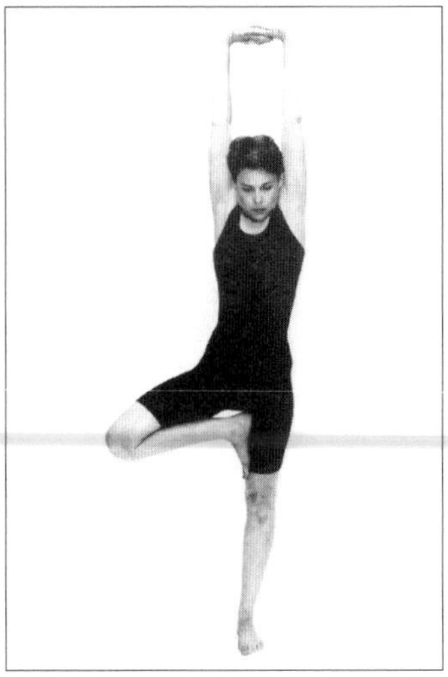

*Bhagīratāsana* (with chin lock)

position is called *vṛkṣāsana,* or tree posture. This *āsana* can be construed as an extension of *tāḍāsana* in which the *pāda-vinyāsa,* or variation in the position of the leg, is attempted. It can be also considered a balancing posture. Switching legs, hold your left big toe with your right hand and raise your left arm overhead as you inhale. Exhaling, balancing on the right leg, slowly bend forward and hold the big toe of your right foot with your left hand and try to touch your knee with your forehead. It is very difficult to maintain balance, but with practice staying in the posture for a length of time, balance will improve. Inhale, raise your trunk, and keep your left arm overhead. As a counterposture, while holding your right big toe with your right hand from behind, slowly inhale and try to sit as if on your haunches, without raising your left heel off the floor. This is called *utkaṭavṛkṣāsana.* The difficult part of the movement is when you are halfway through the trip down. Inhale, come up to *vṛkṣasāna,* and on next inhalation raise both your arms overhead and lower your bent right leg. Return to *samasthiti* as you exhale and lower your arms. Repeat the movement on the other side.

For the next *vinyāsa,* inhale, bend your right knee, and, with your right knee pushed laterally, place your right sole high inside your left thigh with the heel placed firmly in the left groin. Inhale, raise both arms overhead, and keep your palms together. Try to stay for a few breaths. This posture is called *bhagīratāsana,* after the sage Bhagīrata. This *āsana* helps to stretch the pelvis and develops a very good sense of balance. In-hale and lower your right leg. Repeat the movement on the left side.

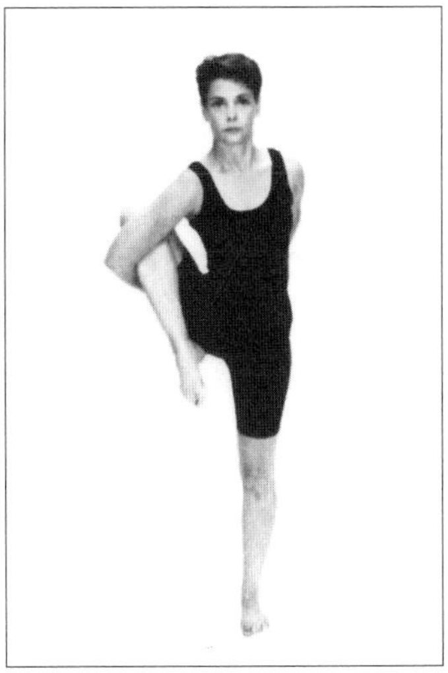

*Ekapādāsana (vinyāsa)*

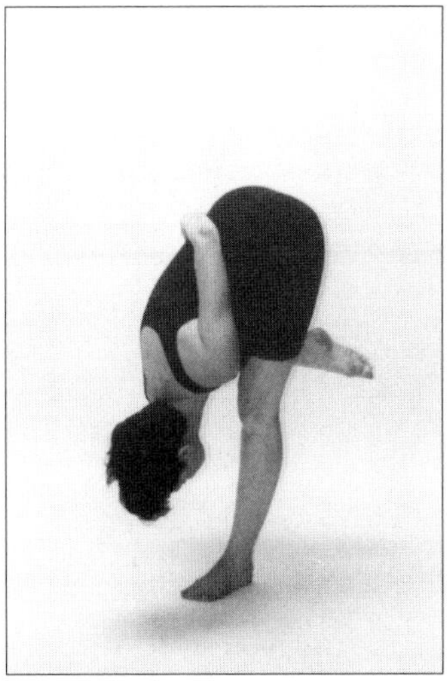

*Uttāna*-ekapādāsana

For another *vinyāsa,* start once again from *samasthiti.* As you exhale, bend your right knee and raise your right leg so that your right knee is close to the chin, your thigh pressing against the chest. Inhale, and on the next exhalation bend forward inside your bent right leg and bring your right arm around your bent right leg. On the next inhalation, bring your left arm behind your back and hold your right hand from behind. Your right leg, which is bent and encircled by your right hand, is pressed tightly against the right side of your torso. Stay for a few breaths. Here again the *utkaṭāsana* and *uttānāsana* movements can be tried. As you exhale, balancing on your left leg, slowly bend forward to the farthest extent possible, up to touching your knee with your forehead. Inhale and come back. During the next exhalation, try to sit on your haunches, balancing on your left foot. Your heel should not be allowed to rise. These postures are extremely good for balance and also work on the lower abdominal muscles and the pelvic organs. Inhale and come back. You may repeat it on the other side as well.

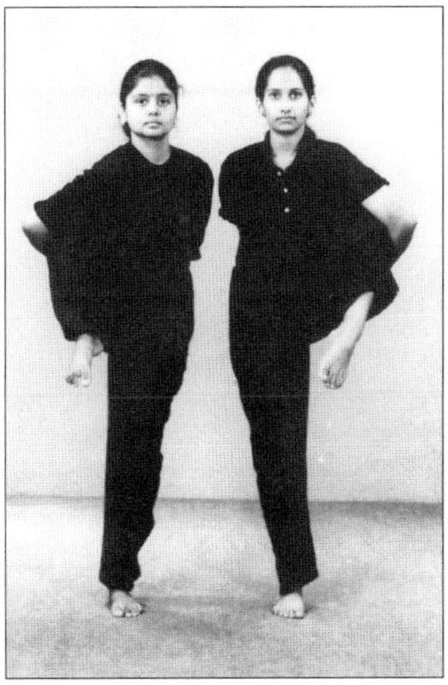

Ekapādāsana (vinyāsa)

The next *vinyāsa* is an extension of the previous one. As you inhale in *samasthiti,* bend your right knee, bring it up, and hold your right foot around the sole. As you exhale the next time, stretch your leg up as high as possible and keep it straight up, holding it with both hands. This is a very difficult posture. Stay in the posture for a few breaths. Inhale, bend your knee, lower your leg and bring it down, and keep your arms by your sides in *samasthiti.* This posture is called *trivikramāsana,* named after an incarnation of Lord Viṣṇu. Repeat it on the other side. This posture is supposed to facilitate arousal of *kuṇḍalinī* and align the *cakras.*

All the *vinyāsas* described so far involve keeping one leg on the floor and moving the other in front or to the side of the body. There are others in which one leg is brought behind the body and held in different positions. There are two important *āsanas* in which a leg is taken behind while balancing on the other leg. In *tāḍāsana*, exhale, slightly bend your right knee, take your right leg around your back, and place your right foot behind your neck. This is called *dūrvāsāsana* after a *ṛṣi* named Durvāsā. Exhaling, you may bend forward and touch the floor with your hands. This is an extremely difficult posture.

The next *āsana* is *naṭarājāsana*, named after the dancing Lord Śiva. Stand in *tāḍāsana* and stretch your right arm in front of your body as you inhale. On the next inhale, bend your left knee, hold your big toe with your right hand, and push the leg up as high as possible, touching the back of the head. You may repeat *naṭarājāsana* on the other side.

It is now time to talk about resting. When one feels the need to take a break from *āsana* practice, one can lie down and slowly allow all the joints to relax. All the joints should be kept loose. Start at the toes, then turn your attention to the ankles, then the calf muscles, and let go. Then move on to the knees, the hamstrings, the huge thigh muscles, the hips, and pelvis, and then on to the entire backbone and neck. Then turn your attention to the shoulders, the elbows, wrists, and knuckles, each side separately. Allow all the joints to relax, as well as the muscles. This is called *śavāsana*, or corpse posture. Don't allow your mind to wander or go to sleep. Turn your attention to the breath. Watch it as it becomes shallower and smoother, until your breath is normal and you feel refreshed. Rest for a brief period, then proceed with further yoga practice.

The standing postures with the feet kept together are comparatively strenuous. It is therefore necessary that those with heart ailments use discretion in doing such postures, especially the difficult *vinyāsas.* These postures are, however, particularly beneficial to teenagers and young men and women, since they help to develop the skeletal muscles, tendons, and joints, and thereby improve the overall blood circulation. Since these postures are done with corresponding modulated deep breathing, respiration and circulation also improve, and these are necessary for achieving and maintaining good health.

## *Trikoṇāsana*

Another group of *āsanas* and *vinyāsas* involves postures in which the legs are spread apart. Those who have difficulty maintaining good balance find doing yogic standing exercises easier with feet spread apart. This *sthiti* is called *trikoṇāsana sthiti*, as the leg position forms a triangle *(trikoṇa).* For some, better stretching becomes possible in specific *vinyāsas.* Start with *samasthiti.* Inhale, and raise your arms outstretched to the sides up to shoulder level. Exhale, jump, and spread your legs three to three and a half feet. Take a few normal breaths and get a "feel" for the posture. Now exhale, turn your head and neck to the left side so that you are looking over your left shoulder, and, bending at the hip, lower your trunk to the right side, keeping your right palm by the side of your right foot. Your feet should be pointing forward and not be turned to the right side. Those who cannot bend all the way down may hold the right leg a little higher. After some practice, many may be able to bend so low as to press their palm on the floor, by the side of the foot. You should not feel tight in the neck or flushing in the face, which indicates that you are straining. With longer and finer exhalation, or the capacity for good *recaka*, it will become easier to do this posture. You may stay in the posture, called *utthita-trikoṇāsana,* for a few breaths and then inhale, rising back to the starting position, which is called *trikoṇāsana sthiti.* Now repeat it on the other side as well. Keep your knees and elbows straight in this posture.

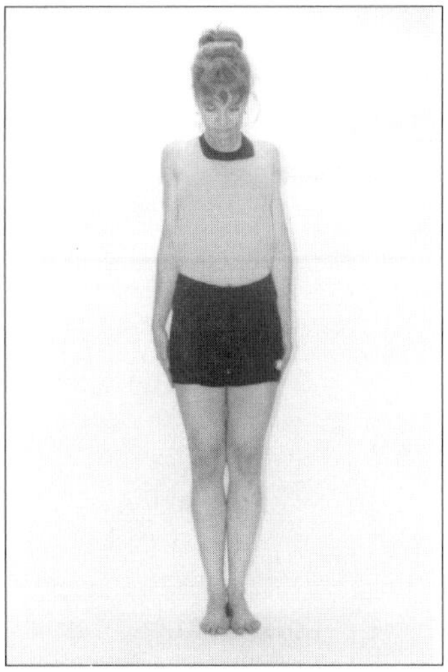

*Samasthiti*

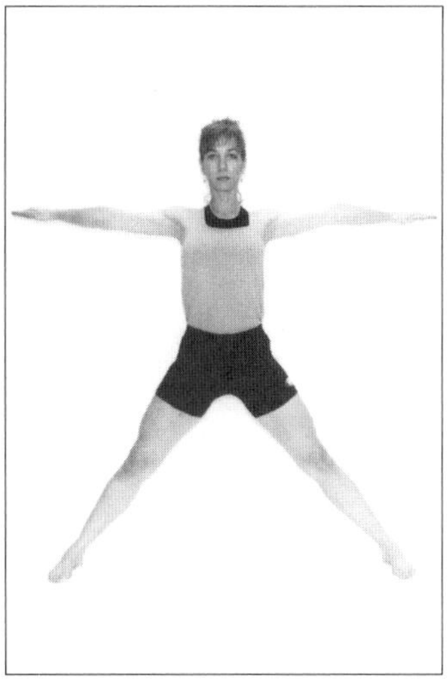

*Trikoṇāsana sthiti*

In this *āsana*, back, hips, arms, neck, and the soles of the feet are flooded with blood. If practiced consistently, one's physical condition will improve, and rheumatic pain in the hips, back, knees, and elbows will gradually decrease. This is one of the best postures for obese people to reduce fat in the arms, back, waist, and lower abdomen and back regions. Those who are unsteady while standing erect may do the posture while lying down, keeping the back of the neck, back, buttocks, and back of the heels firmly on the floor. After a few days, one may start doing the practice while standing in *trikoṇāsana.*

The next *vinyāsa* in this group requires twisting of the trunk. Stay in *trikoṇāsana sthiti.* Raise your arms sideways and keep them at shoulder level. With feet facing forward, inhale, slowly turn your upper body to the left side, place your right palm by the

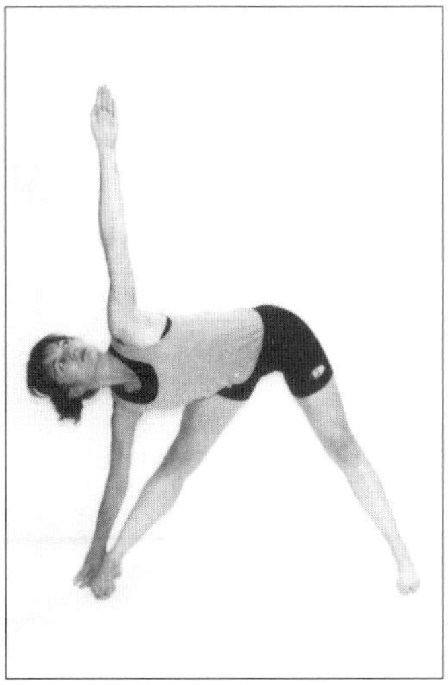

*Utthitatrikoṇāsana*

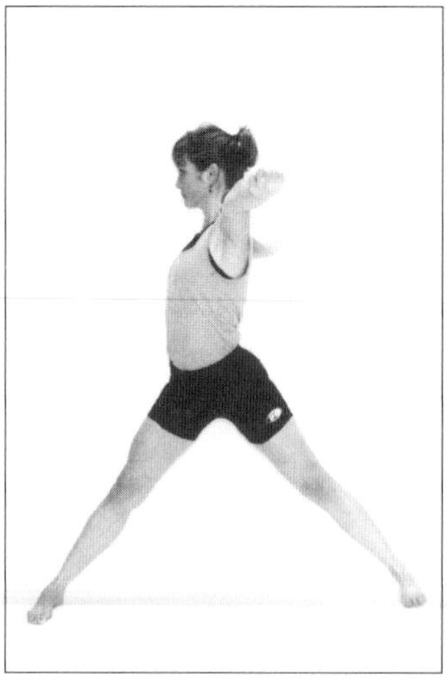

*Parivṛtta trikoṇāsana*
(stage 1)

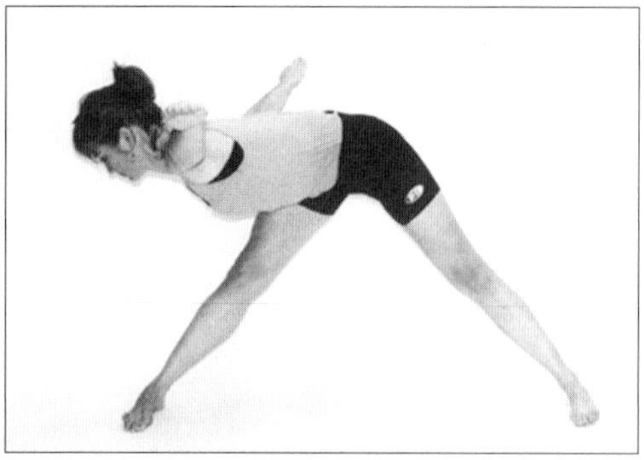

*Parivṛtta trikoṇāsana*
(stage 2)

side of your left foot, and look up. Your arms should be in a straight line. Stay in the posture for a few breaths, and as you inhale come back to *trikoṇāsana sthiti.* This posture is called *parivṛtta* (twist) *trikoṇāsana.* There is a more refined method of doing this posture in three *vinyāsas.* From *trikoṇāsana,* with arms outstretched at shoulder level, exhale and turn to the left side. Then inhale. On the next exhalation, bend forward, keeping your trunk horizontal. Inhale, and during the next exhalation do the third *vinyāsa,* which is turning your trunk and placing your right palm by the side of your left foot and looking up. To return to *trikoṇāsana sthiti,* first inhale and "unwind," bringing your body up and parallel to the floor. Exhale, and in the next inhalation raise your trunk, still turned to the left side, and as you inhale again, turn and face front and enter *trikoṇāsana sthiti.* In this way, the stretching and the efficacy of the posture are enhanced, and the chances of injury (if you do the whole movement in one go) are also reduced. People with lower-back pain, back strain, or a suspected slipped disk will do well not to attempt this involved posture. This is a very graceful but powerful posture. Now you may repeat it on the other side.

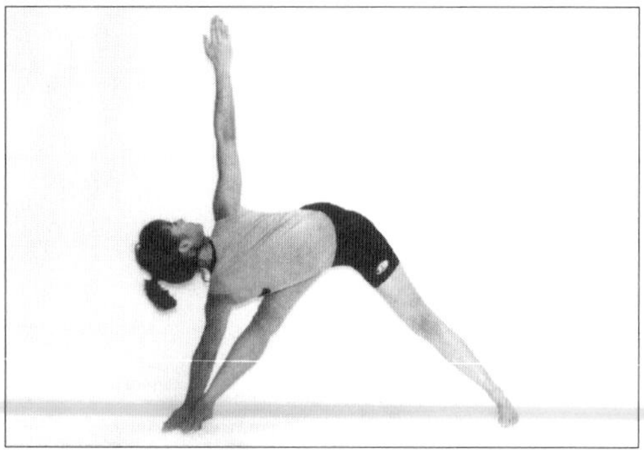

*Parivṛtta trikoṇāsana*

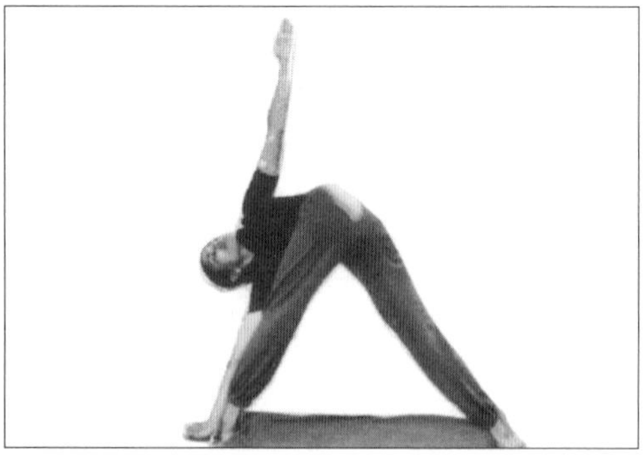

*Parivṛtta trikoṇāsana* (rear view)

In the next *āsana* in this sequence, one knee is bent so that the lateral movement of the hip joint is enhanced. Again, start from *samasthiti* and proceed to the *trikoṇāsana sthiti* on exhalation. On the next exhalation, turn your right side at a ninety-degree angle to your straight left foot. Looking forward, push your trunk to the right side and slowly lower it as you bend and thrust out your right knee, of course while exhaling. As you complete the exhalation, place your right

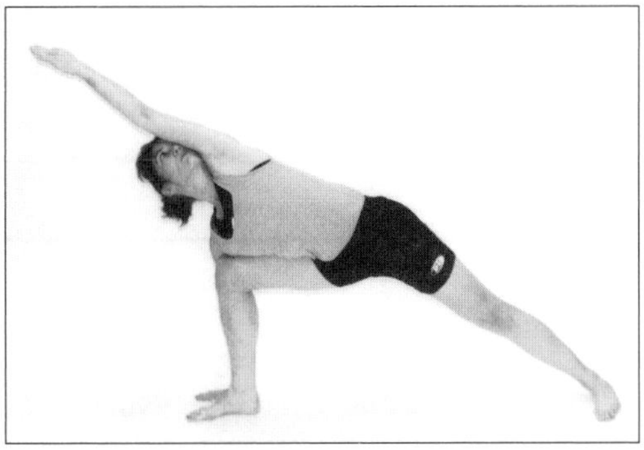

*Utthitapārśvakoṇāsana*

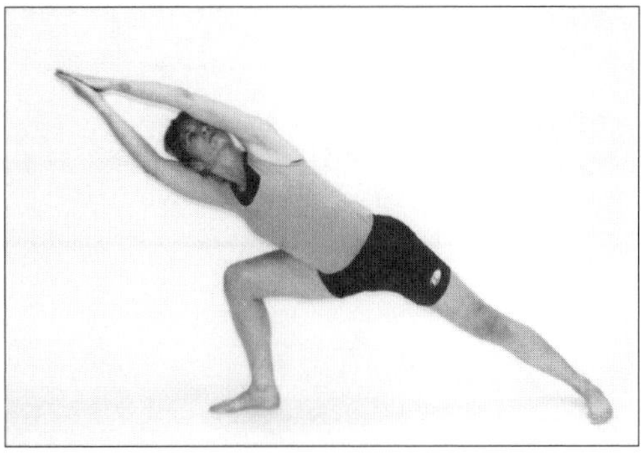

*Utthitapārśvakoṇāsana (vinyāsa)*

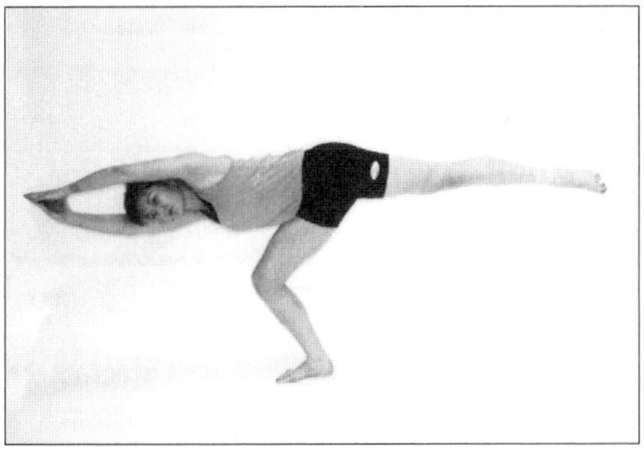

*Utthitapārśvakoṇāsana*
(balancing)

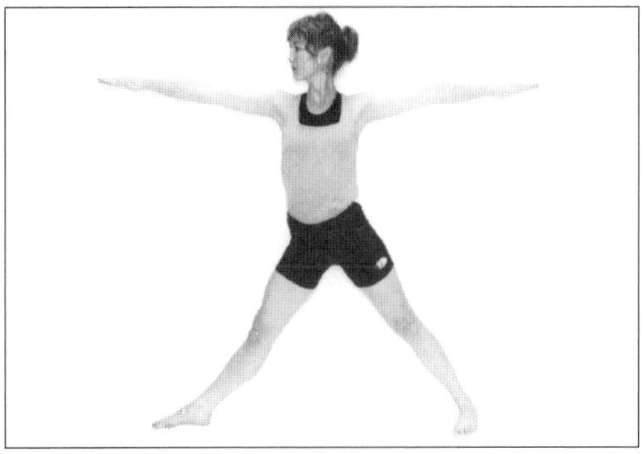

*Utthitapārśvakoṇāsana*
(return)

palm by the side of your right foot. Your left arm also gradually swings overhead so that it is parallel to the floor, and you will be looking straight ahead, even as you bend to the side. Stay for a few breaths. This posture is called *utthitapārśvakoṇāsana*. You have to be careful while lowering your trunk, as you will be looking straight ahead and not at the floor on the side in which you are moving. This posture helps to stretch the hips and the waist, and the groin muscles are also toned up. Constipation and certain types of dysmenorrhea respond well to this posture. This is also a very good practice for athletes, especially those for whom lateral movement is important. Regular practice with appropriate breathing will help reduce chances of sports injuries. Additional

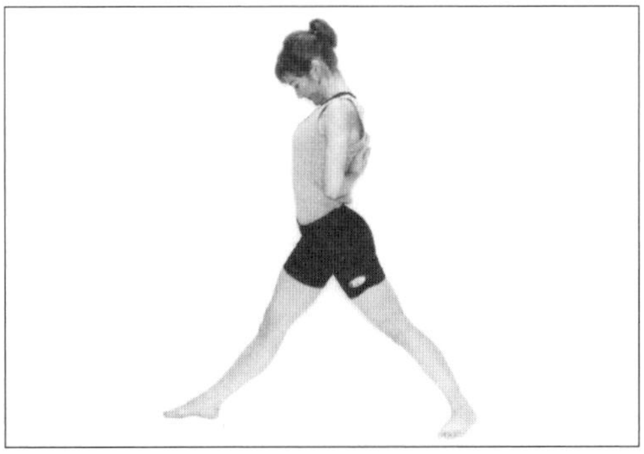

*Pārśvakoṇāsana*
(stage 1)

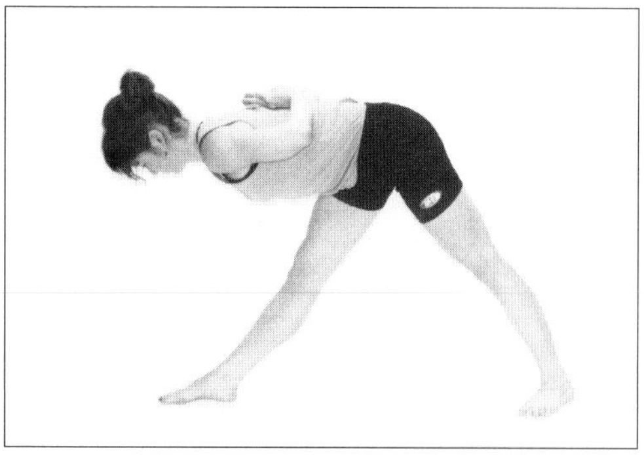

*Utthitapārśvakoṇāsana*
(stage 2)

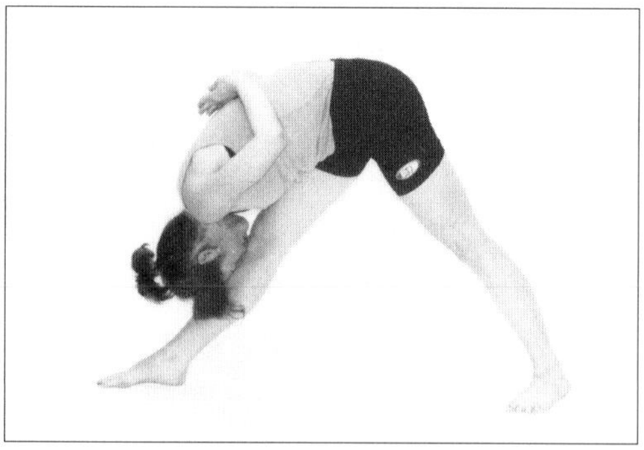

*Utthitapārśvakoṇāsana*

*vinyāsas* here include raising the right hand on inhalation and closing it with the left palm; one may feel this stretch in the thigh and groin. Keeping the right palm by the side of the right foot and leaning on the right side, slowly raise your left leg in the same plane as the body. Stay for a few breaths. The brave ones may now raise the right arm as well, and on the inhale, close both palms overhead. This is a balancing *vinyāsa* of *utthitapārśvakoṇāsana.* With the right knee bent, it gives a tremendous stretch to the thighs and the groin. You have to be careful about the bent knee, and you should find the exact point at which you can stay balanced without straining the knee. Inhale, lower the leg, and place the right hand by the side of the right foot. As you inhale the next time, slide back to *trikoṇāsana sthiti,* raising your trunk from the right side. Repeat the *āsana* and the *vinyāsas* on the other side.

In the last *vinyāsa,* the *trikoṇāsana sthiti,* there was no turning of the trunk (except the *parivṛtta*), and the upper body moved from side to side. One can do the next group of *āsanas* in the same *trikoṇāsana* by turning to either side and doing different *āsanas* and *vinyāsas.* As you inhale, turn the left foot outward ninety degrees, keeping the right foot pointed forward. Inhale, raise both arms overhead, and interlock the fingers. Exhale and turn to the left side. Breathe normally a couple of times and then while exhaling, press the feet and, keeping the knees straight, stretch the back and also the neck and bend forward until the

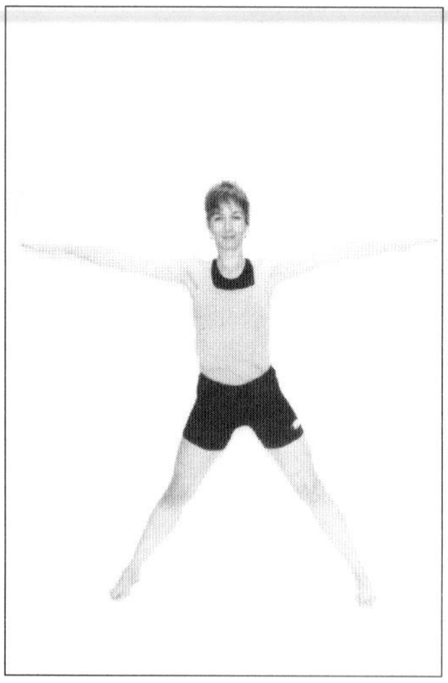

*Vīrabhadrāsana* (start)

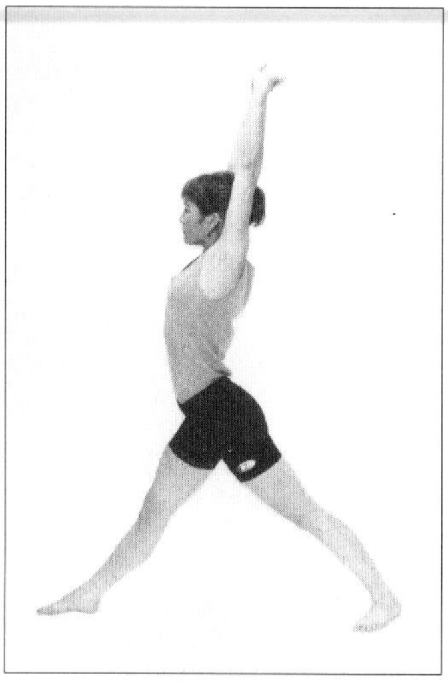

*Vīrabhadrāsana*
(step 1)

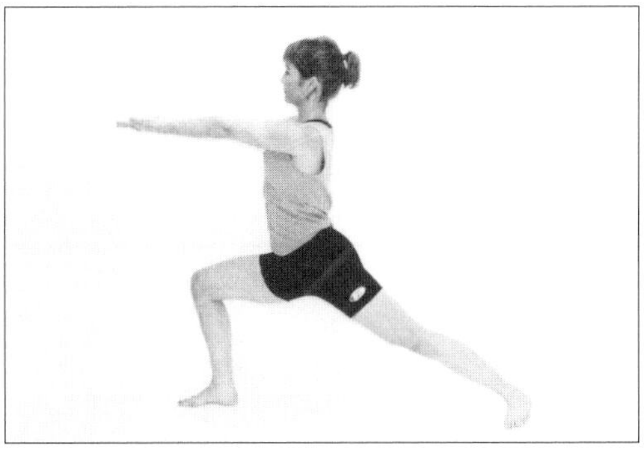

*Vīrabhadrāsana*

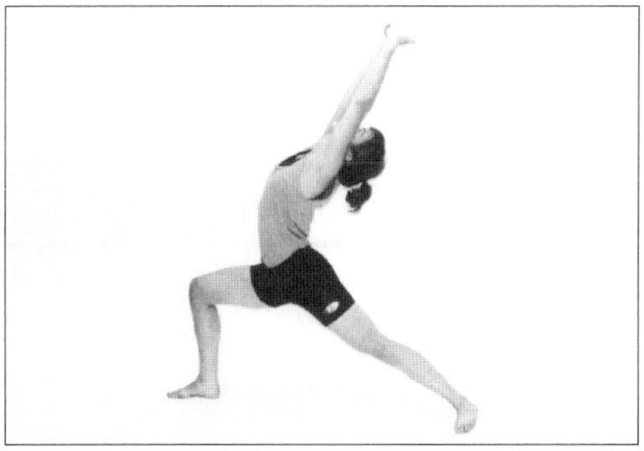

*Vīrabhadrāsana (vinyāsa)*

forehead touches the left knee. Stay in this posture for a few breaths, and while inhaling return to *trikoṇāsana sthiti.* This is called *pārśva-uttānāsana (dakṣiṇa)* and the right side of the body is stretched. The same movement can be repeated, which is known as *vamapārśva-uttānāsana.* In this posture, the hip and the pelvic joints are twisted or rotated. The knees and the ankles experience an angular stretching, and this posture, therefore, helps in improving the flexibility of these joints. It can be practiced by all. There are a few different *hasta vinyāsas* (positions of the arms). You can keep the palms halfway between the extended legs. Thereafter, pressing both the palms and the front leg to the floor and keeping the forehead on the knee, the back leg can be lifted up (and stretched) as high as possible, balancing on one leg and the palms. Exhaling, return to *pārśva-uttānāsana sthiti.* The forward movement can be done keeping the arms stretched wide at the level of the shoulders, or keeping the palms together behind the back in *pṛṣṭāñjali.*

The next *āsana* on this side in *trikoṇāsana* is called *vīrabhadrāsana*, named after a warrior-devotee of Lord Śiva. This is a *vinyāsa* of *pārśva-uttānāsana.* From *trikoṇāsana sthiti*, exhale and turn your right foot outward. Stretch your left leg, keeping your left knee straight, and bend your right knee, pushing it forward and lowering your body. Now inhale deeply and stretch your upper body, keeping your arms overhead with fingers interlocked and turned outward. Stay for a few breaths. This posture is *vīrabhadrāsana.* Now inhale, bend forward, and touch your bent right knee with your forehead and place your palms by the sides of your right leg. Stay for a few breaths. Then as you inhale, raise your left leg and keep it horizontal, and raise your upper body to horizontal, keeping your arms stretched overhead. This is another variation of *vīrabhadrāsana* in which the right knee is still kept bent. In another variation, straighten the right knee and keep the right leg straight (on inhalation), and the upper body and the left leg will be in one line horizontally. Exhale and lower your arms and left leg. Inhale to return to *trikoṇāsana sthiti.* Repeat this set of *vinyāsas* on the other side as well. It could be observed that this aggressive posture requires further stretching of the thighs and calf muscles, and the turn in the hip joint is further accentuated. Athletes and sportsmen who require agility may benefit by this group of *āsanas.* This is not to say that yoga encourages sports. On the contrary, it is the contention of yogis that games, since they waste energy, are a hindrance to the realization of the higher benefits of yoga. Sports are considered *aṅgabhāṅga sādhana* (injurious to one or another part of the body), whereas yoga is *sarvaṅga sādhana,* or the system that is beneficial to all parts of the body, including the internal organs. But, then, those who care only for sports activities may still benefit from these *āsanas* with *vinyāsas.*

From *trikoṇāsana sthiti,* if you spread your legs so your feet are about five feet apart, this is known as *prasāritapāda-uttānāsana sthiti.* Keeping your knees straight, inhale and bend forward as far as possible, pushing the hips back. Inhale, raising up your trunk. Now raise your arms overhead, keeping your palms facing front, then exhale, bend forward, and hold your toes with the fingers of the corresponding hands. Inhale, straighten your back, and look up, arching your back a little. Return to the standing position with arms overhead. Exhale, bend forward, and, keeping your palms between and in line with your feet, push your hips, press your palms, lower your trunk, and touch the floor between your palms with the top of your head. This posture is known as *prasāritapādāsana.* Inhale and return to the starting position. After the *prasāritapāda sthiti,* one may spread the legs farther on inhalation and sit on the floor with the legs spread on either side of the body, which is called *samakoṇāsana.* This is a very difficult posture, but youngsters with supple hip joints, good muscle tone, and groin flexibility will be able to do it.

We have broadly covered the *āsanas* and *vinyāsas* that can be done while standing. These *āsanas* are basically done with the feet together, or *samasthiti,* or with a broad base, like *trikoṇa* and *prasāritapāda sthitis.* Each group has its own benefits. People with vertigo, abnormal blood pressure, or heart ailments should not attempt these standing *āsanas* and *vinyāsas* requiring bending of the body. Youngsters will find that the *tāḍāsana* group improves poise and sense of balance and will help them carry themselves well and also have a better sensitivity and awareness of their own bodies. The *trikoṇāsana* and others that provide a broader base between the feet will give strength and help improve circulation and one's sense of well-being. It is time to lie down and take rest in *śavāsana.*

## Transition Postures

It has been noted that all *āsanas* in this *vinyāsakrama* start with *samasthiti* and end with it. But we also need some intermediate or transition postures to reach other postures, whether in sitting, supine, or prone position.

*Caturaṅgadaṇḍāsana* is an important intermediate posture. It also forms the centerpiece in the well-known sun salute or *sūryanamaskāra. Catur* means "four," *aṅga* is "limb," and *daṇḍa* is "stick," making this a "four-legged stick posture." It is done by following the *vinyāsa* sequence. First, stand in *samasthiti*, with arms overhead. Exhaling, proceed to *ardha-uttānāsana* and *uttānāsana,* in that order, and place your palms by the sides of your feet as mentioned earlier. Then press your palms, inhale, raise your head, and, while exhaling, proceed to *utkaṭāsana*, but without raising your arms. Do a few inhalations and exhalations in that posture. Then, holding the breath after the exhalation, press your palms slightly and lift your feet off the floor. Then gently jump back and land on the tips of your big toes, dropping your body horizontally like a stick, so that the body rests about four inches above the floor and parallel to it. In this position only your palms and big toes rest on the floor, and your entire body is above it. It is said that the body should be truly horizontal. You may stay in the posture for a few breaths. In the initial stages, your hands and legs are likely to tremble, but in due course you will overcome this deficiency. For a number of people, it may not be possible to jump back as mentioned, out of fear of falling down on one's face, or from sheer weakness of the limbs. It is all the more so with obese people—some of whom may have difficulty in keeping their belly from touching the floor and keeping their back straight. For beginners, therefore, rather than jumping up, it

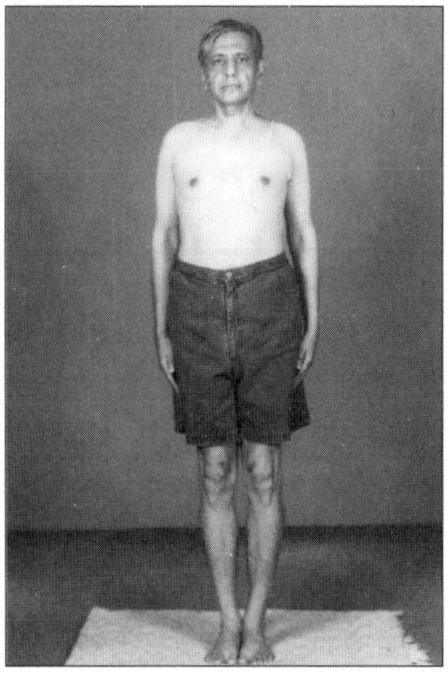

*Samasthiti sūryanamaskāra,*
steps 1 and 12

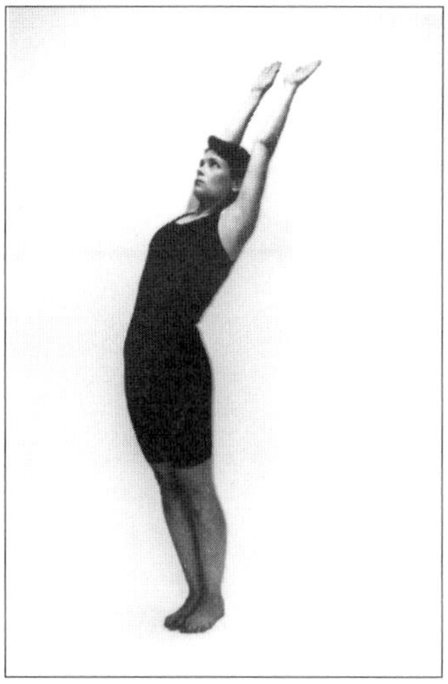

*Sūryanamaskāra,*
step 2

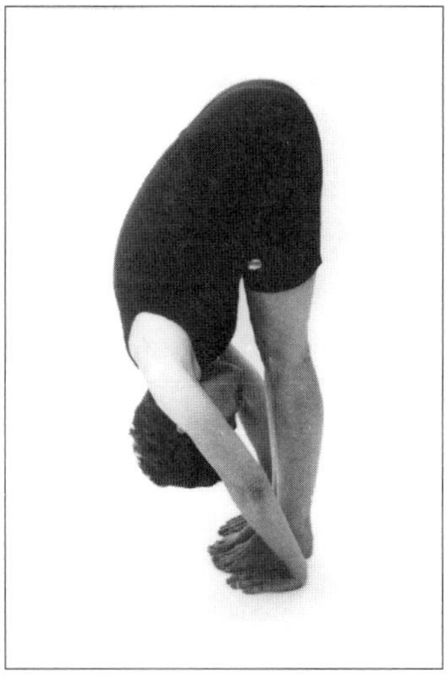

*Uttānāsana sūryanamaskāra,*
step 3

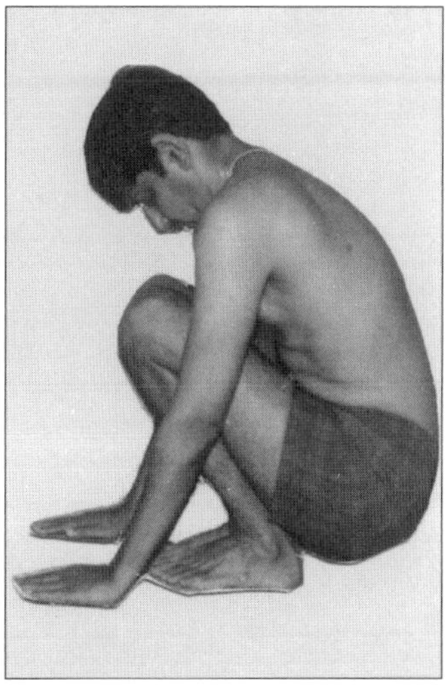

*Utkaṭāsana sūryanamaskāra,*
step 4

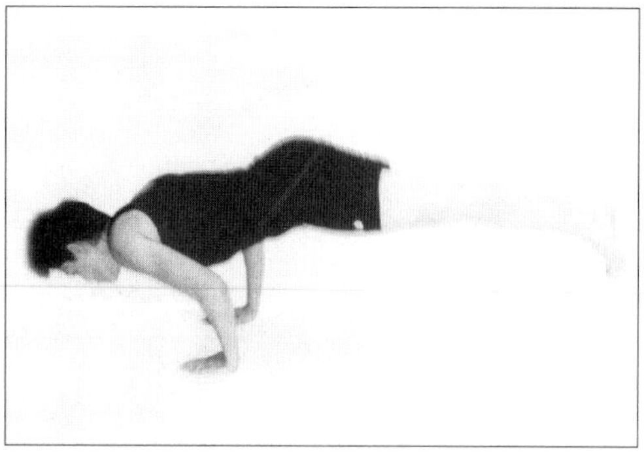

*Sūryanamaskāra*,
step 4 to step 5

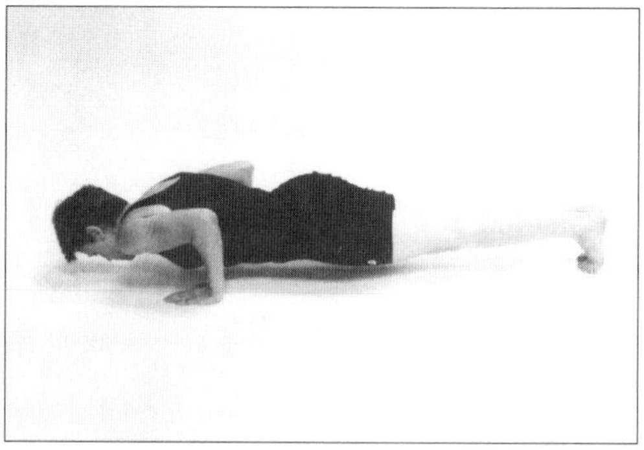

*Caturaṅgadaṇḍāsana sūryanamaskāra*,
step 5

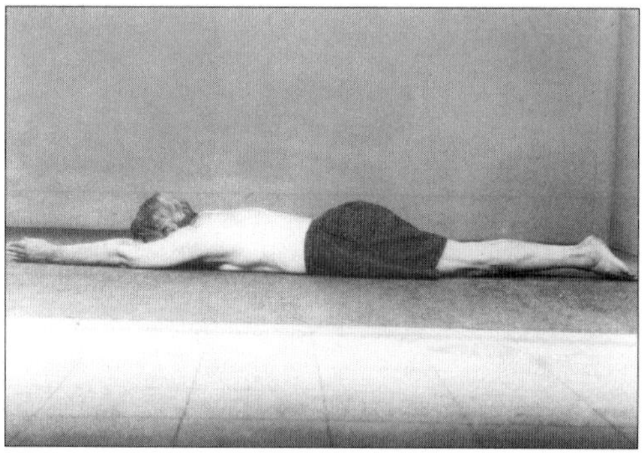

*Daṇḍa samarpaṇam sūryanamaskāra*,
step 6

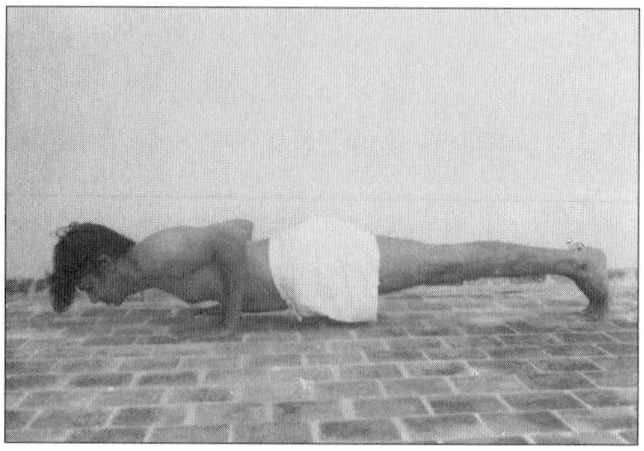

*Caturaṅgadaṇḍāsana sūryanamaskāra*,
transition between steps 6 and 7

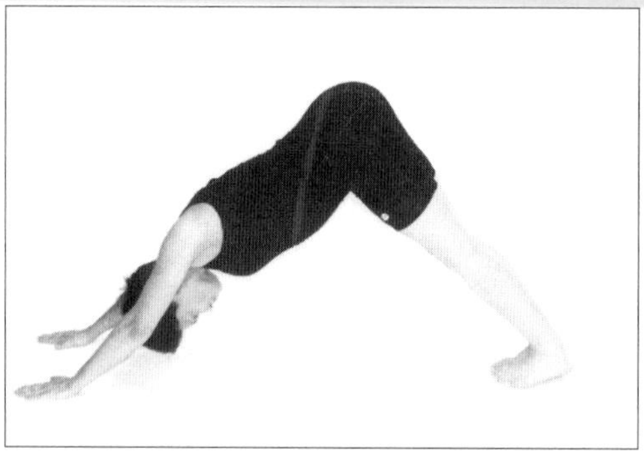

*Adhovamukhaśvānāsana sūryanamaskāra*,
steps 7 and 9

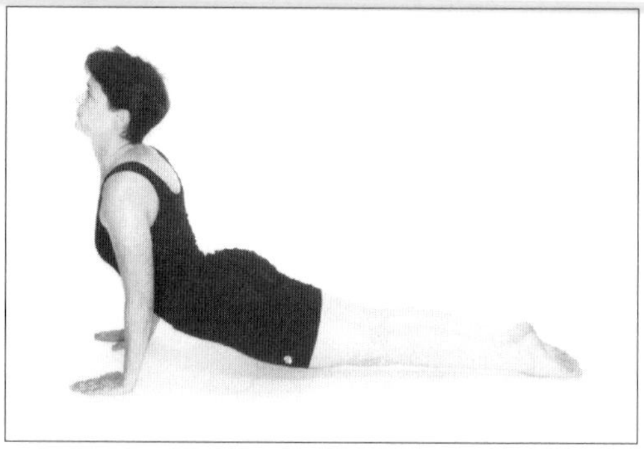

*Ūrdhvamukhaśvānāsana sūryanamaskāra*,
step 8

may be better to proceed from *utkaṭāsana* step by step. First, just raise your heels and then stretch one leg back and then the other as you inhale. This is a good posture to strengthen the forearms and shoulders and improve their tone.

The next *āsana vinyāsa* in this sequence is *ūrdhvamukhaśvānāsana,* or upward-facing dog posture. This *āsana* gets its name because it resembles a dog stretching up on its four legs. First assume *caturaṅgadaṇḍāsana.* Stretch your ankles and rest on the tips of your toes. Then, inhaling, press your palms, stretch your upper body, and raise it up, but keeping your legs (and thighs) parallel to the floor. This can be achieved by stretching your feet, legs, thighs, and knees and by pushing your pelvis forward so that your navel is in line with your hands. The recommended *dṛṣṭi* (gazing) is at the tip of the nose. Stay in the posture for a few breaths. This helps to correct the postural defect of desk workers (and computer addicts) who tend to crouch. Exhaling, you may return to *caturaṅgadaṇḍāsana.*

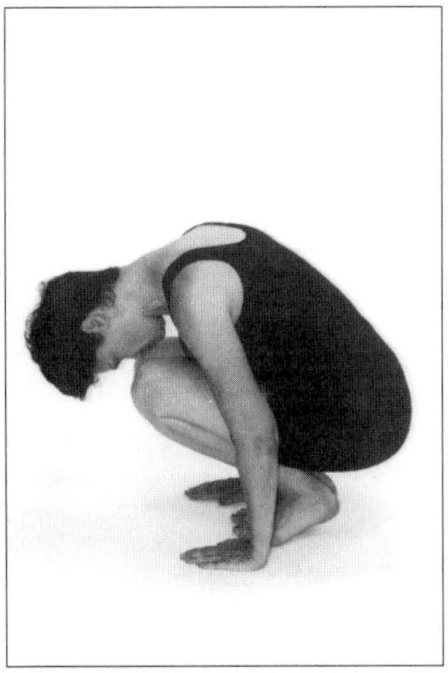

*Utkaṭāsana sūryanamaskāra,*
step 10

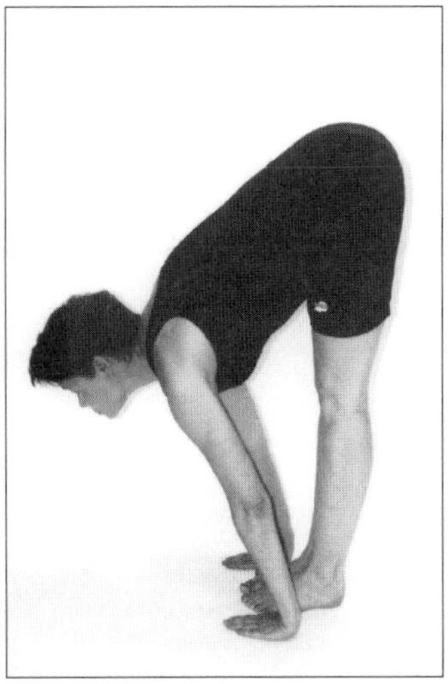

*Uttānāsana sūryanamaskāra,*
step 11

A countermovement in this sequence will be to perform *adhomukhaśvānāsana,* or downward-facing dog posture. Proceed from *caturangadaṇḍāsana,* which position you have reached after doing *ūrdhvamukhaśvānāsana.* While pressing your palms and exhaling, push your hips back and up as far as possible. In the final posture, your feet (including your heels) are fully on the floor. Then breathe normally a few times. It is easier in this posture to work on the lower abdomen and stomach. After exhaling, draw in your rectum and also your lower abdomen *(mūla* and *uddīyāna bandhas)* and hold for a few seconds. This may be repeated after every exhalation. Also, stretch the back of your neck and lock your chin against the breastbone *(jālandhara bandha).* This is a very good posture to help relieve flatulence and help digestion. The two *śvānāsanas* act as counterposes to each other. You may do a few cycles of this three-*āsana* sequence, or stay in each posture one after the other for a few breaths. From *adhomukhaśvānāsana,* you may return to *tāḍāsana* by retracing the steps. From *adhomukhaśvānāsana,* you may press your palms and, after exhaling and holding your breath, slightly raise your heels and jump forward (with palms still on the floor) and land your feet between your palms. This posture, as you know, is *utkaṭāsana.* Do a few normal breaths and, keeping your forehead on the knees, inhale, press your palms and feet, raise your hips, and come to *uttānāsana.* Then after a few breaths, inhale, raise your arms, and straighten your body to come to *tāḍāsana.* Then, lower your arms upon exhalation and reach *samasthiti.* For those who are unable to come to *utkaṭāsana* from *adhomukhaśvānāsana* by jumping forward, the easier method of returning by bringing in one foot after the other may be better. And again, if it is not possible to go to *uttānāsana* from *utkaṭāsana*, you may raise your arms in *utkaṭāsana* and then return to *tāḍāsana sthiti.* You may have observed dogs doing beautiful stretching exercises. One should relax with the help of long deliberate exhalation *(recaka)* to do these postures.

## *Sūryanamaskāra*

As mentioned earlier, the sun salute, or *sūryanamaskāra,* is a very popular and dynamic group or sequence of exercises. Actually the dog postures are important *vinyāsas* in *sūryanamaskāra.* The following table outlines the *vinyāsas* and mantras used in the sequence of the *sūryanamaskāra.* The sixth *vinyāsa* is the actual *namaskāra*, in which one lies down prone (prostrate) with the arms stretched overhead in total surrender to the deity, here the sun, considered a visible aspect of God. The twelve *vinyāsas* can be done with mantras also. Thus, as one completes the appropriate aspect of the breath, the mantra is mentally chanted and then the next *vinyāsa* is done and the appropriate mantras used. The mantras used are *bījākṣara*, Vedic, and *laukika* mantras. It is also a custom to chant all three mantras one after the other. Again, those who are unable to do the whole *vinyāsakrama* of the *sūryanamaskāra* can merely chant the mantras and prostrate themselves in the direction of the sun in the east. Those who do the *aruna* chanting or Vedic prayer of Surya (mentioned in the chapter on mantrayoga) would do the *vinyāsakrama sūryanamaskāra* at the end of each of the thirty-two *anuvākas,* spread over an hour of chanting of the *sūryanamaskāra* chapter. Here are the *vinyāsas* and their associated mantras.

| | Vinyāsa | Bījākṣara mantra | Vedic mantra | Namaskāra mantra |
|---|---|---|---|---|
| 1. | *Samasthiti* with folded hands | *Om hrām* | *udyannadya mitramahaḥ* | *mitrāya namaḥ* |
| 2. | Inhale, bend back, arms overhead | *Om hrīm* | *arohannuttārā am divam* | *ravaye namaḥ* |
| 3. | Exhale, *uttānāsana* | *Om hrūm* | *hrudrogam mama sūrya* | *sūryāya namaḥ* |
| 4. | Inhale, exhale, *utkaṭāsana* | *Om hraim* | *harimaṇanca nāśaya* | *bhānave namaḥ* |
| 5. | Inhale, hold breath, *cāturaṅgadaṇḍāsana* | *Om hraum* | *sukesu me harimanam* | *khagāya namaḥ* |

| | | | | |
|---|---|---|---|---|
| 6. | *Daṇḍa samarpaṇam* (prostrating before sun) | *Om hraḥ* | *ropaṇākāśu dhadhmasi* | *pūṣṇe namaḥ* |
| 7. | Exhale, *adhomukhaśvānāsana* | *Om hrām* | *atho haridraveṣume* | *hiranyagar bhāya namaḥ* |
| 8. | Exhale, inhale *urdhvamukhaśvānāsana* | *Om hrīm* | *harimananni dhadhmaśi* | *marīcaye namaḥ* |
| 9. | Exhale, *adhomukhaśvānāsana* | *Om hrūm* | *udagādayam ādityaḥ* | ādityāya namaḥ |
| 10. | Inhale, exhale, *utkaṭāsana* | *Om hraim* | *viśvena sahasa saha* | *savitre namaḥ* |
| 11. | Inhale, *uttānāsana* | *Om hraum* | *dviṣantam mama randhayan* | *arkāya namaḥ* |
| 12. | Exhale, inhale, *samasthiti* | *Om hraḥ* | *no aham dviṣato ratam* | *bhāskarāya namaḥ* |

*OM Śāntiḥ Śāntiḥ Śāntiḥ*

# 8 Supine Postures

## *Bandhas* and Breathing

Before discussing the supine postures, it may be good to introduce the *bandhas,* or locks. In chapter 7 some important standing postures and their variations, counterposes, and accompanying breathing patterns were described, along with some of the benefits that accrue from their practice. If one practices them regularly at a fixed time each day, one's body should become lighter *(laghu)* and one's circulation, respiration, and digestion should improve, leading to better health and a positive sense of well-being. One's breathing should also become longer, smoother, and more vital, thereby giving one a sense of calm. It is the uniqueness of the system of my *ācārya,* based on the *śāstras* that he inherited, that one is imperceptibly led to control of the breath, or *prāṇāyāma*, even while doing the *āsanas.* Synchronous and long breathing also helps relax the muscles and joints and helps one attain a posture smoothly and with less effort. Regular practice results in both more tranquillity—and paradoxically—improved stamina, as revealed in one's capacity to do the postures more deliberately and with slow stretching, and in one's ability to stay in the final posture longer and for a greater number of breaths.

The four aspects of yogic breathing were also discussed in chapter 7. To repeat, the first is *recaka,* or long and smooth exhalation. The second is *pūraka,* or long inhalation. It is, however, possible to hold in the breath after inhalation, which is known as internal holding, or *antaḥ-kumbhaka,* and is the third aspect. Holding the breath out during the time interval between the completion of exhalation *(recaka)* and the beginning of inhalation *(pūraka)* is *bāhya-kumbhaka*, the fourth aspect.

Readers may recall mention in chapter 7 of the *bandhas,* or the contraction of certain groups of muscles. It is now time to introduce the use of *bandhas* in the practice of *āsanas.* There are three important *bandhas.* The first is *jālandhara bandha*, or locking the chin against the breastbone. This may be done during both *kumbhakas* and whenever the postures require the chin to be locked, which is normally the case during forward bends and when keeping the back erect. In back bends and twisting postures it is not possible to do *jālandhara bandha.* The other two *bandhas,* however, should be practiced in most of the *āsanas,* especially after exhalation. The first is *mūla bandha,* which means "constriction of the anus." It is done after a complete exhalation. After the exhalation is over, the *abhyāsī* should anchor the body in the *āsana* he or she is in and then slowly and deliberately close the anus and draw in the rectum by contracting the perineal and surrounding muscles of the pelvic floor. Then as if in a continuous movement, the abdomen, including the navel, is drawn in, pushing up the diaphragm into the now almost empty chest cavity, which is then called *uddīyāna bandha* (drawing in of diaphragm). The two *bandhas, uddīyāna bandha* and *mūla bandha,* make use of both the pelvic diaphragm and the diaphragm, which separates the chest from the stomach. This technique is one of the specialties of yogic breathing. It is not possible to do the *bandhas* initially without practice of long inhalation and exhalation, so that the strength of one's *prāṇa* is first enhanced. If one has practiced the standing postures mentioned in chapter 7 in tandem with the correct breathing patterns as well as with dietary restrictions *(tapas),* and one has reduced one's waistline to its healthy level, then the *bandhas* can be attempted.

The one standing posture in which all three *bandhas* can be effectively practiced is *utkaṭāsana,* and its variation, *ardha-utkaṭāsana.* After regular practice of the dynamic movements in the standing postures, one should attempt to stay in *utkaṭāsana* or *ardha-utkaṭāsana* for a few breaths, say, three to six complete cycles. In the initial stages one may barely be able to accomplish the posture. When one is able to stay in the posture comfortably for three to six breaths, then one should slowly increase the time to complete a stipulated number of breaths. Thereafter, one should remain in the posture for a predetermined number of breaths chosen by the practitioner or teacher, or for a fixed period, say three to five minutes. Then one's practice should be aimed at reducing the number of breaths while remaining in the posture for the same duration. For instance, one may take a total of twenty breaths while in the posture. Later on, it may be possible to remain in the posture steadily and comfortably *(sthira* and *sukha)* for five minutes with perhaps only ten breaths. This is one method of attaining *āsana siddhi* (perfection in posture) that one can test for oneself. Having achieved this level of comfort in the posture, one can then introduce the *bandhas,* which will increase the time taken for each breath. It obviously requires not only stamina, or *prāṇāyāma bala*, to hold the breath for the duration of the *bandha* but also a healthy stomach, digestive system, and pelvic organs. No *bandha* is possible with an ulcer, constipation, colic pain, prostatitis, urinary tract infection, dysmenorrhea, obesity, or weakness arising out of indiscriminate sexual activity. It should be noted here that the *bandhas*, in many places, are often taught after one learns *prāṇāyāma*. But in the system of my guru, based on a proper interpretation of the *Yogasūtras*, because breath practice is introduced early, the *bandhas* can be introduced while practicing *āsanas* with several *vinyāsas*. Because the *bandhas* help to exercise and stimulate the internal organs, they provide great benefits, especially in the therapeutic application of yoga.

## *Taṭākamudrā*

The next group of *āsanas* are those done lying down with face upward, the *suptāsanas*. First is *taṭākamudrā* (pond gesture), which makes effective use of the *bandhas*. Start with *samasthiti*. Inhale, raise your arms overhead, and interlock your fingers. Exhale, do *utkaṭāsana*. Do a few breaths with or without the *bandhas*. Exhale, keeping your palms a few inches behind your back. Now sit down. Inhale, stretch your legs forward together, raise your arms overhead, and lie on your back. Exhaling, lower your arms along the sides of your body and place your palms flat on the floor. This is the starting position for all supine postures. One may start straightaway lying down, but the advantage of starting from *samasthiti* is that one can limber up a bit, and also be sure that the body is straight by making use of one's sense of balance. In addition, this is the traditional method. The lying posture is called *śavāsana* by some authorities. Now, keep your feet, ankles, and knees close. Stretch your thigh and calf muscles. Press your heels, buttocks, palms, shoulders, and neck to the floor and stretch your spine while inhaling, so that your entire back tends to be flat on the floor. By doing this it may be possible to stretch your neck and do *jālandhara bandha*, but it is preferable to

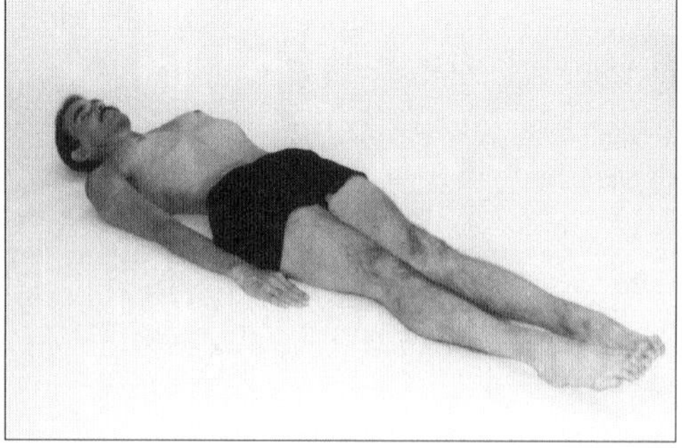

*Taṭākamudrā*

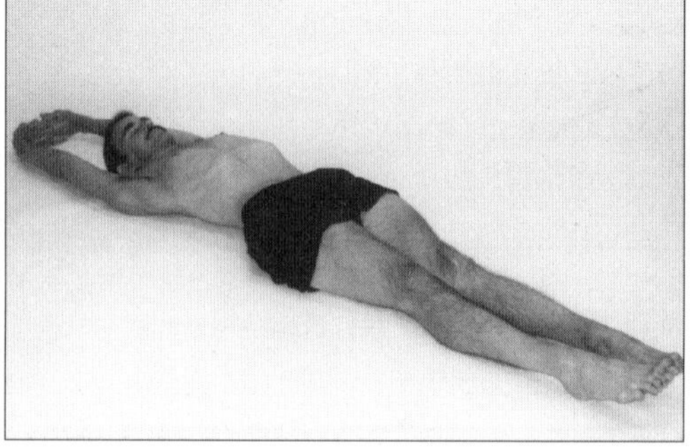

*Taṭākamudrā (vinyāsa)*

use a small pillow to raise the head and lock the chin. Do a few deep breaths.

After a deep and complete exhalation, and while pressing your heels, knees, buttocks, palms, shoulders, and neck and stretching other body muscles, do *mūla bandha* and *uddīyāna bandha*, so that your entire abdominal portion is drawn in completely, making it scaphoid. It should resemble a small, beautiful pond formed by the pelvic bones and the lower ribs. Stay with the *bandha* for at least a few seconds. This is *taṭākamudrā*. Now relax the drawn muscles and then inhale. Repeat for about six breaths. Inhale, raise your arms overhead, exhale, and do *taṭākamudrā* six more times. The *mudrā* can be done easily for some if they keep their legs bent and feet on the ground, close to the buttocks. Obviously it is not possible to do the *bandhas* without adequate preparation of the body through modulated breathing in *āsanas*, as has been explained already. A person suffering from acute abdominal diseases will not be able to do the *bandhas* at all and thus derive benefit; they are more a preventive exercise than a curative one. But with *āsanas*, breathing, a proper diet, and a few other *yamaniyamas,* a patient could become fit enough to start the practice of the *bandhas* and then begin to derive immense benefits. It may be noted that those with conditions such as the early stages of hemorrhoids, prostatitis, prolapse—both rectal and vaginal—incontinence, constipation, indigestion, and so on would respond well to *taṭākamudrā*. Some yoga therapists claim that this *āsana* activates the liver and pancreas, so some diabetics could also benefit. There are yogis who claim that they can draw the diaphragm in so much as to massage the heart. Since its effects on the sex organs are clearly felt, people who practice from early in life will maintain their youth for a longer period—or so it is said. *Taṭākamudrā* is also helpful after childbirth, if it has been practiced from early in one's life. Pregnant women may practice *mūla bandha*, but not *uddīyāna bandha*.

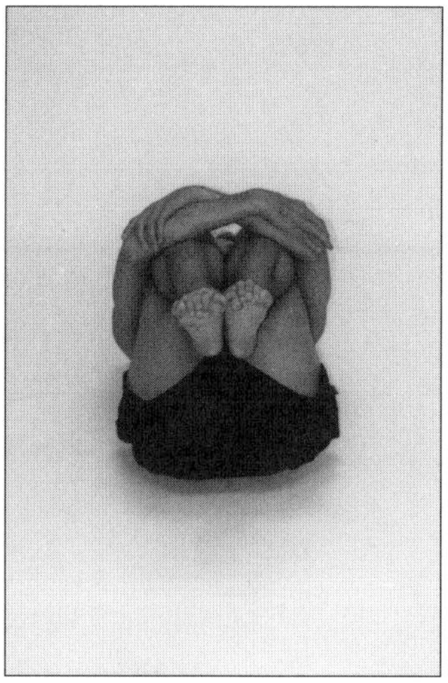

*Apānāsana*

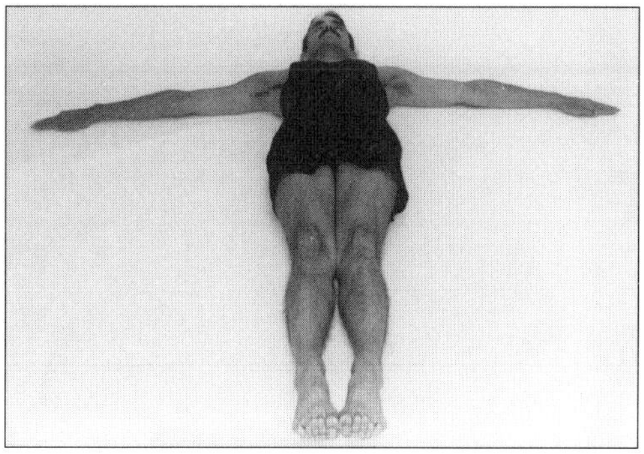

*Jaṭharaparivṛtti* (preparation)

From the lying-down position (as for *taṭākamudrā*), inhale and raise your arms to shoulder level. Inhale, raise your head slightly, and turn your head to the left side. Exhale and, while pressing your palms and shoulders and pivoting your lower back, take your right leg away from your left at a thirty- to forty-five-degree angle. On the next exhalation take your left leg and, while stretching it, move it beside the right leg, so that both feet are together. Take six to twelve long breaths, doing the

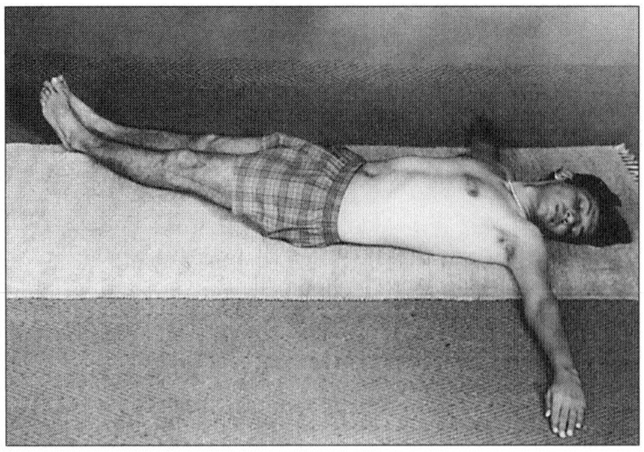

*Jaṭharaparivṛtti*

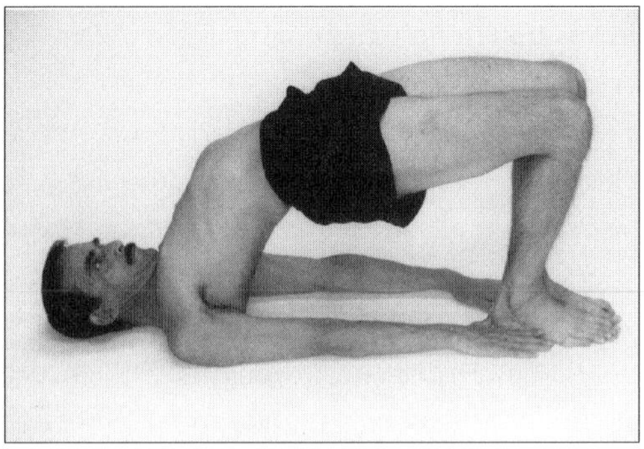

*Dvipāda pīṭham*

*mūla* and *uddīyāna bandhas,* if possible. Your upper body should be straight. You should feel the stretching all along your ribs, hips, and left leg. The stomach muscles on the left side are also stretched. This is called *jaṭharaparivṛtti,* or abdominal stretching posture. When done with the *bandhas,* this pose is extremely effective in reducing the waistline, especially on the sides, increasing the appetite, and generally helping the digestive system. It is useful in correcting stiffness in the lower back, as the sacroiliac joint is made supple. It enhances the effects of *tāḍāsana,* in this case laterally. This is the first twisting of the spine. After the required number of breaths, inhale and return to the starting position. Breathe normally a few times and do the posture on the other side.

## *Dvipāda Pīṭham*

Many *yogāsanas* aim at maintaining the suppleness of the spine. It is said that a man is as old as the condition of his spine. The desk pose, or *dvipāda pīṭham,* is a simple, effective *āsana* that works on the backbone. Proceed from *samasthiti* and reach the *suptāsana sthiti,* or supine position. Further *vinyāsas* will follow. Lie on your back on a soft carpet. In the initial stages you may want to support your neck and head with small soft pillow. Exhale and place your arms alongside your body. Keep your knees, ankles, and feet together and slowly stretch them. Exhale, bend your legs at the knees, and draw up and place your feet close to your buttocks. Do a few modulated breaths. Now hold your ankles with your palms, only if possible; otherwise, keep your palms on the floor. Inhale, press the back of your head, your neck, your hands, and your feet; then raise your trunk slowly as high as you can, arching and stretching your spine, neck, shoulders, and arms in the process. Stay for two seconds. Exhale, lowering the body. Repeat three times. This is *dvipāda pīṭham,* or desk pose. As for the variations, inhale and stretch the right leg while keeping the left leg bent, as in the previous position. Inhale again and arch the back and raise the hip while pressing the left foot. Stay for two seconds. Exhale and return to the starting position. Inhale, press the back of the neck and left foot, and raise the right leg as high as you can, stretching especially the neck and the right hip joint. Stay for two seconds. Exhale and return to the starting position. Exhale, bend your right leg at the knee, and place your right foot at the root of your left thigh in the half-lotus position. Inhale and raise the trunk and your bent right leg. Stay for two seconds. Exhale and return to the starting position. Repeat the same movements with the right leg bent. Stretch both legs on inhalation and return to the starting point, which is the lying-down position. Now inhale, press the back of your neck and your heels, and arch your body between the neck and heels. You may stretch your ankles so that your feet are flat on the floor. This is known *madhyasetu,* or bridge pose. Stay for a few seconds, exhale, and return to the starting position. Older and obese people should perform the trunk-raising movement on exhalation and the return movement on inhalation. This is *langhana kriyā.*

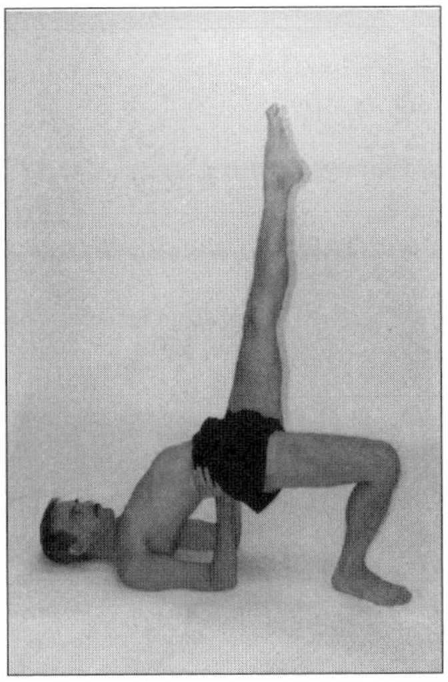

*Dvipāda pīṭham (vinyāsa)*

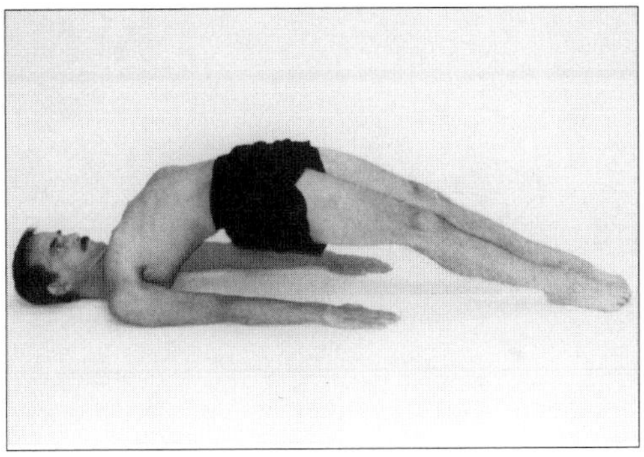

*Madhysetu*

The desk pose is a convenient exercise for arching and hence strengthening the spine. Since the feet and neck are anchored, this posture is easier for beginners when compared with many other back-arching *āsanas.* It helps relieve the pain of a stiff neck, which is common enough among machine operators, drivers, typists, and so on. It is also useful to relieve lower-back pain, especially that experienced by pregnant women. They should, however, do only the first two *vinyāsas,* and then only after getting clearance from their obstetricians. Because the feet, neck, and head are anchored, the back stretch can be controlled and done to the greatest extent possible without straining.

## Other *Suptāsana* Variations

The following group of *āsanas, vinyāsas* that resemble the letters L, U, and V, require lower-back strength and bring into play, as well as tone, the lower stomach muscles. These *āsanas,* in which the arms and legs are stretched out and up, are known as

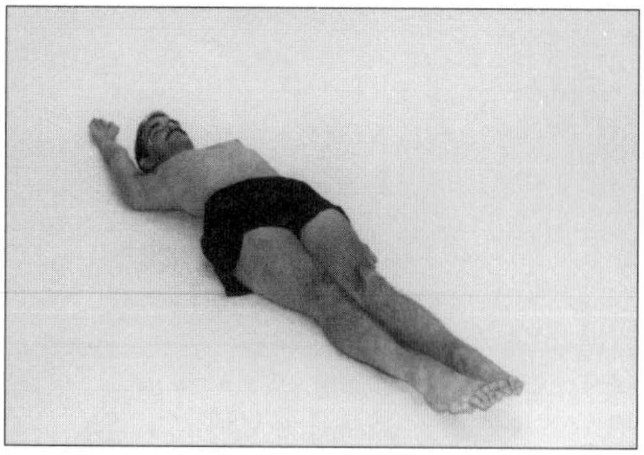

*Ūrdhvaprasāsana*
(preparation)

*urdhvaprasāritapādahastāsanas.* To begin, lie on your back on a soft carpet. Support your neck and head with a small soft pillow during the first few weeks of practice. Place your arms alongside your body and keep your knees, ankles, and feet together. Slowly stretch them while taking a few modulated breaths. Inhaling, raise and stretch your right arm overhead. Exhaling, raise your right arm and right leg from the hip as high as you can, the goal being to make a ninety-degree angle to the floor. In the beginning, you may first bend your right knee as if kicking high toward your face and then straighten it. Stay for a few seconds. Inhale and return to the starting position. Now exhale and raise your right arm and left leg. Stay for two seconds. Inhaling, return to the original position, stretching your right arm and left leg, and feeling the stretch across your body. Exhaling, lower your right arm to the side of your body. This posture is *ūrdhvaprasāsana.* Repeat the movements with your left arm raised. Exhale deeply, press your palms, and raise both legs together from the hips as high as possible, up to ninety degrees from the floor. Stay for two seconds. Inhale and lower your legs. This posture resembles the letter L and is known as *ūrdhvaprasāritapādāsana.* Inhale and raise both arms overhead. Exhale and raise both arms and both legs so they are perpendicular to the floor. Stay for two seconds. Inhale, stretch both of your arms and legs, and return to the starting position. This resembles the letter U and is known as *ūrdhvaprasāritapādahastāsana.* Inhale and raise both your arms overhead. Exhale, as in the previous *vinyāsa*, and raise both your arms and legs but take your legs a bit further and hold your big toes with your thumbs and first two fingers. Inhale and spread your legs so that they resemble the letter V; this is known as *ubhayapādāṅguṣṭhāsana.* These postures will be easier to perform with longer and smoother exhalations. These exercises are a very good preparatory *vinyāsa* for doing another important combination lying-down and inverted posture known as

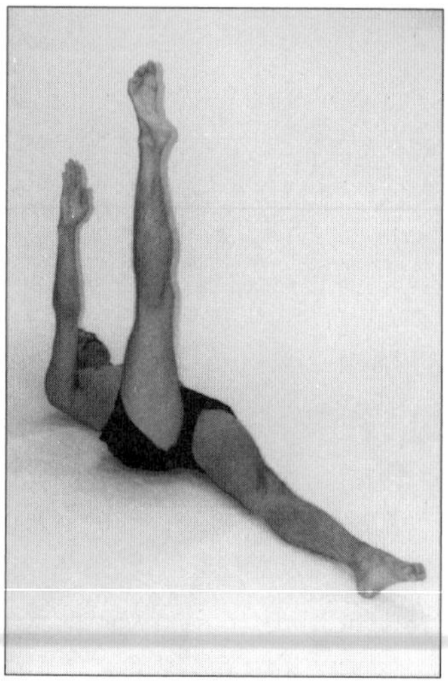

*Ūrdhvaprasāsana*
(preparatory *vinyāsa*)

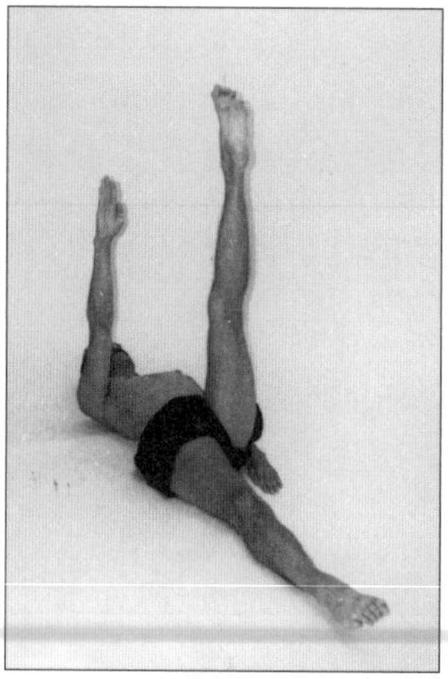

*Ūrdhvaprasāsana*

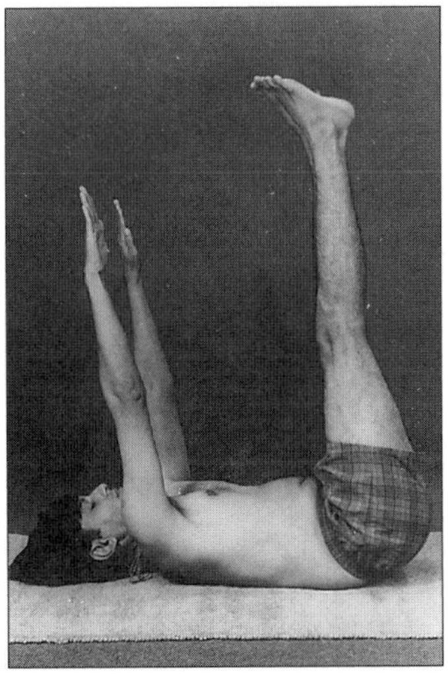

*Ūrdhvaprasāritapādahastāsana*

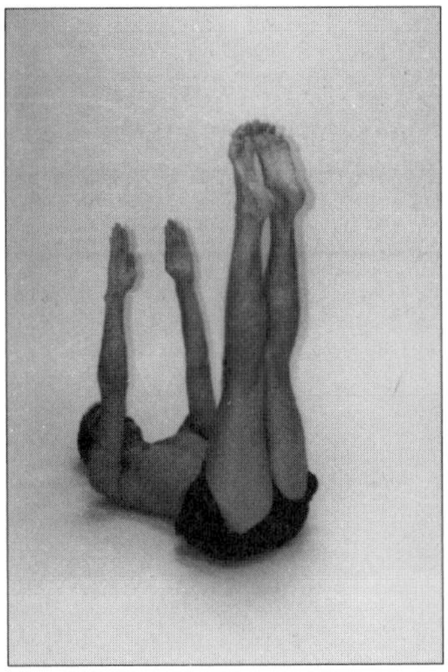

*Ūrdhvaprasāritapādahastāsana*
(back view)

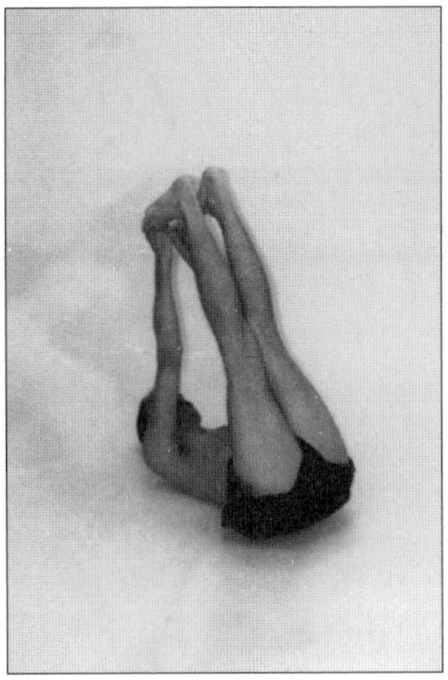

*Ūbhayapādāṅguṣṭhāsana*

*sarvāṅgāsana. Dvipāda pīṭham* helps to make the hips and lower back more flexible, and other arm- and leg-raising postures prepare the legs for the *viparītakarnanī,* or inverted postures.

Another variation may be attempted after one gains familiarity with the *vinyāsas* in *suptapādāṅguṣṭhāsana.* From *suptāsana sthiti,* mentioned above, slightly stretch your right leg, bring it forward, and hold your big toe with the fingers of your right hand. Keep your left hand on your left thigh and do a few modulated breaths. This is *suptapādāṅguṣṭhāsana.* Now slowly exhale and, pressing the left side of your body, leg, and heel, lower your right leg, with your arm to the right side, holding your toe all the while. In the final position, your right leg is stretched on the floor to the right of the body and held by your right hand at about shoulder level. This is *suptapārśvapādāṅguṣṭhāsana.* Repeat the movements on the other side. As mentioned, this group of *āsanas* helps to strengthen lower abdominal muscles and effectively checks

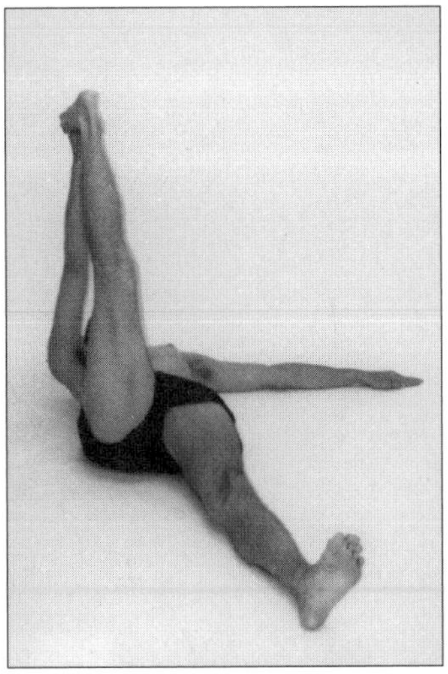

*Suptapādāṇguṣṭhāsana*
(preparation)

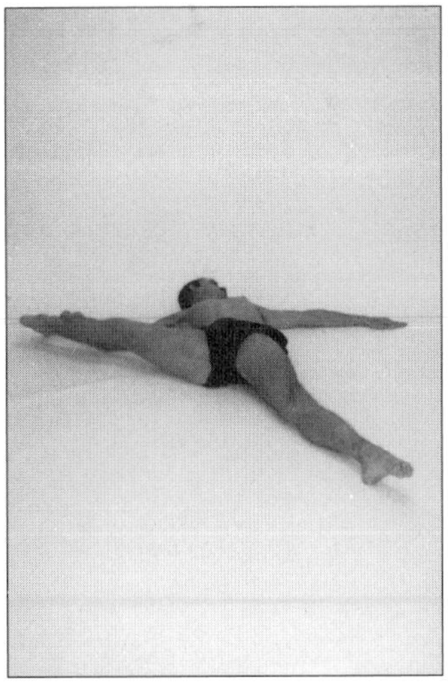

*Suptapārśvapādāṅguṣṭhāsana*

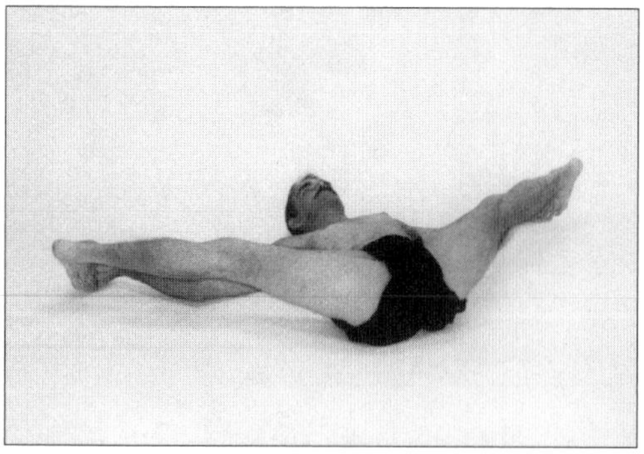

*Suptapārśvapādāṅguṣṭhāsana*

obesity; tuberculosis and the early stages of hemorrhoids respond well to these exercises. People who spend long hours standing and tend to develop varicose veins will also benefit. Girls, if they practice from puberty, will improve the tone of their pelvic muscles.

# 9 *Sarvāṅgāsana* and *Śīrṣāsana*

*ŚĪRṢĀSANA* AND ITS CLOSE ALLY, *sarvāṅgāsana*, hold pride of place among the *āsanas.* Yoga teachers, ancient and modern, have much good to say about these postures. Even a novice experiences the tonic effects of *sarvāṅgāsana* when starting to practice it. Medical practitioners and researchers interested in yoga give considerable importance to these *āsanas* and have studied their effects on the whole system. One should surely include *sarvāṅgāsana* in one's daily practice. It is common knowledge that in the normal erect posture, the main organs of perception—ears and eyes as well as the brain—do not get a copious supply of blood, being located above the heart. And when we breathe in normally, which breathing is partly diaphragmatic, the vital organs—liver, spleen, kidneys, diaphragm, and so on—get pressed and displaced from their position, albeit to a small extent. According to yogic theory, disease results from the displacement of vital internal organs and muscles, and yogic practice aims to return them to their original positions. The *ṛṣis* have sought to remedy this displacement through the practice of inverted postures, of which *śīrṣāsana* and *sarvāṅgāsana* are the most important.

## *Sarvāṅgāsana* and Variations

Sarvāṅgāsana is one of the most difficult postures because one has to prepare the body, especially the neck, before beginning its practice. *Dvipāda pīṭham* and

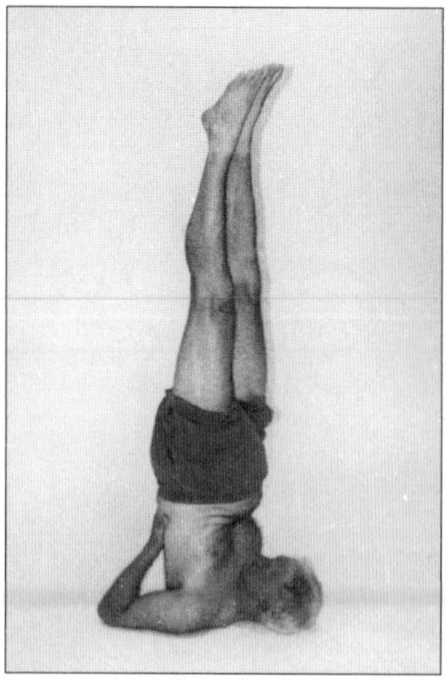

*Sarvāṅgāsana*

*ūrdhvaprasāritapādāsana* are two postures that prepare the body for *sarvāṅgāsana*. As its name implies, *sarvāṅgāsana* (whole-body posture) tones up all centers, nerves, organs, joints, and muscles. The technique described here is not for absolute beginners. But those who have practiced the *āsanas* already discussed, and who have attained a certain proficiency in staying in postures with the proper yogic breathing described earlier, can attempt to do this *āsana*.

Assume the lying-down position following the *vinyāsakrama*. Lie flat on a soft mat, keeping your legs stretched out and feet together, and place your arms alongside your body with palms flat on the floor. Exhaling, slowly raise your legs without bending the knees, pressing the palms, back, neck, and head, until the legs are straight up from your hips. This is *ūrdhvaprasāritapādāsana*. Stay there for a few breaths. Then, exhaling, raise your legs further up, lifting your hips and back from the floor. When your whole trunk is raised and vertical, place your palms behind your back, thereby supporting your body with your hands. Your chest should be pressed against your chin, which covers the neck pit between your collarbones, thereby ensuring that your body is not tilted to either side. This *āsana* also allows one to do *jālandhara bandha*. Your body should be straight. After a few breaths, adjust your palms so that they are as low as possible, until, say, they are supporting your floating ribs. Your elbows should not be spread far, and the ideal position is to keep them about the same distance apart as your shoulders. After a few more breaths, slowly and deliberately stretch your back, spine, hips, and thigh and calf muscles, as well as your relaxed knees, ankles, and feet, pointing your toes. Your eyes should be closed and your vision directed toward the middle of the eyebrows *(bhrūmadhya dṛṣṭi)*. This is *sarvāṅgāsana*. It is better to keep the full surface of your palms on your back rather than holding the side of your ribs and pressing with your thumb, which is the normal practice and tendency. One should attempt to maintain the posture for at least five minutes, which can be achieved gradually, with practice. This is a

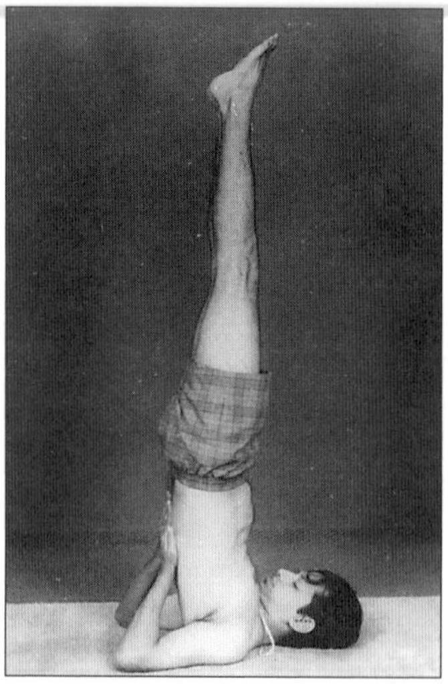

*Sarvāṅgāsana* with *bandhas*

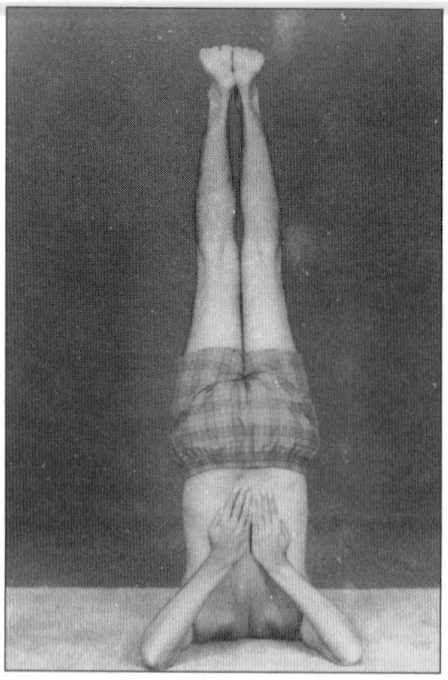

*Sarvāṅgāsana*
(proximate hands position)

posture to stay in and from which one can do *vinyāsas*. One can stay in this posture for a long time, up to a half hour. The effects start building after about five minutes or so. A simple *vinyāsa* involves spreading one's legs apart while exhaling. This is called *ūrdhvakoṇāsana*, or upward triangle pose in *sarvāṅgāsana*.

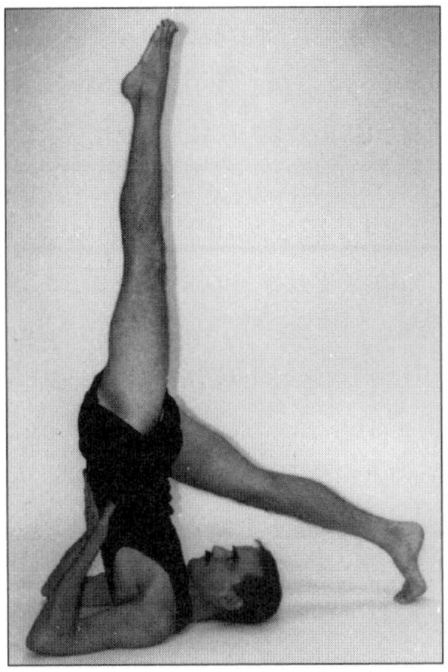

*Ekapāda sarvāṅgāsana*

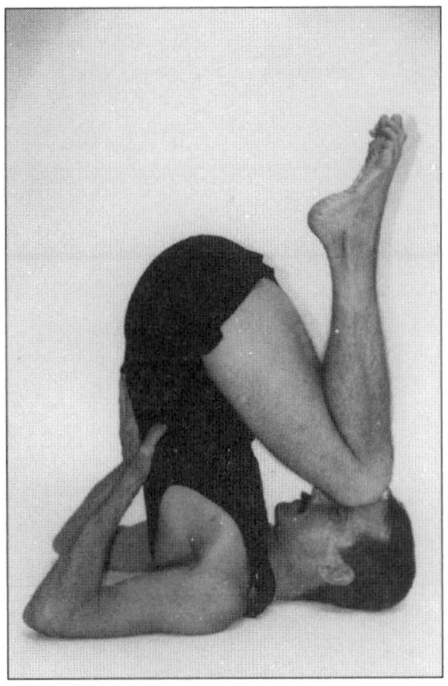

*Ākuñcanāsana*

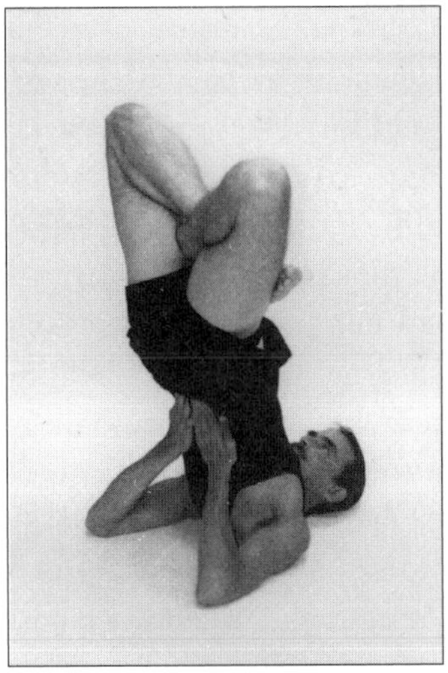

*Ūrdhvapādmāsana*

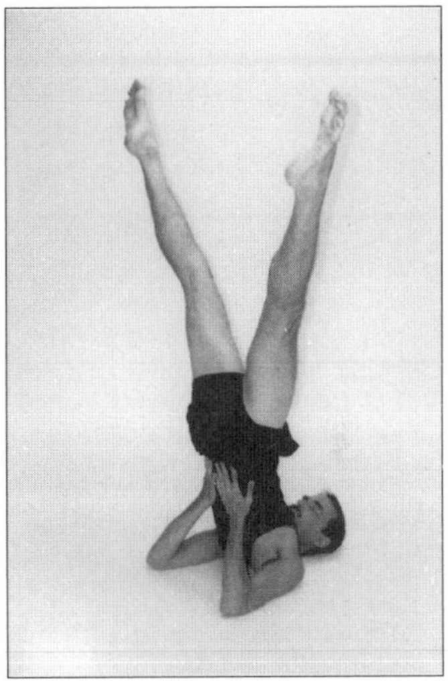

*Ūrdhvakoṇāsana*

One's breathing should be with the throat constriction that produces a hissing sound. One need not attempt to retain the breath after inhaling, but it may be attempted after exhaling. After some weeks of practice, when the posture is steady and one's waist has been reduced, one may attempt *mūla bandha* and *uddīyāna bandha*, the beneficial effects of which are enhanced with the help of gravity. After staying in the posture for the required length of time, upon inhalation return to the starting position without raising the head and with a slow rolling motion. The stretching of each vertebra feels good as one returns to the starting point. *Sarvāṅgāsana* tones up the system, and many who start the practice of this *āsana* feel its beneficial effects within a short period of time. One starts feeling light, one's joints become flexible, and muscles achieve better all-around tone. Its effects on the thyroid and parathyroid have been studied, and it is of considerable help in certain cases of hypothyroidism. In this posture, there is good return of venous blood to the heart, and there is a significant drop is the blood pressure in the legs after five minutes of practice. The neck and back also get a copious supply of blood.

Those suffering from respiratory ailments, especially asthma and bronchitis, respond well to *sarvāṅgāsana.* A medical doctor has suggested that the posture, if done for up to three minutes, seems to act as a bronchodilator, and because of the effects of gravity, there is better draining of bronchial secretions. The posture also provides great relief to those suffering from sinusitis and bronchial congestion. The cerebrospinal fluid circulation is increased, and thus there is an all-around toning up of the entire nervous system. *Sarvāṅgāsana* keeps the spine supple, and when done with the *vinyāsas,* the spine is exercised to the fullest possible extent. As mentioned above, the thyroid gland is also well massaged and its arterial supply enhanced, which helps to improve its functional capacity, its internal secretions being important for the proper metabolism and growth of the body. The larynx also gets massaged in this posture, and it could be that the asthmagenic area below the glottis is exercised and thus normalized. The sympathetic nervous system and the entire spinal cord are toned up. The blood supply increases to the chest and to the organs. Varicose veins tend to disappear. The posture has a tonic effect on the testes, ovaries, and pelvis by removal of congestion. Gastrointestinal diseases are also helped. The liver and spleen are also exercised with gravity and the *bandhas.* Leg muscles and sluggish knee joints become more supple over the course of time. *Sarvāṅgāsana* truly benefits all parts of the body. Some important variations tend to enhance the effects of *sarvāṅgāsana.* A few are mentioned below.

After remaining in *sarvāṅgāsana* for some time, slowly exhale, and by gently taking your legs a little farther, raise both arms and place your hands alongside your raised legs. This is *nirālamba sarvāṇgāsana.* Stay for a few breaths. You should gaze at the spot between your eyebrows. Your arms should be stretched, and also your legs. This *āsana* helps to correct indigestion and to reduce one's waistline. According to our *ācārya,* if one practices this late in the evening for fifteen minutes, one will cure insomnia and enjoy restful sleep. People who are on their feet for long periods—sportsmen and athletes—will find this *āsana* exceedingly soothing. Pregnant woman may do this *āsana* up to the end of the first trimester. Those who suffer from frequent nocturnal emissions would also benefit, since it reduces pelvic congestion in general.

From *sarvāṅgāsana,* slowly exhale and place your left foot in your right groin and then your right foot in your left groin. Then extend your crossed legs straight up and stretch your back and pelvic region. Do a few breaths. Repeat, flexing the right knee first. This is called *ūrdhvapadmāsana,* or upward-looking lotus. Proceeding from *ūrdhvapadmāsana,* exhale and bend and lower your crossed legs from the hip and then extend them over your head. Slowly release the hands from the back and clasp your crossed legs, gripping one wrist with the other hand. This is *piṇḍāsana,* or fetus pose. These two *āsanas* make use of gravity to stretch the knees and hips in the opposite direction from the normal upright position.

*Padmāsana* and the subsequent bending to *piṇḍāsana* help work on the spine, back, and stomach even more. The benefits of *sarvāṅgāsana* are enhanced. Your breath may be short, but in time it will stabilize. These are fairly advanced postures and may be attempted only after one feels steady in *sarvāṅgāsana* and in *nirālamba* (unsupported) *sarvāṅgāsana. Sarvāṅgāsana* and *śīrṣāsana* are to yoga as head and heart are to an individual. Yes, they improve physical and mental well-being.

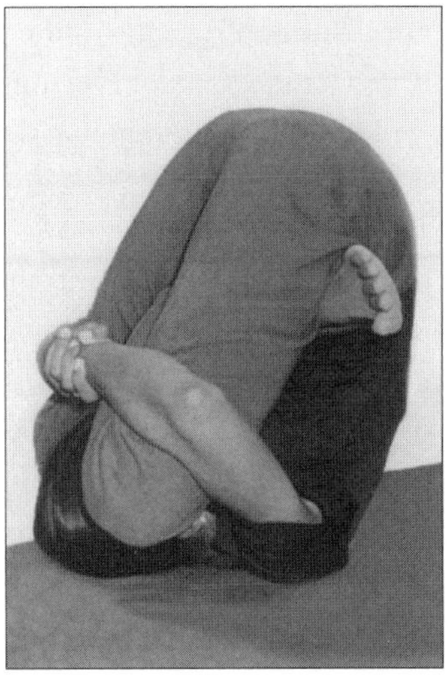

*Piṇḍāsana*

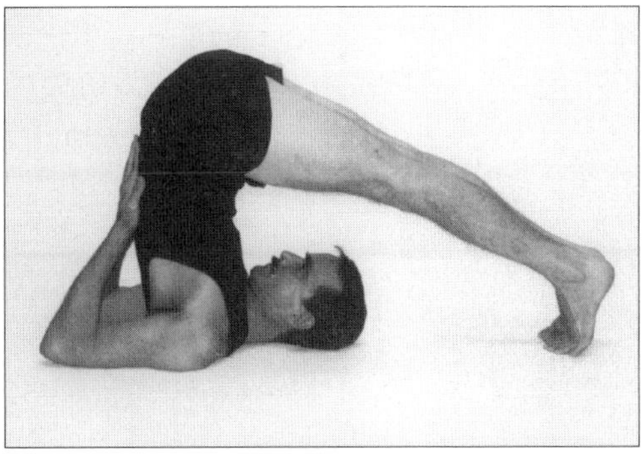

*Halāsana*

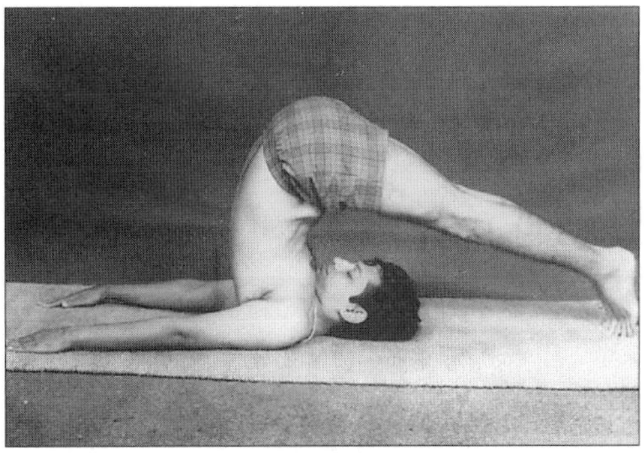

*Halāsana (nirālamba)*

*Halāsana*, or plow posture, which is an extension of *sarvāṅgāsana*, is also a well-known posture. The procedure is the same as for *sarvāṅgāsana.* Thereafter, slowly exhale and lower your legs over your head and place your toes on the floor. Stretch both arms and press your palms on the floor. Your knees and ankles should also be stretched. You may stay for a few breaths. Your inhalations will be short, but you may practice long exhalation in the posture, and also do the *bandhas* after exhaling. After staying for a few breaths, or up to three minutes, return to the lying-down posture by slowly rolling back, consciously stretching

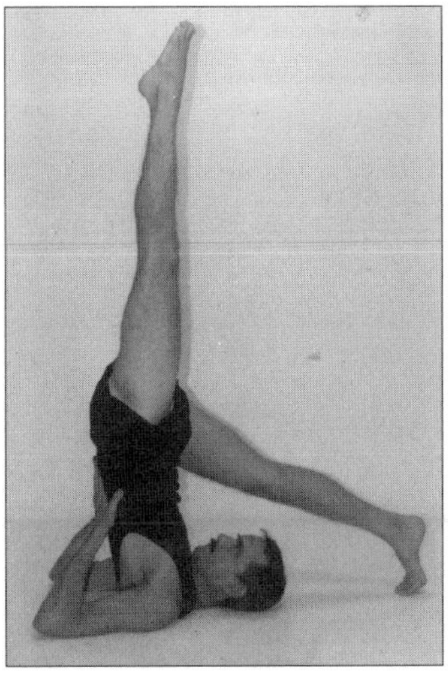

*Ekapāda halāsana*

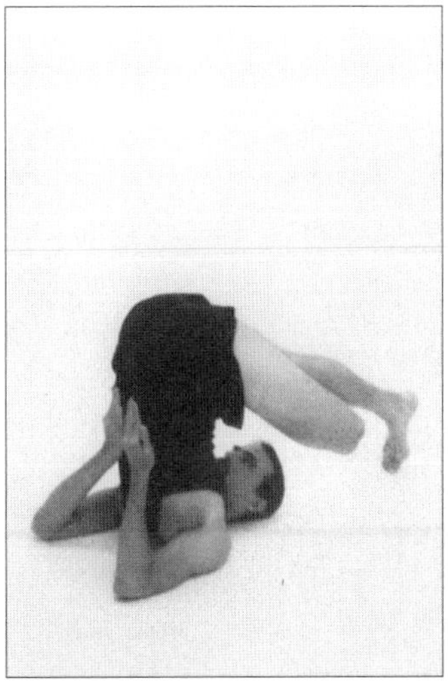

*Ardhapadmahalāsana*

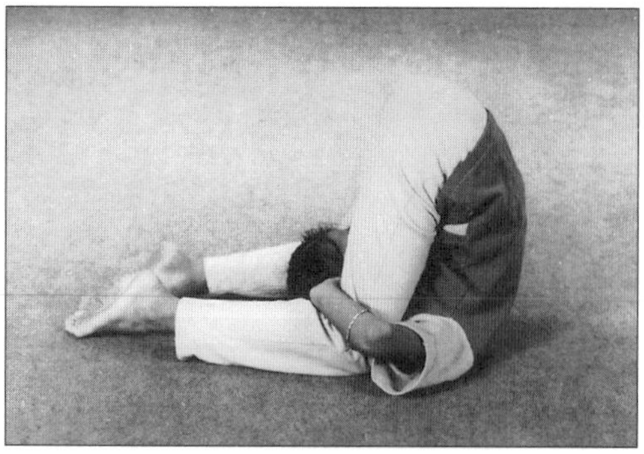

*Karṇapīḍāsana*

every intervertebral ligament, as well as your thighs, knees, ankles, feet, and toes.

There are a number of *vinyāsas* possible in *halāsana*. One of them is *ardhapadmahalāsana*. The starting point is again *sarvāṅgāsana*. Exhaling, place your left ankle over your right thigh, and then on the next exhalation, slowly lower your right leg as in *halāsana*, with your left foot pressing against your thigh and lower abdomen. Stay for a few breaths. Return to the starting point on inhalation, also stretching your left leg. Repeat on the other side. Keeping the arms overhead and holding the toes and spreading the legs at an angle overhead are two of the variations. It should be noted that *halāsana*, because it requires further stretching of the posterior muscles and abdomen, helps the functioning of the pelvic and other internal organs. The neck and shoulders are also stretched considerably. Those who are prone to hypertension should avoid pressure on the back of the head, which may lead to flushing of the face. They may, however, lower their legs, allowing the torso to be a little away from the chin. The correct position for such people could be achieved by trial and error, and a comfortable, balanced position could thus be maintained. One should concentrate on fine breathing and, with eyes closed, direct the visual attention to between the eyebrows. *Sarvāṅgāsana* and *halāsana* should be followed by counterposes, such as *bhujaṅgāsana* and *śalabhāsana*.

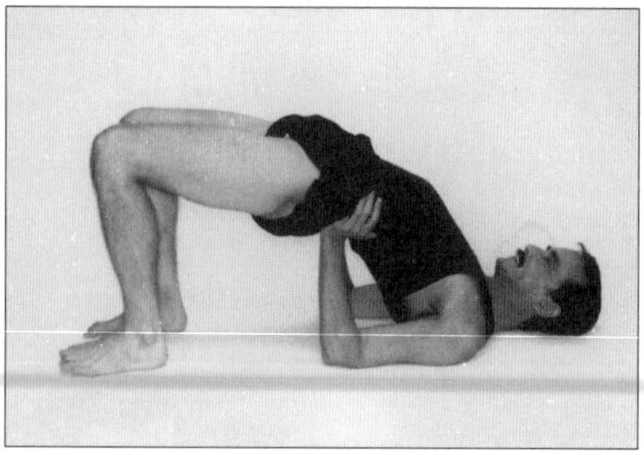

*Uttānamayūrāsana* (preparation)

*Uttānamayūrāsana*, or stretched peacock pos-

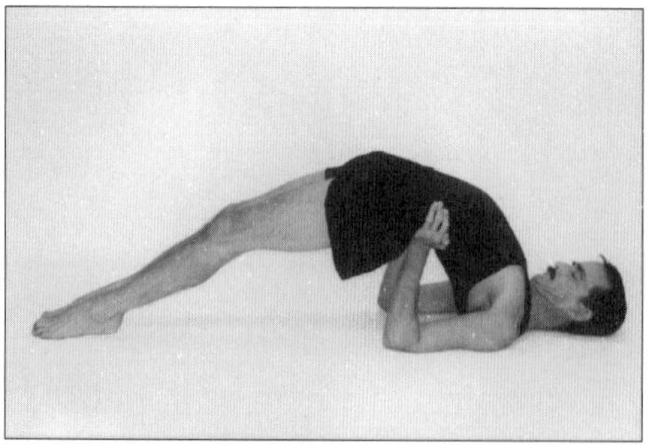

*Uttānamayūrāsana*

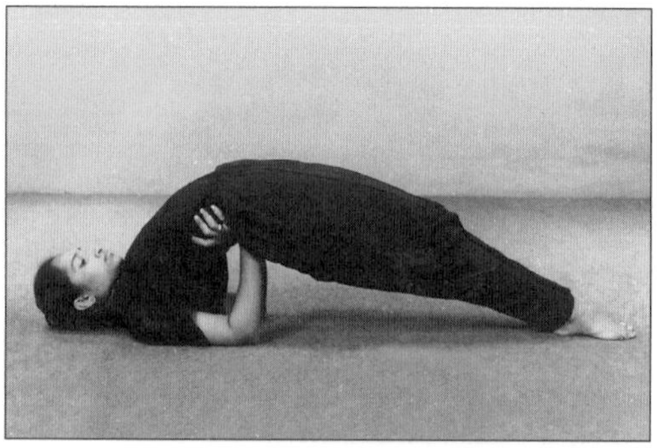

*Uttānamayūrāsana*
(with *jālandhara bandha*)

ture, can be practiced by youngsters. It considerably strengthens the torso, shoulders, and neck. *Uttānamayūrāsana* is also known as *madhyasetu,* which can be approached from *dvipāda pīṭham,* explained earlier. The starting point is *sarvāṅgāsana.* Exhale, and keeping your palms firmly on your back, slowly drop the legs to the ground, stretching the front portion of your body. Stretch your legs, keeping your head, neck, and shoulders on the floor. Stay for a short period, say, up to one minute. Exhale, press your elbows and head, slightly bend the knees and return to *sarvāṅgāsana.* After considerable practice it may be good to follow *halāsana* with *uttānamayūrāsana* and then return to *halāsana,* with the appropriate breathing. This sequence may be repeated three to six times.

## *Śirṣāsana* and Variations

The ability to stand on one's head unaided for the first time brings the same sense of elation as a child seems to feel when it stands unaided on its feet for the first time. *Śirṣāsana,* or headstand, is arguably the first among all *āsanas.* Yoga teachers and practitioners, ancient and modern, have spent considerable time on the practice and study of its physiological and mental effects. Medical practitioners and researchers interested in yoga give considerable importance to this posture and study its effects on the whole system. Unable to get large numbers of subjects who practice *śīrṣāsana,* some researchers have even gone to the extreme of using mice turned upside down in glass tubes, or novices strapped inverted on inclined planes, to study the effects of *śirṣāsana.* The best research in yoga is for one to experiment on oneself and feel the effects.

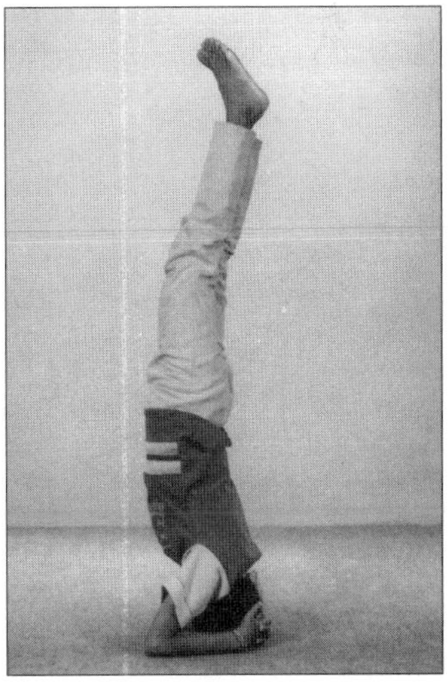

*Śirṣāsana* by a 12-year-old girl

In *śīrṣāsana,* gravity aids in the free flow of blood to the organs of perception. It has both curative and preventative properties. *Śirṣāsana* requires considerable preparation of the body, however. Especially for those who are obese, it is imperative that the body acquire some flexibility *(laghava)* through the practice of *mudrās* (especially *mahāmudrā*) and *prāṇāyāma* in such postures as *padmāsana, vajrāsana,* and so on, before attempting *āsanas* like *śīrṣāsana.* Several renowned commentaries on Patañjali's *Yogasūtras* give considerable details that are helpful in the practice and mastery of many *āsanas.* The main objective of *śīrṣāsana* is not merely to arrange for a copious blood supply to flow to the head and upper limbs of the body, but also to slow down the respiratory rate. It is the contention of yogis that one's predetermined life span is measured in terms of breaths, and not in time. Thus yogis have always attempted to prolong the life span by reducing the number of breaths per unit of time. The word *prāṇāyāma* means both "breath" and also "lengthening the life span." In that, *śīrṣāsana* has a very important role to play. Thus when *śīrṣāsana* is mastered *(āsana siddhi),* the breath rate, which is normally about fifteen to twenty breaths per minute, automatically comes down. Such a reduction is within the capacity of anyone who spends the time necessary to achieve it. The aim should be to reduce the breath rate to about two breaths per minute while doing *āsanas;* at this rate it is normal to do twenty-four breaths over twelve minutes while practicing the *āsana.*

*Śīrṣāsana* should always be done in the morning, as is laid down by authorities on yoga. And as a counterpose, it should be followed by an equal length of time in the practice of *sarvāṅgāsana.* The procedure is thus to do *śīrṣasanam* for twenty-four breaths, followed by a two-minute rest in *śavāsana.* Then one should do *sarvāṅgāsana* for the equal number of twenty-four breaths, followed by a sitting posture such as *padmāsana* for a few breaths, until one feels normal and relaxed. This is the method of progression, or *vinyāsa.* Even then, *śīrṣāsana* should be done only after a few preparatory exercises, such as *sarvāṅgāsana,* and certain *bandhas* and *mudrās,* as mentioned earlier.

In *śīrṣāsana,* the brain and the glands in the brain get a better supply of blood, and the body's internal organs get displaced upward. The two-minute rest is used to normalize. Similarly, the organs are displaced upward in *sarvāṅgāsana,* but the flow of blood to the head is restricted (especially if one does *sarvāṅgāsana* properly, with the chin pressing against the chest making a *bandha*). But the thyroid and the upper part of the body get an extra supply of blood. Again, a rest period helps to normalize. Then when a sitting posture is taken up, the internal organs retain their proper position. This group of *āsanas,* therefore, helps to restore the state of equilibrium of the vital organs such as the liver, kidneys, and prostate. This is the reason for doing those postures in that particular order.

The breathing pattern in *śīrṣāsana* requires some attention. As mentioned, there are four distinct steps in breathing in *yogāsana* practice. One should practice normal inhalation *(pūraka),* with no deliberate holding after inhalation in the initial stages of practice, and then a long exhalation *(recaka).* During the changeover from *pūraka* to *recaka,* however, there is an interval of about two seconds when there is a pause in the *gati* (movement or flow) of *prāṇa.* After some practice, *kumbhaka,* say, for up to five seconds after inhalation and for up to ten seconds after exhalation *(bāhya-kumbhaka),* may be practiced. During *bāhya-kumbahka,* one should slowly start practicing *mūla bandha* and *uddīyāna bandha* as well. If one is steady *(sthira)* and comfortable *(sukha)* in *śīrṣāsana,* then the effects of the *bandhas* are accentuated owing to the effects of gravity. Actually, after a few minutes of practice, the muscles of the legs and thighs, the gluteal muscles, and even the chest, back, shoulders, and neck relax, and with these muscles not being required to maintain their tone, the perineal and rectal muscles can also be drawn in to get good *mūla* and *uddīyāna bandhas*. *Śīrṣāsana*, which is also known as *kapālāsana* and *brahmāsana*, depending upon which part of the head touches the floor (and which are, however, only learned from great yogis who can tell the difference), lends itself to a variety of *vinyāsas*.

Research done so far on the headstand confirms most of the views expressed in the traditional books, though some claims appear to be inconclusive, since adepts in

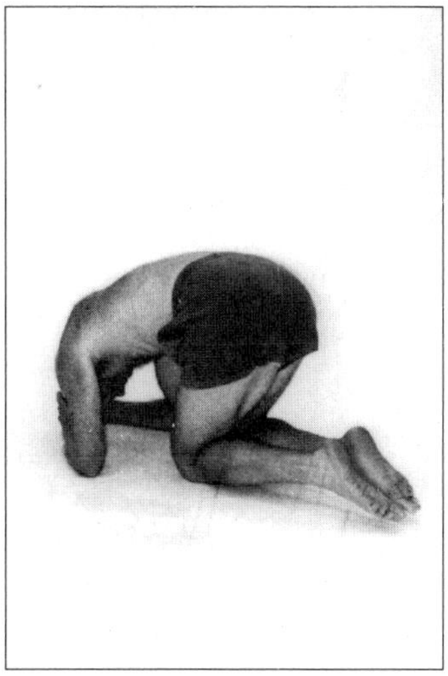

*Śīrṣāsana* (at age 75) Step 1

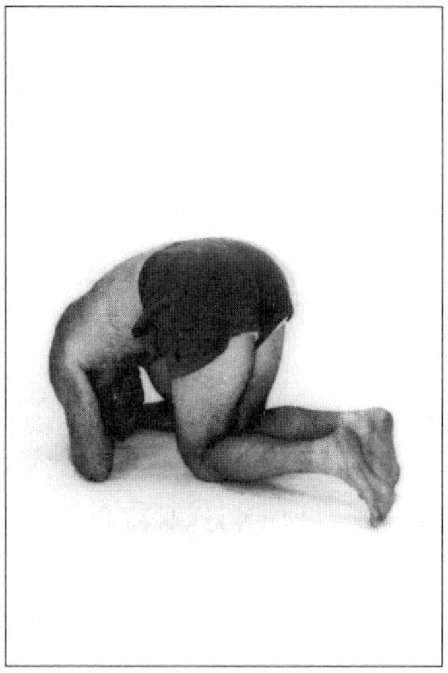

Step 2

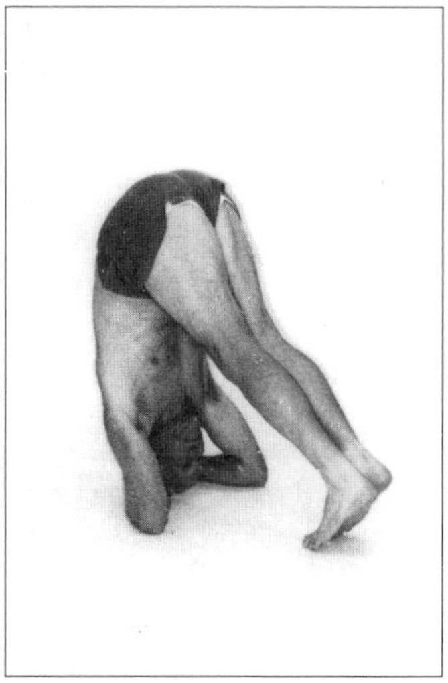

Step 3

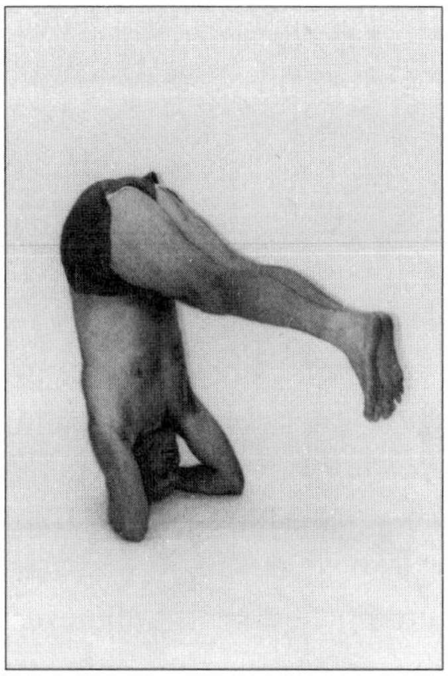

Step 4

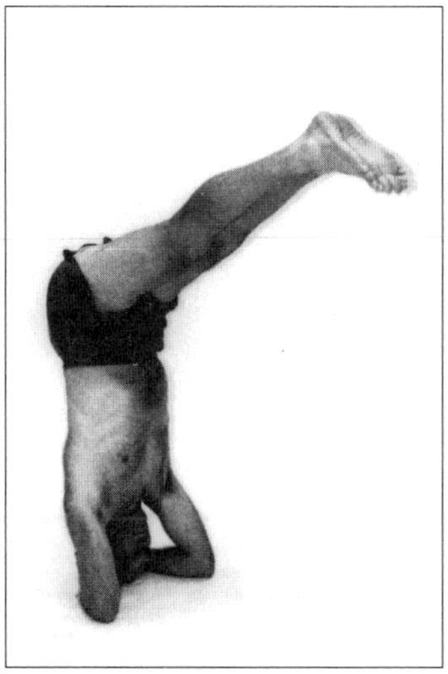

Step 5

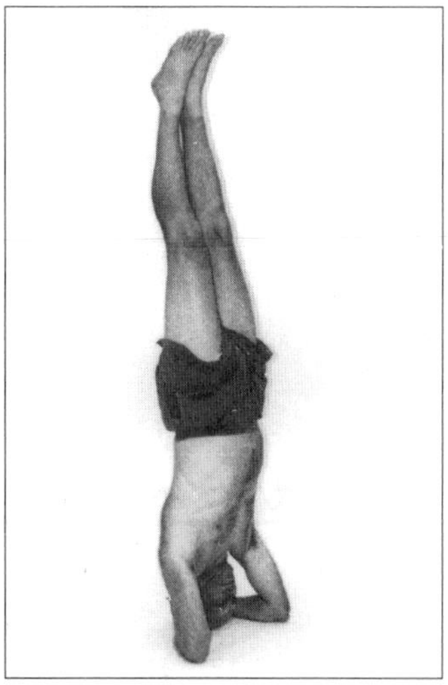

Step 6

yoga are not readily available for study. It has been found that, owing to the inverted nature of the posture and the relaxation in the leg muscles, the pressure in the legs drops to about twenty or thirty milligrams. There does not seem to be a great rush of blood to the head, however, as is normally believed. In fact, a few years back, when yoga was not as popular as it is today, many people were advised not to do *śīrṣāsana* because it was thought it could precipitate a stroke as the result of the increased flow and pressure in the brain vessels. But now we know that the blood flow to the head is not appreciable enough to cause any serious damage, and, because of autoregulation, the body adjusts the flow by constriction. But it is sufficient to dilate many capillaries that are normally closed, and it helps to improve the oxygen supply to many cells that normally are not sufficiently oxygenated. Thus different parts of the brain that are never helped during normal standing or sitting appear to be helped in *śīrṣāsana*. One has to admit that people with high blood pressure or retinal problems are well advised to be cautious and to do the posture under expert guidance. In cases of mild heart condition, because it appears to help increase pressure on the shoulders, the brain acts to reduce the blood pressure. It is therefore found that if one practices *śīrṣāsana* regularly, one's pulse rate lowers significantly, thereby reducing the strain on the heart. There is also a reduction in blood pressure.

The circulation of cerebrospinal fluid is also increased to a greater degree than in any other exercise. If properly done, *śīrṣāsana* increases brain capacity and memory power. It also has some sedative effect, and many people suffering from insomnia respond well to *śīrṣāsana*. It has a tonic effect on the testes, ovaries, and pelvis because it removes congestion. Gastrointestinal diseases are also treated by the posture, and varicose veins tend to disappear. The liver and spleen are also exercised by the effects of gravity and the *bandhas*. The leg muscles, knee joints, and stubborn hip joints became more flexible in due time. Some of the variations of *śīrṣāsana*, such as *ūrdhvapadmāsana*, tend to enhance its effects.

Research has also suggested that *śīrṣāsana* seems to stimulate the nerve centers responsible for bronchial-tube dilation, and as such it is highly beneficial to asthmatics. There is a draining of the bronchial tubes, and thus the posture is beneficial to those suffering from all respiratory ailments. The *bandhas* in *śīrṣāsana* help in eradicating hemorrhoids in the early stages and both rectal and vaginal prolapse, especially in their early stages. It is also a good postnatal exercise. Even in certain prenatal cases, if the patient had been practicing the posture before pregnancy, it may be continued under proper guidance during pregnancy, for it helps improve circulation. Certain cases of retroversion of the uterus can also be helped, in the early stages. Some women are known to have practiced all through their pregnancy. I have seen students of my *ācārya*, encouraged by him, doing *śīrṣāsana* during advanced stages of pregnancy.

Even though *śīrṣāsana* is an exceptionally great yogic posture, many find it very difficult to attain it and become steady and comfortable enough to derive its full benefits. Some have a natural tendency and a good sense of balance, and they attain the posture easily; but many others have considerable difficulty. It is better to practice *śīrṣāsana* under proper guidance. Having prepared one's body well, especially the neck and shoulders, with *sarvāṅgāsana* and other arm movements, one may attempt to do *śīrṣāsana*. Use a soft carpet, folded into four. In the initial stages it is advisable, or, rather, necessary, to use a wall for support.

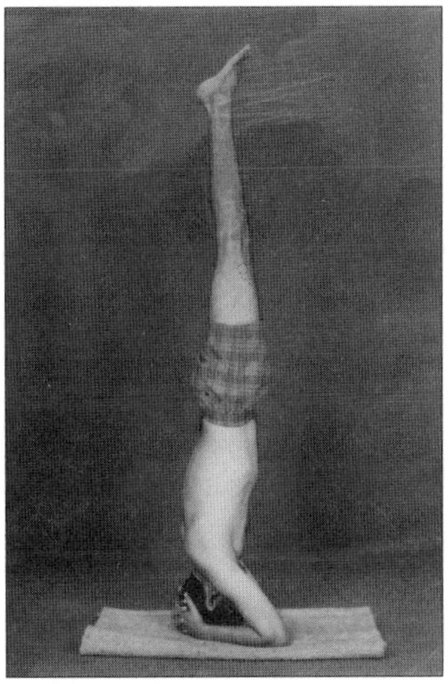

*Śīrṣāsana* with *mūla* and *uddīyana bandhas*

Start with *samasthiti*. Exhale and proceed to do *utkaṭāsana* and then *vajrāsana* (explained in chapter 12). Then, exhaling, bend forward, keeping your elbows and hands on the floor, with fingers interlocked but turned inward, the sides of the little fingers remaining on the floor. Keep your head between the cupped palms, the head itself remaining about two to three inches away from the wall. Slowly exhale, press your elbows, hands, and little fingers, and stretch your legs, pushing your back toward the wall, arching it in the process, and using the top of your head as the fulcrum. In the process, your legs and feet are also drawn a little toward your body, "walking" on your big toes in the process. Stay for a few breaths, then, as the small of your back touches the wall, hold the breath after exhalation and with a slight push transfer the weight of your body to the head, placing your back against the wall and taking your feet off the floor. Your legs may also be bent in the process, so that your knees are a few inches above your chin (called *ākuñcanāsana*). Stay for a few breathes, getting a feel for your balance. Then slowly stretch your legs on inhalation and keep your heels on the wall. One should keep the neck, body, and legs straight, and the thighs, knees, and ankles together. This is *śīrṣāsana*. Stay for a few breaths. Now again on exhalation, bend your knees, return to the intermediate stage of *ākuñcanāsana*, and stay for a few breaths. On the next exhalation, lower the legs and return to *vajrāsana*. This process may be repeated a few times.

After some practice, try to pull your body (back, buttocks) away from the wall, keeping only your heels on the wall for support. Try to keep your ankles stretched. After gaining some confidence, draw one leg completely away from the wall, stay for a few breaths, and return the leg to the wall. Repeat on the other side. Thereafter, one should attempt to take both heels away from the wall and to practice true *śīrṣāsana*, repeatedly returning to the wall for support. Day by day, one will be able to maintain good balance. After a few days' practice (some may take weeks or even months), one should try to go up into the posture purely on the strength and control of the elbows, with the shoulder and neck muscles barely touching the wall while one is going up or coming down. After repeated practice, one may attempt to do the posture without a wall. There are advantages to practicing in the corner of a room: It helps to prevent lateral movements of the body and legs and to avoid distortions and consequent pain in the neck and shoulders. It is better, however, to learn the posture from a teacher.

In *śīrṣāsana* the head point should be the top (crown) of the head; however, one has to make minor adjustments almost continuously. The elbows should be used, especially in the initial stages, to attain and maintain balance. Later on, it may be possible to take the arms away from the head for *nirālamba* and other variations of *śīrṣāsana*, which depend on the variations in the arm positions. Then there are *vinyāsas* that vary the positions of the legs, spine, and so on. For the *yogābhyāsī*, *śīrṣāsana* affords perhaps the maximum number of variations and movements. A few of these variations will be described here. Bending and lowering the legs into *ākuñcanāsana* is good for exercising the shoulders and for getting good control over the headstand posture. *Ākuñcanāsana* is done on exhalation, and one may return to *śīrṣāsana* upon inhalation. Further, one may stay in *ākuñcanāsana* for a few breaths, say, up to six or so. Another variation would call for exhaling and rounding the back so as to lower the legs so that they are straight and parallel to the floor. Good control of the elbows and shoulder muscles is required for this movement, which is known as *ūrdhvadaṇḍāsana*, and which has a very good effect on the abdominal muscles, helping to strengthen them. Inhale and return to *śīrṣāsana*. Perhaps one of the more fascinating variations is *ūrdhvapadmāsana* in *śīrṣāsana*. In *śīrṣāsana*, exhale and spread the legs, which is known as *ūrdhvakoṇāsana*. Then exhale, and bend your left leg, keeping your foot on the right thigh. On the next exhalation, complete *padmāsana* while in *śīrṣāsana*. This is *ūrdhvapadmāsana*.

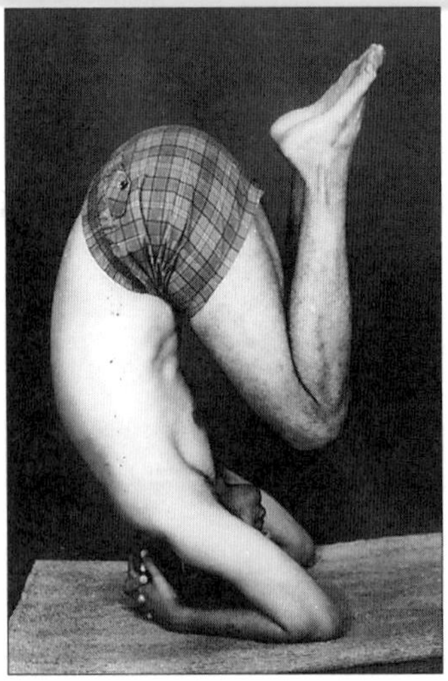

*Ākuñcanāsana*

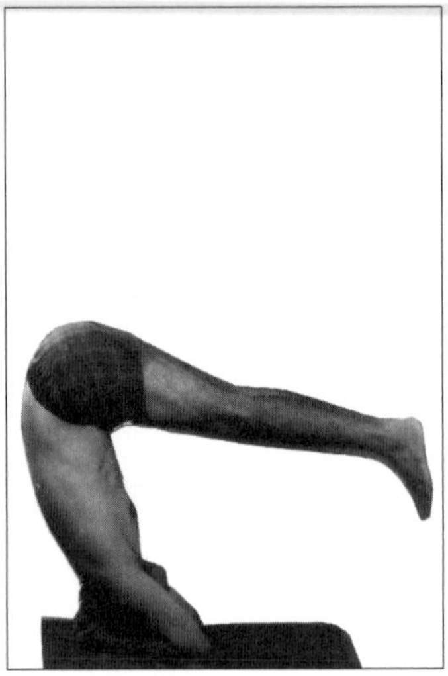

*Ūrdhvadaṇḍāsana*

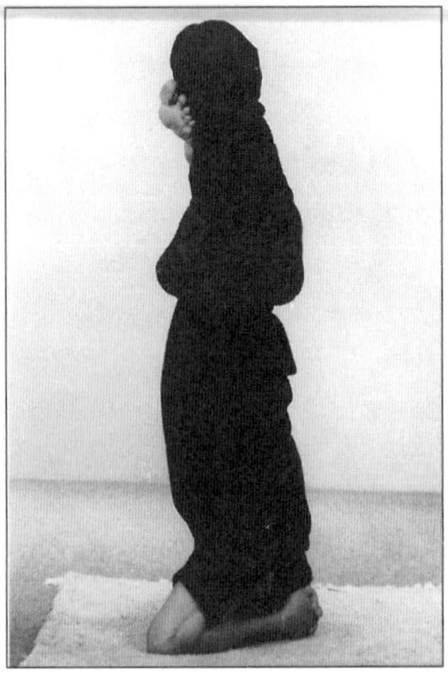

*Ūrdhvapadmāsana*

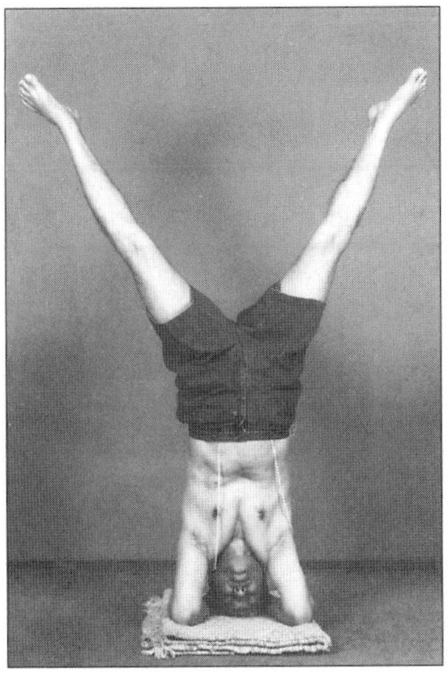

*Ūrdhvakoṇāsana*

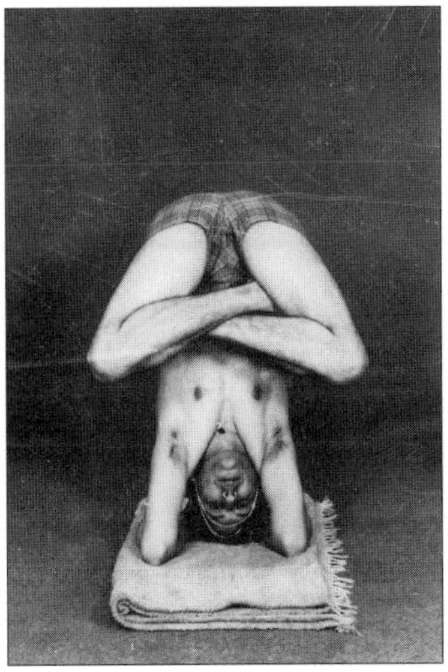

*Ākuncita-ūrdhvapadmāsana*

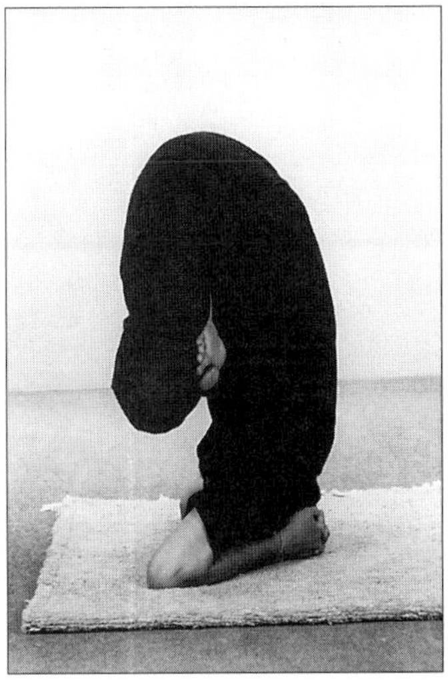

*Ākuncita-ūrdhvapadmāsana*
side view

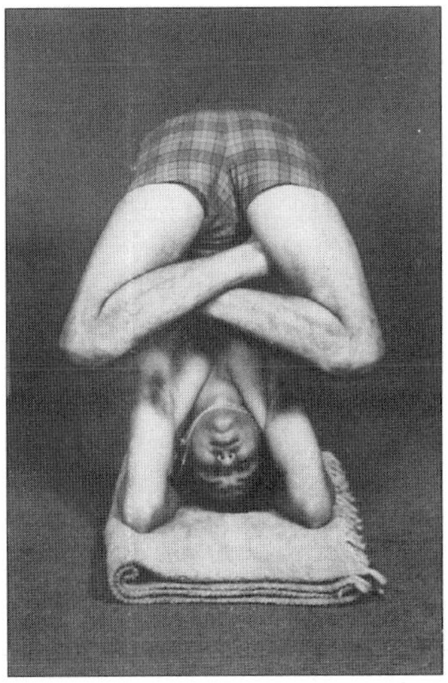

*Viparīta yogamudrā*

Now exhale, bend at the hips, and fold the *padmāsana* by bringing your knees toward your body, bending at the hips. This is *ākuncita-ūrdhvapadmāsana.* Then, exhaling further, round your back and lower your legs in *padmāsana* so that they are in front of the chest. According to a few authors, this is called *piṇḍāsana* in *śīrṣāsana,* as it resembles a fetus (refer also to *piṇḍāsana* in *sarvāṅgāsana*). It is also known as *viparīta yogamudrā.* Inhale, return to *ūrdhvapadmāsana,* and then with your right leg crossed first for *padmāsana* repeat the movements. *Śirṣāsana* could be the transition posture for some of the balancing postures. Keep your forearms, elbows, and palms on the floor by releasing the interlocking of the fingers. Now, as you inhale, press your forearms and raise your head, even as your body is arched back and your legs are pushed back to maintain balance. This is called *pincamayūrāsana,* or dancing peacock pose. If on the next inhalation, you bend your knees and bend your body a little more and raise your head, you may be able to place your feet on top of your raised head even as you balance on your forearms. This balancing pose is called *vṛścikāsana,* or scorpion pose. There are several other balancing postures that can be reached form *śīrṣāsana.*

One may go up into *śīrṣāsana* by bending the knees as described earlier, or by keeping them straight as well, reaching the *ūrdhvadaṇḍāsana* halfway through. It is also possible to go up into *ūrdhvapadmāsana* straight from *padmāsana.* One may also return to *padmāsana* by retracting the steps from *ūrdhvapadmāsana* and *ākuncita-ūrdhvapadmāsana* and then touching the ground with the knees, releasing the head from *śīrṣāsana* and moving back to *padmāsana* or *parvatāsana*. Youngsters love to do *āsanas* when they are interspersed with such variations; through them, they get to appreciate what a beautiful, versatile, and dexterous piece of equipment the body really is. Only a few variations have been covered here.

It is nice to stand on one's own head, after all.

# 10 Prone Postures and the Spine

POSTURES STARTING FROM THE PRONE POSITION, lying facedown, form another important group of *āsanas* that are especially useful for the spine and lower back. When done with *vinyāsas,* they are easy to make progress in and have very important benefits. The main prone-position *āsanas* are *bhujaṅgāsana* (serpent), *śalabhāsana* (locust), and *dhanurāsana* (bow posture). And some of these could be used as counterposes, or *pratikriyās,* following *sarvāṅgāsana.*

## *Bhujaṅgāsana*

For *bhujaṅgāsana,* start with *samasthiti.* Inhale, raise your arms overhead, and interlock your fingers, turning them outward. Exhale, proceed to *utkaṭāsana,* and place your palms by the sides of your feet. Take a few breaths. Then, holding your breath after exhalation, press your palms and jump back to *caturaṅgadaṇḍāsana.* Then lie down on the floor, facedown. This procedure may be adopted for starting any of the prone postures. Keeping your palms at your sides and in line with the diaphragm, inhale and raise your upper body by pressing your palms,

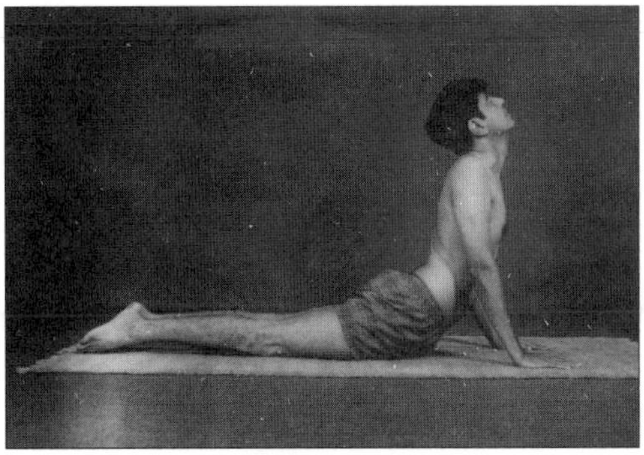

*Bhujaṅgāsana*

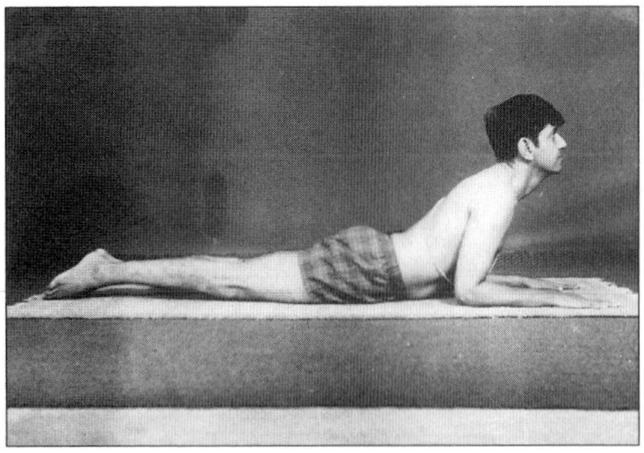

*Makarāsana*

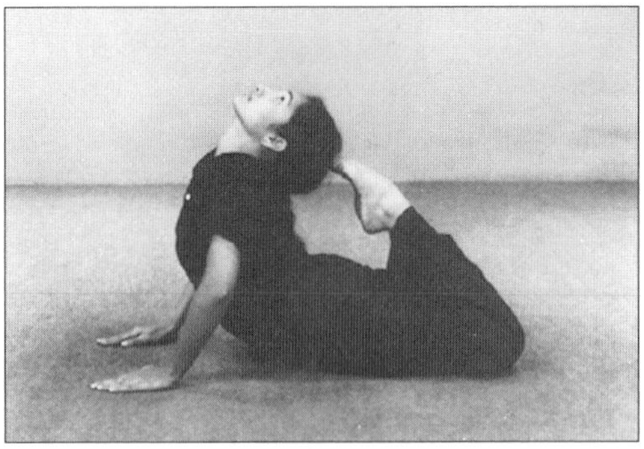

*Rājakapotāasana*

pelvis, and legs. Arch your back up to your navel, keeping your eyes open. This is *bhujaṅgāsana,* or serpent posture. Stay for a few seconds and return to the starting position on the exhale. You may also just keep your forearms on the floor and raise your upper body. This is a very simple and effective posture to relieve strain in the neck. Some authors call it *makarāsana,* or crocodile posture. The next step will be to raise your upper body and arch your spine, raising your trunk up to your pubis while inhaling. Press your pubis and contract your anal and gluteal muscles. This is another variation of *bhujaṅgāsana.* Exhaling, return to prone position. Repeat a few times. *Bhujaṅgāsana* is especially useful for relieving lower-back pain, and, if done carefully and under proper supervision, it can be very beneficial for those suffering from slight displacement of a disk. It strengthens the ligaments and muscular supports of the spinal column.

*Bhujaṅgāsana*, as the name indicates, should be done purely with the strength of the spine, dispensing with the aid of one's hands altogether. The posture then resembles a limbless reptile, the snake. One's palms are kept either by the side of the thighs, or on the back, or in a back salute. A further variation requires bending the knees on exhalation, so that the thighs are parallel to the floor and the chest above the floor is slightly arched. There is a tremendous contraction of the lower back that helps to relieve lower-back pain. Some authors refer to *this* variation as *makarāsana,* or also as a variation of *śalabhāsana.*

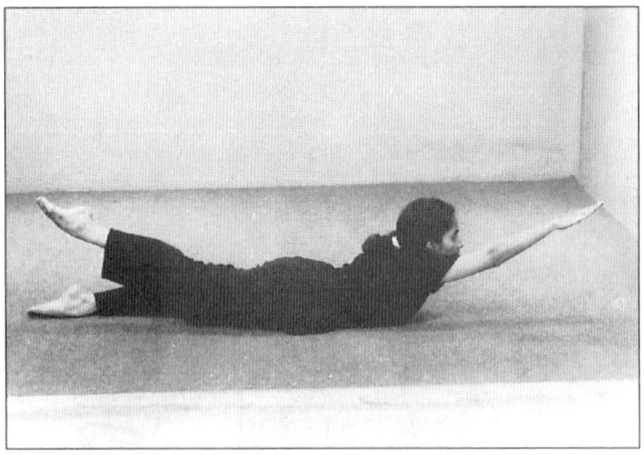

*Śalabhāsana (vinyāsa)*
(preparatory)

# *Śalabhāsana*

*Śalabhāsana* is an improvement on *bhujaṅgāsana* in that not only is the chest raised and the spine arched but the legs are also raised, so that the body is balanced on the stomach. To explain this pose and its variations, a step-by-step approach is best. Start from *samasthiti.* Inhale, raise your arms overhead, interlock your fingers, and turn them outward. Exhale, and proceed to *utkaṭāsana.* Then, keeping your palms at the sides of your legs, press your palms, exhale, and jump back to *caturaṅgadaṇḍāsana.* Stay for a few breaths. Exhaling, lie down on the floor, face-down; keep your arms stretched alongside your body, palms facing upward. Close your left fist. Inhale, and raise your right arm overhead, sweeping it along the floor. Inhaling, raise your right arm and your head, chest, shoulders, and right leg, from the pelvis, so that your right thigh is clearly above the floor. Don't tilt to the left side. Your shoulders should be at the same level. Exhale and return to the prone position. Inhale, and raise your right arm and your head, chest, shoulders, and left leg, from the pelvis, stretching all the way from your fingertips to your toes along the spine and across to your left leg. Return to the starting position. Exhale and lower your right arm. Repeat with your left arm raised overhead.

Raise both arms overhead while inhaling, and keep both palms together as if doing *prāṇam.* Inhale and raise both arms and both legs so that you are balanced on your navel region. The stretching is felt all over your body, from your fingertips to your outstretched

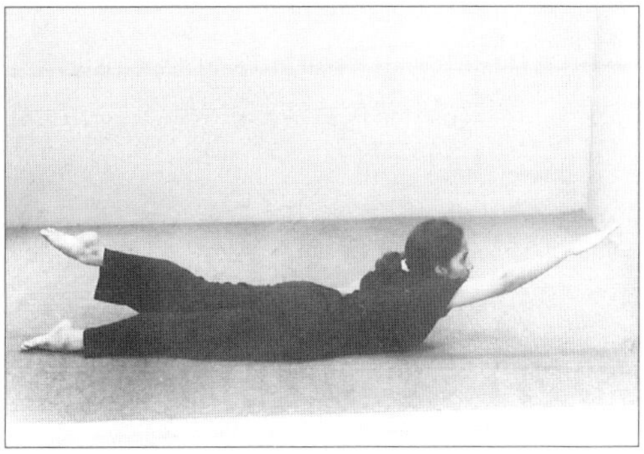

*Śalabhāsana (vinyāsa)*

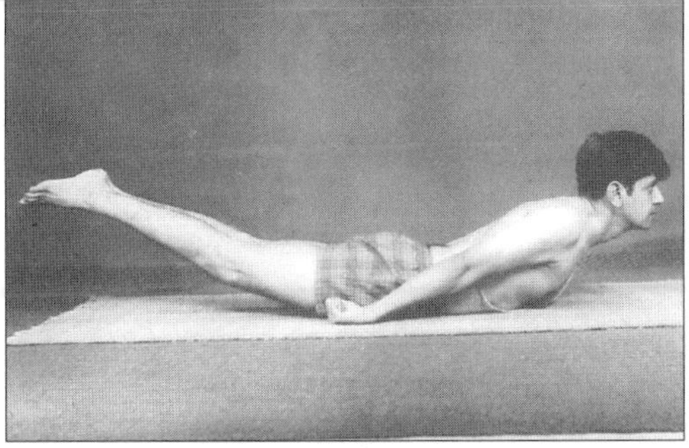

*Śalabhāsana*

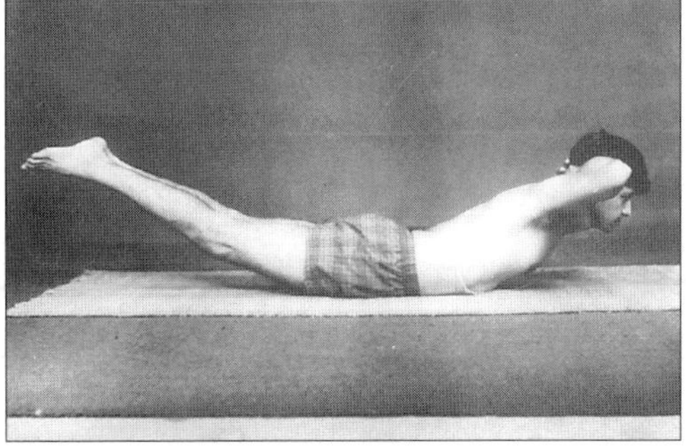

*Śalabhāsana (vinyāsa)*

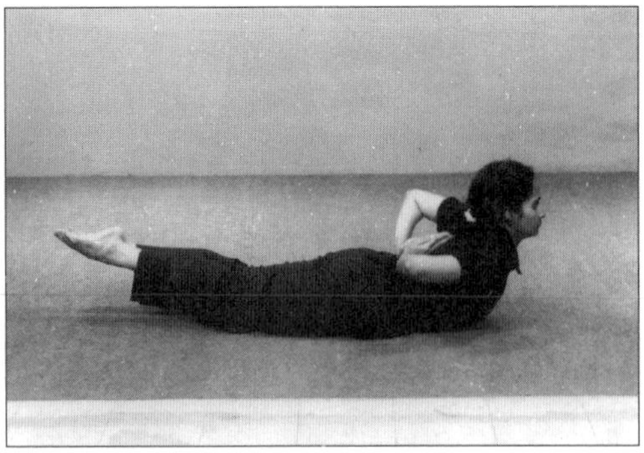

*Śalabhāsana pṛṣṭañjali*

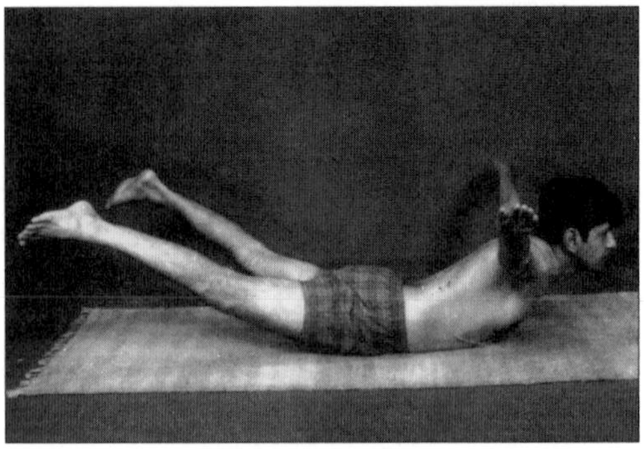

*Vimānāsana*

ankles, feet, and toes. Your shoulders should be thrown slightly backward, forming a canal along the spine; your gluteal muscles should be contracted to enhance the stretching of the spine and legs. Return to the starting position. Keep your arms alongside your body and repeat. This is *śalabhāsana.*

Further variations are possible. Keep your palms with fingers interlocked on the back of your neck. Inhale, raise your head, chest, arms, and also your legs, keeping your knees together and straight. Some authors call this posture *makarāsana*, but it is basically a variation of *śalabhāsana.* Inhale and return to the prone position. Inhale and spread your arms, keeping them at shoulder level, with palms on the floor. Exhale, and on the next inhalation raise your head, shoulders, and your stretched hands. Also raise your legs and spread them apart as much as possible, balancing on the navel region. Exhale and return to the starting position. This is known as *vimānāsana,* or aircraft pose. Keeping your palms on your back in the *añjali* position, inhale and raise your head and shoulders, arch your spine, and raise your legs, again balancing on the lower abdomen. Raising the trunk, which is the operating movement, can be done on exhalation. This *langhana kriyā* will be helpful for obese, stiff, and older people in doing these *vinyāsas.*

## *Dhanurāsana*

Having made the shoulders, lower back, and spine more flexible, one may attempt *dhanurāsana,* both to enhance the effects of these easier *āsanas* and to give strength to the shoulders and the back. *Dhanurāsana* can be done with various preparations and *vinyāsas.*

As in *bhujaṅgāsana*, move into the prone position from *samasthiti.* Inhale and raise your right arm overhead, making a sweeping movement along the floor.

Exhale, bend your left knee, and hold it, with the left hand, behind your back. Initially it may not be possible to do this variation. But the preparatory *āsanas*, especially *śalabhāsana,* will be helpful for preparation. After one or two breaths, inhale and raise your head and right hand and arch your spine, simultaneously pulling your left leg and thigh up, as high as possible, keeping your right leg on the floor. Exhale and return to the starting position. Exhale, lower your right arm, and hold your left ankle with both hands. On the next exhalation, raise your head, chest, and shoulders and pull your left leg upward as high as possible, arching the spine. Exhale and return. Now inhale, holding your left ankle with your right hand, and raise your left arm overhead. Exhale, and then inhaling, raise your head, chest, and shoulders, and left arm and also pull your left leg up with your right hand, keeping your right leg on the floor. Inhale and return. Repeat for the other side.

Exhale, bend both knees, and hold both ankles with their respective hands; inhale and raise your head, chest, and shoulders and pull your legs up as high as possible, arching the back and pulling the thighs to form a bow. Stay a few seconds

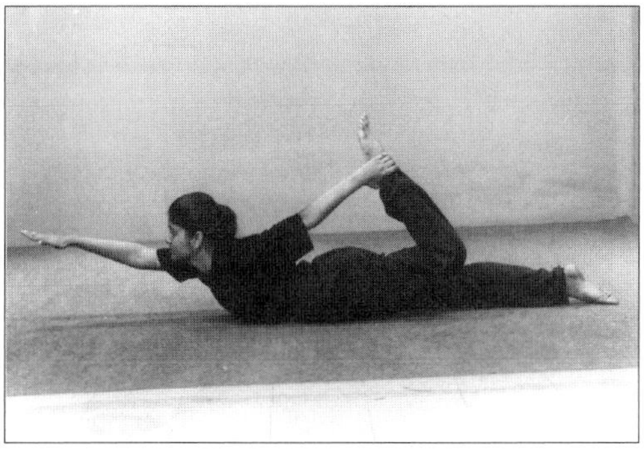

*Dhanurāsana* (*vinyāsa* 1)
preparatory

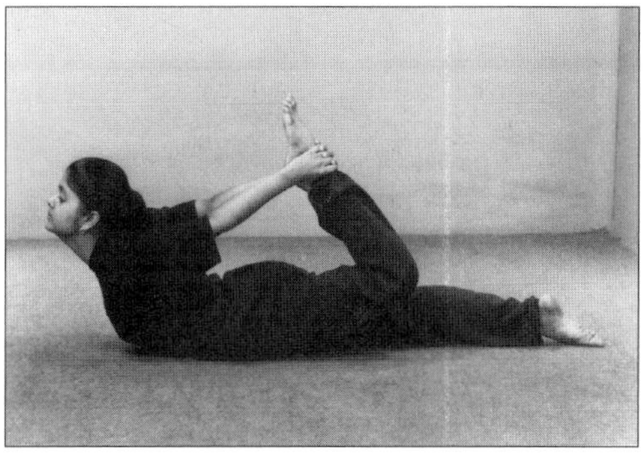

*Dhanurāsana* (*vinyāsa* 2)
preparatory

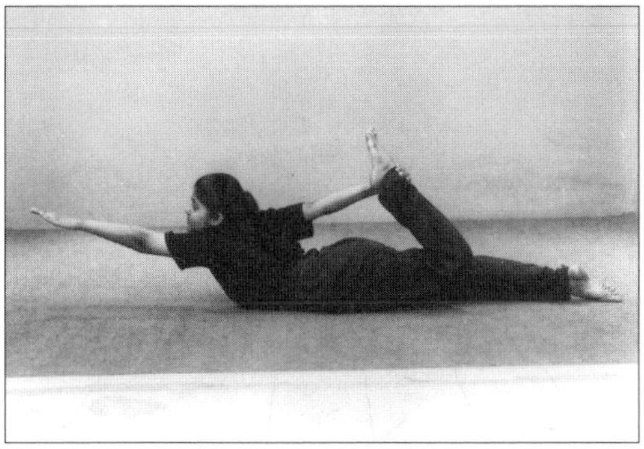

*Dhanurāsana* (*vinyāsa* 3)
preparatory

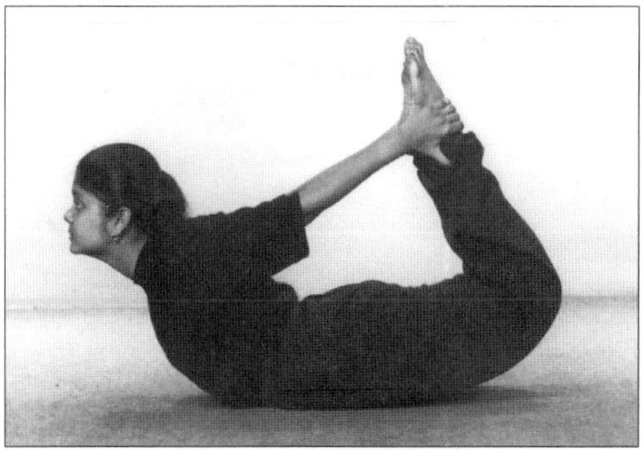

*Dhanurāsana*

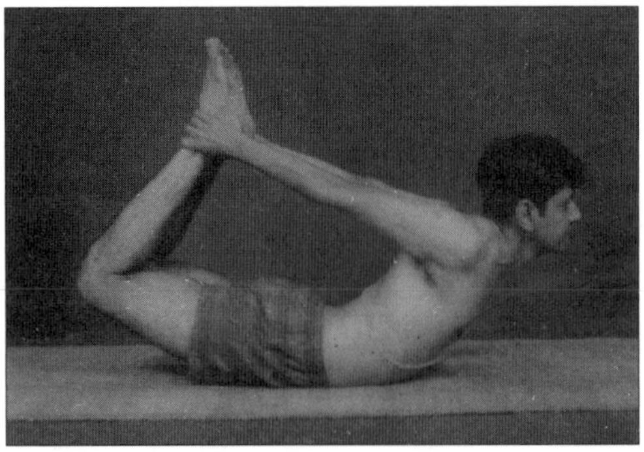

*Dhanurāsana (pūrṇa)*

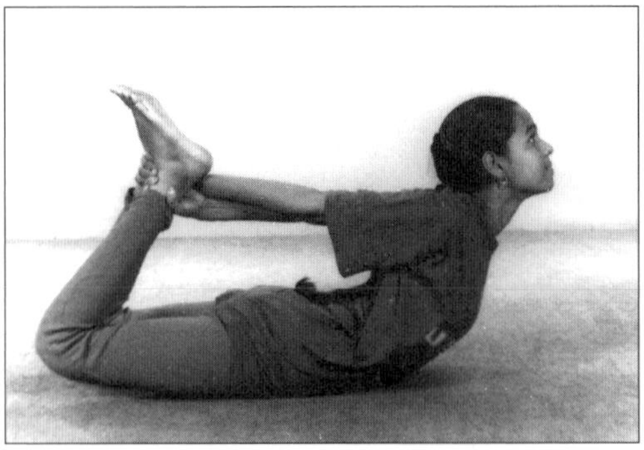

*Dhanurāsana (vinyāsa)*

and return to position. Repeat a few times. The knees and ankles should be kept close together. This is *dhanurāsana*, or bow posture. With some practice, after achieving *dhanurāsana*, one can inhale and roll over to one side, keeping the body arched. On exhalation, return to *dhanurāsana*. Repeat on the other side. Now hold your right ankle with your left hand and your left ankle with your right hand on exhalation. On inhalation, arch the trunk. This is one variation of *dhanurāsana* that works more on the shoulders, forearms, and wrists. The shoulder blades press against each other and form a canal along the spinal column.

With age, the spine becomes rigid, and *dhanurāsana* helps to keep the lower back flexible; thus one is supposed to be kept young by the regular practice of *dhanurāsana*. Apart from strengthening the spine, it works on the abdominal organs and improves their function. Along with the practice of *śalabhāsana*, people who suffer from slight slipped disks could benefit considerably from *dhanurāsana*. With our unnatural upright position, aggravated by sedentary habits and other activities requiring long periods of crouching, we can feel the tonic effects of this robust backbending exercise. *Śalabhāsana* is also a very useful counterpose for many forward-bending exercises and those requiring the forward curving of the spine, such as *sarvāṅgāsana* and *halāsana*. Gheraṇḍa refers to these postures in his *Saṃhitā*, and he lists the following as the benefits. *Makarāsana* and *śalabhāsana* are supposed to increase body heat by improving circulation, digestion, and metabolism. Regarding *bhujaṅgāsana*, he says,

*Aṅguṣta nābhi paryantam*
*Ādhi bhūmau Vinyāset*
*Karatalābhyām dharam dhrutvā*
*ūrdhvaśirsa phanaiva hi*
*Dehāgniḥ vardhate nityam*
*Sarvāroga vināśanam*
*Jāgarti bhujaṅgī devi*
*Bhujaṅgāsana sādhanam.*

Gheraṇḍa explains that "the part of the body between the navel and the toes is kept on the floor. Place the pelvis on the ground, raise the head [and upper portion of the body] like a serpent. This is called the serpent posture. This posture always increases body heat and eradicates all ailments, and through practice of *bhujaṅgāsana* the goddess Bhujaṅgī (the serpent goddess, or *kuṇḍalinī*) becomes alive or is awakened."

*Dhanurāsana* is simply explained as follows:

*Prasārya padau bhuvi daṇḍarūpau*
*Karān ca dhṛtapādayugamam*
*Kṛtva dhanustulya parivartitāṅgam*
*Nigadya yogī dhanurāsanam tat.*

"Stretching the legs on the ground, straight as a stick, and catching hold of the feet with the hands, thus making the body bent or arched like a bow, is known by yogis as *dhanurāsana*."

# 11 Paścimatānam

ONE OF THE *ĀSANAS* THAT COMPREHENSIVELY test the willpower, perseverance, and endurance of an *abhyāsī* is *paścimatānam*, or the posterior-stretching *āsana*, along with its *vinyāsas*, in which the stretching extends from the toes to the fingertips in one continuous movement. A highly beneficial posture, it improves circulation and muscle tone in a large group of posterior muscles, especially when it is combined with its counterpose, or *pratikriyā*, *pūrvatānāsana*. Almost all texts on yoga refer to this *āsana*. It is also known as *paścima-uttānāsana*, the preposition *ut* indicating an upward pull of all posterior muscles. Another name by which it is known is *ugrāsana*, which is indicative of the tremendous effort necessary to achieve it and the benefits in the areas of muscle tone and strength it bestows. *Brahmacaryāsana* is yet another name given to it. Evidently it helps in maintaining *brahmacarya* and is foremost among those that awaken *kuṇḍalinī*.

*Paścimatānāsana* is yet another posture that brings out the unique character of our *ācārya's* yogic system. It does not involve merely sitting, stretching one's legs, and touching one's toes, as is generally understood. When done with *vinyāsas* and proper breathing, the *paścimatāna* group works on the complete system, as is reported in the yoga texts. *Vinyāsas,* with corresponding breathing and *pratikriyās,* are essential for *āsana siddhi.*

A stanza appearing in the Triśikhibrāhmaṇa Upaniṣad of the Śukla Yajur Veda merely gives the basic description of the posture. It says to sit and extend the legs, keeping them straight. Then, extending the arms, one should hold one's big toes with the hooked fingers. Stretching the torso, one should then bend down and place one's forehead on one's knees. There are many variations of *paścimatānam*. The most popular one described in the above Upaniṣad can be done in steps, or *vinyāsas*.

Start from *samasthiti*. Breathe normally a few times. While inhaling, raise your arms overhead. Exhale, and while stretching from the hips, bend forward and keep your palms by the side of the feet, touching your knees with your forehead. This is *uttānāsana*. Some people do *utkaṭāsana*. Now keep your palms by the side of your feet. Inhale and hold your breath. Press your palms, and after slightly bending your knees, jump back to attain *caturāṅgadaṇḍāsana*, as described in chapter 7. One may also reach this position from *utkaṭāsana*, by gently raising the buttocks and attaining a position halfway between *utkaṭāsana* and *uttānāsana*. From *caturāṅgadaṇḍāsana*, inhale. While pressing your palms, stretching your ankles, and arching your back, bring your pelvis between your palms, supporting your body on your palms and toes. This is called *ūrdhvamukhaśvānāsana*. Proceed to *adhomukhaśvānāsana* on the exhale. Slightly bending your knees and holding the breath after inhalation,

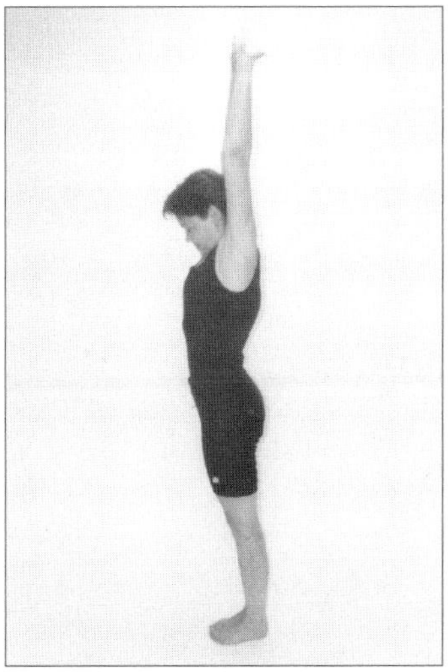

Samasthiti

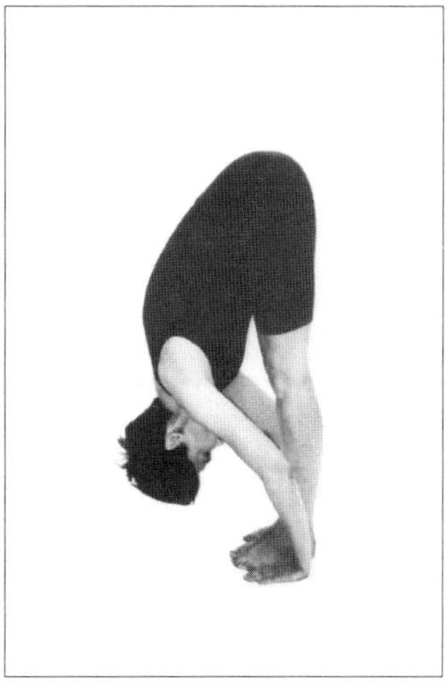

*Uttānāsana*

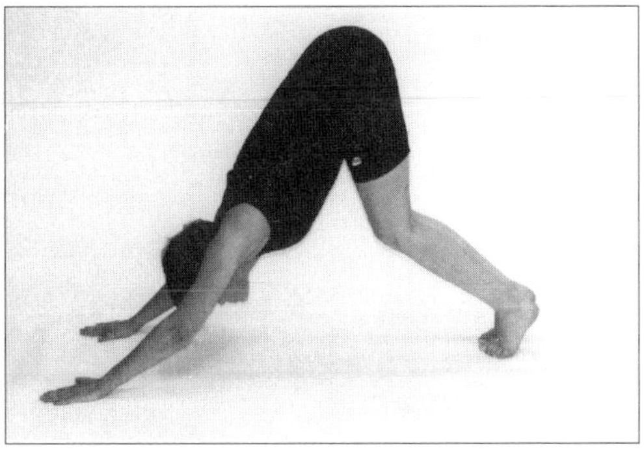

Preparation for *daṇḍāsana*

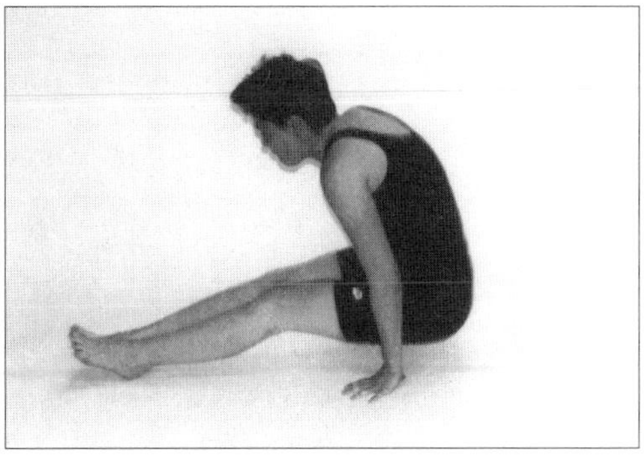

Jumping to *daṇḍāsana*

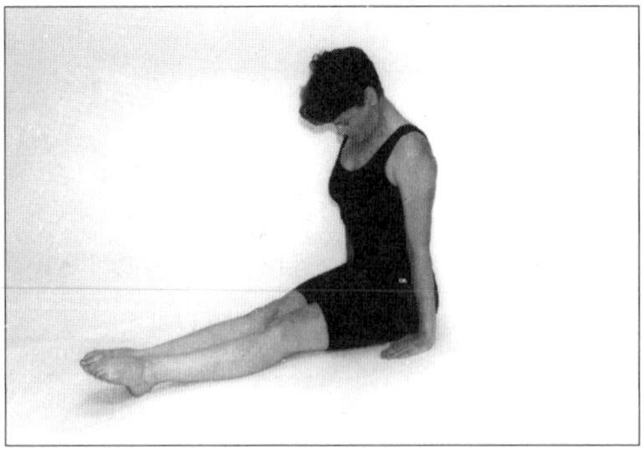

*Daṇḍāsana*

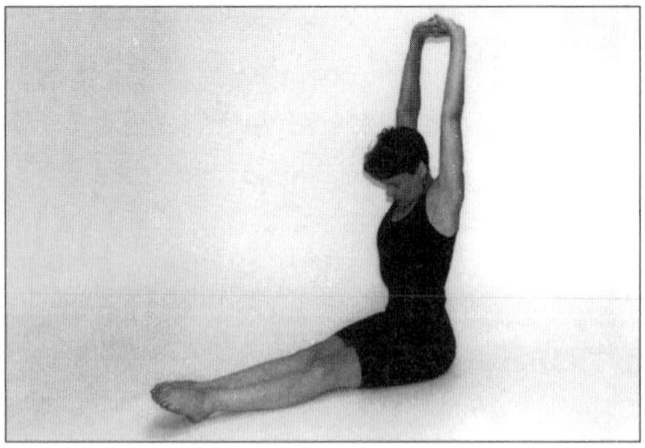

*Daṇḍāsana (nirālamba)*

swing forward, first completely flexing the knees and extending them after crossing the supporting arms. Land on the floor with legs extended and your buttocks between your palms. This is *daṇḍāsana*, mentioned in Vyāsa's commentary on Patañjali's *Yogasūtras.* Now inhale and raise your arms, stretching your shoulders and neck in the process. Stay for a few breaths, focusing your attention on the tip of your nose. Exhaling, extend your arms forward, pushing your pelvis and spine, and hold your big toes with your thumbs and next two fingers, which form a hook, all the while pressing the back of your legs against the floor. After a few breaths, further extension may be attempted. Exhaling and spreading the elbows, you should lower your torso so that the forehead is placed between your knees, which should be straight. This is *paścimatānāsana.*

*Prasārya padau bhuvi daṇḍarūpau*
*Sanyasṭa bhalancita yugma madhye* ।
*Yetnena pādam ca dhrutau karābhyām*
*Yogindra pītam paścimottānamāhuḥ* ।

This stanza from Gheraṇḍa admits the necessity of repeated efforts *(yetna)* to achieve the posture. In the initial stages, it may be difficult even to sit in *daṇḍāsana* with your arms raised. Back, thighs, the stubborn hamstrings, and the ankles refuse to budge. But with deeper exhalation, relaxed concentration, perseverance, and some coaxing by the *abhyāsī*, the muscles slowly yield and after considerable practice the posture may be achieved fairly comfortably.

One may stay in this *āsana* for a few breaths, or even up to a few minutes. It will be possible only when one begins to enjoy the posture, as is evidently the case in Svātmārāma's description in the *Haṭhayogapradīpikā:*

*Prasārya padau bhuvi daṇḍarūpau*
*Dorbhyān pādāgra dvitayan gṛhītva* ǀ
*Janūpari nyasta lalaṭadese*
*Vasetidam paścimatānamahuḥ* ǀ

Here, the author recommends the *abhyāsī* stay in the posture. By his use of the word *vaseth* one should infer a considerable length of time. Adepts may proceed to a further extension of the posterior muscles. After some practice, one may keep one's chin on one's knees. Further extension will require keeping one's forehead on one's shins, about three inches beyond one's knees. Variations of hand positions are also possible by keeping one's palms fully on the floor, or by holding one's heels while keeping the fingers interlocked and turned outward around one's soles. Keeping one's palms on the floor and clasping one wrist with the other hand is yet another *vinyāsa*. The stretch can be also done without the support of one's arms *(nirālamba)*, such as if one keeps one's arms extended at shoulder level, or keeps one's palms clasped behind one's head, as mentioned in the Śiva Saṃhitā, or keeps them together in the *añjali* position behind the back, and so on. One may attempt to balance in the posture by keeping one's palms by the side of the thighs and raising the body. Readers may find a similarity with certain exercises using the parallel bars in gymnastics. Our *ācārya* contended that yogis had actually invented many gymnastic aids, and thus it is highly probable that gymnastics is basically an offshoot of yoga, or at least its basis was provided by yoga, even though gymnastics these days appears to be far different from yoga. This exercise is known as *utpluti* and may be attempted in different sitting postures, such as *padmāsana* and *siṃhāsana*. Keeping your palms on the floor by the side of your hips, return to *caturāṅgadaṇḍāsana*. The next *vinyāsas* actually retrace the path via *ūrdhvamukhaśvānāsana, adhomukhaśvānāsana, utkaṭāsana, uttānāsana, tāḍāsana,* and *samasthiti.*

This *āsana* is highly beneficial for general improvement in circulation, muscle tone, and strength, and it improves the function of all abdominal and pelvic organs, the kidneys, and the spine. It is said to improve vitality, correct certain cases of impotency resulting from increased vascularity of the organs of the genitourinary tract, and, paradoxically, helps control the sex drive *(reta-skhalanam)*, whence derives its name of *brahmacaryāsana*. A friend once told me at the end of a class in which several variations of *paścimatānam* were done that he had experienced a free flow of urine for the first time in several years; he appeared to suffer from some degree of prostatitis. All the posterior muscle groups and joints, including the heels, calf muscles, hamstrings, and knees, and the thigh, gluteal, and lumbosacral muscles, as well as the spine, shoulders, neck, arms, wrists, and even knuckles, get stretched. There is hardly a yoga text that does not refer to this posture and describe its benefits, of course using the peculiar language used by ancient yogis. This important *āsana* *(āsanamāgrayam)* makes the wind, or force *(pavana)*, flow through the *suṣumṇā* and stimulates the gastric fire *(jāṭharānala)*, reduces the abdomen *(kārṣyam udre)*, and makes one free of disease *(arogatām)*.

Stretch out your legs and keep them slightly apart. Firmly take hold of your head with your hands and place it between your knees. This is called *ugrāsana*, said to be the best among *āsanas*, for it improves the movement of bodily forces (*anila*). Known also as *paścima-uttānāsana*, it removes lethargy and weakness *(deha avasanahāranam)*. Discriminating *abhyāsīs* should master this beneficial posture by daily *(pratyahan)* practice. It makes *vāyu* (energy) flow in the posterior regions and makes one strong. Those who practice it with diligence find all the *siddhis* generated in themselves. Thus, through his or her own effort, the yogi should master the posture. These benefits should be treated with great care and not given out indiscriminately. For through it, *vāyusiddhi*, or activation of all the *prāṇas* (metabolism, circulation, respiration), takes place and it destroys multitudes of miseries. Gheraṇḍa refers to this as the king of all sitting postures *(yogindrapīṭham)*.

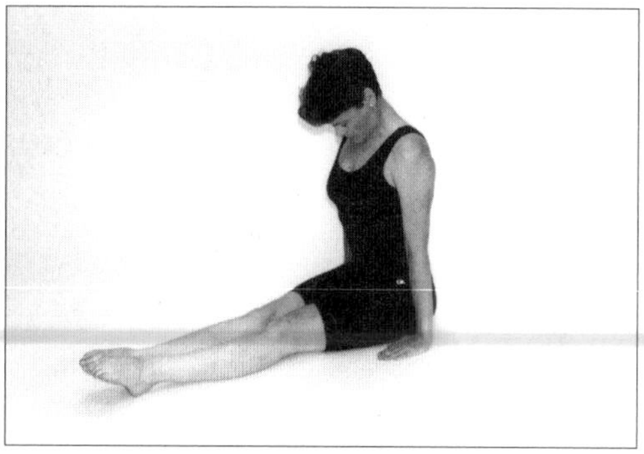

*Daṇḍāsana*

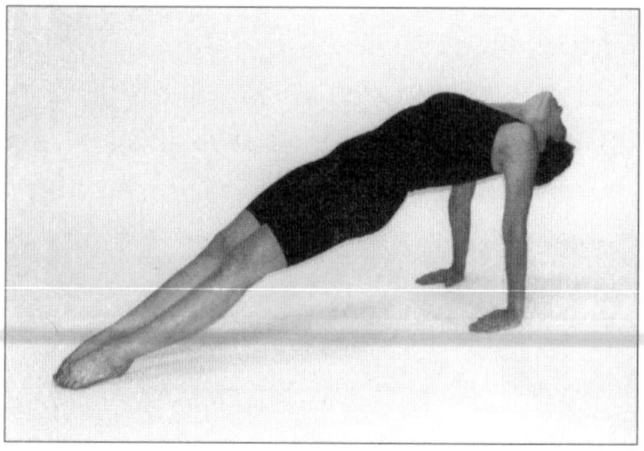

Anterior stretching pose

Since this posture is strenuous exercise, it requires a counterpose to normalize the body. *Pūrva-uttānāsana*, or anterior-stretching pose, not only helps relieve strain but also stretches the anterior muscles, and thus completes the involvement of all the major muscle groups. Proceed from *daṇḍāsana*. Keep your palms by the sides of your buttocks or about a foot behind them. Pressing your palms and heels, inhale and raise your trunk as high as possible, stretching your ankles and keeping your feet on the ground, and also keeping your knees straight and stretched. Exhale and return to the starting position. You may repeat the posture a few times, and later, stay in the posture for a few breaths. It is a very good stretching movement involving the front portions of the ankles, shins, knees, thighs, pelvis, abdomen, chest, neck, shoulders, arms, and wrists. For obese people, the raising of the trunk may be done in *langhana kriyā*. Since in both postures the knees are kept straight, to release knee strain another posture, *catuṣpādapīṭham*, can be included in the same group of *āsanas*. From *daṇḍāsana*, exhale and bend your knees. Then inhale, pressing your palms and feet, and raise your trunk, keeping it parallel to the floor. Exhale and return. Repeat a few times. One may also remain in the posture for a few breaths. With this *āsana*, a better stretching of the shoulders and neck is possible; the hip joints are also exercised better. It may be done as *langhana kriyā*. Since it resembles a table, it is called *catuṣpādapīṭham*, or four-legged seat. From the starting point of *catuṣpādapīṭham*, inhale, press your palms, and stretch your legs, making a sixty-degree angle to the floor. Balancing on your buttocks, lift your hands and stretch them in front, stay for a few seconds, and then return to the original position. Repeat a few times. This is known as *nāvāsana*, or boat posture.

This group of postures can be done in one continuous stretch, and then one may rest in *śavāsana*. For the majority of people who have difficulty in doing *paścimatānāsana*, a few methods are suggested to get more mobility out of the stubborn hip joints. You may start from the lying-down posture. With arms overhead, exhale, pressing your heels and buttocks, and raise your trunk, bending forward as far as you can, and hold the ankles or toes. Inhale and return to lying position. This may be repeated a few times. One may also start from *halāsana*. From *halāsana*, inhale, raise your arms overhead, and then touch your toes. While inhaling, roll back to lying position and, in a continuous motion, exhale and do *paścimatānam*, as

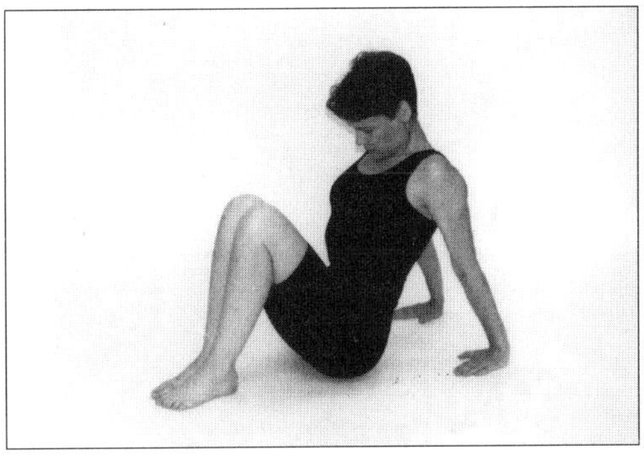

*Catuṣpādapīṭham* (preparation)

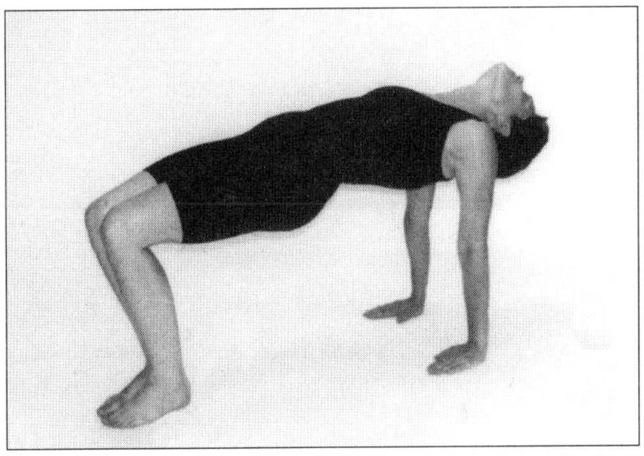

*Catuṣpādapīṭham*

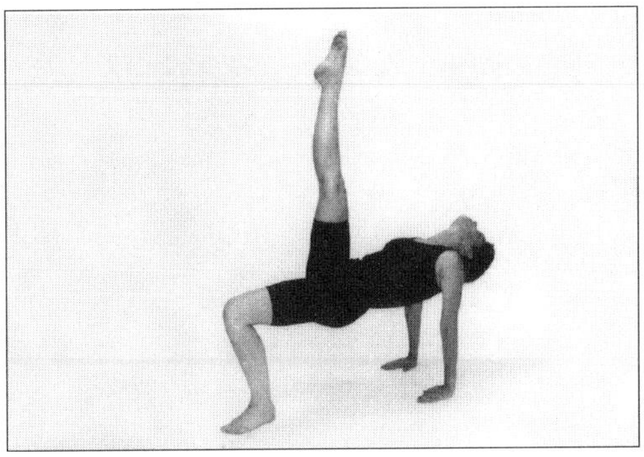

*Catuṣpādapīṭham (vinyāsa)*

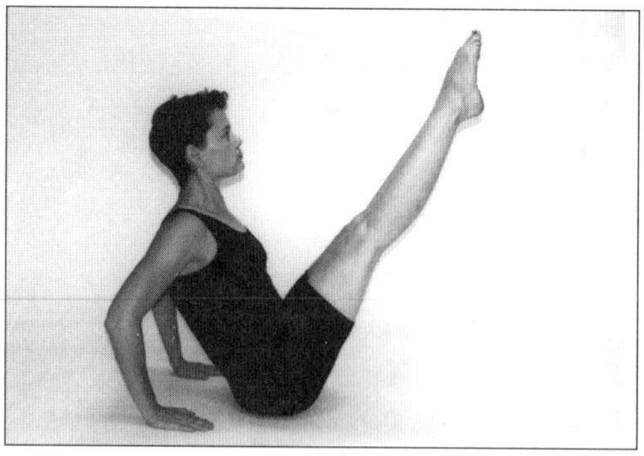

*Nāvāsana (sālamba)*

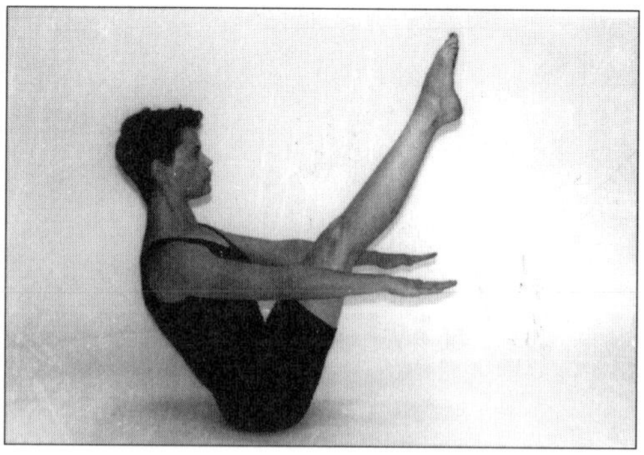

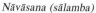

*Nāvāsana (nirālamba)*

described earlier. One may repeat a few times. These dynamic movements help to exercise the posterior muscles, paving the way for achieving the posture. Children love these dynamic movements.

Because there are a number of muscles and tendons that are seldom exercised, yogis have invented several hybrid postures to stretch and exercise them. Many such postures are in vogue. Combining *paścimatānāsana* and *baddhapadmāsana* gives *ardhabaddhapadmapaścimatāna,* a *vinyāsa.* Similarly, there is *mahāmudrā,* which can be looked upon as a combination of *baddhakoṇāsana* and *paścimatāna.* When continued with *vīrāsana,* we have *triyaṅgmukha-ekapādam,* and so on.

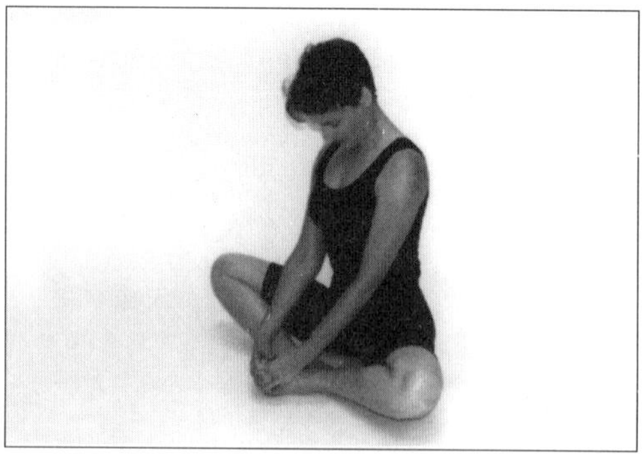

*Baddhakoṇāsana*

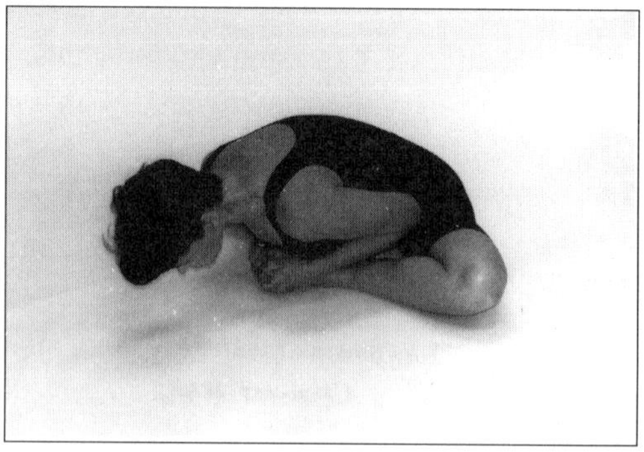

*Baddhakoṇāsana* (forward bend)

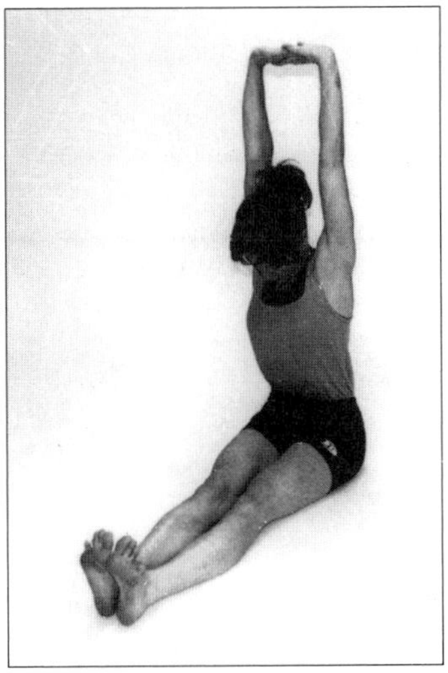

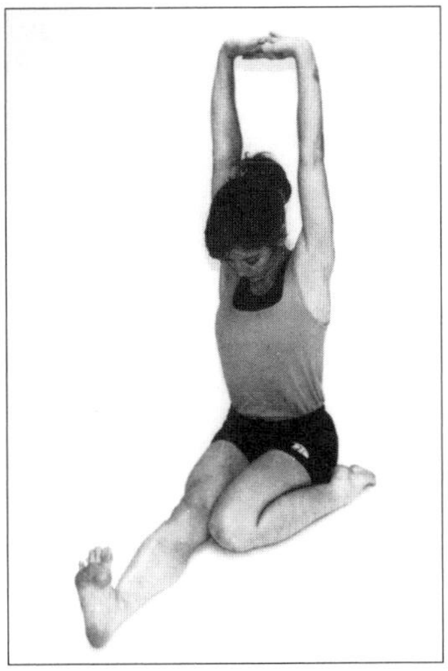

*Daṇḍāsana*
(preparation for *triyaṅgmukha*)

*Triyaṅgmukha sthiti*

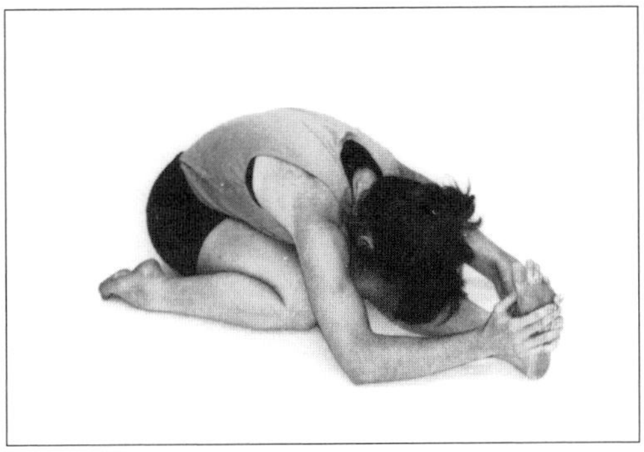

*Triyaṅgmukha-ekapāda-paścima-uttānāsana*

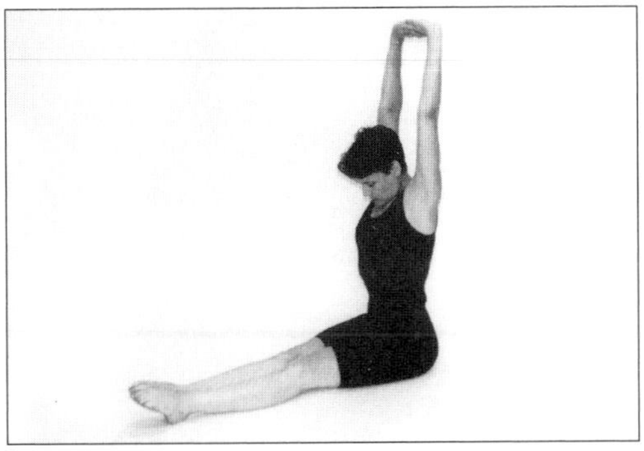

*Daṇḍāsana*
(Stage 1 for *prasāritapāda*)

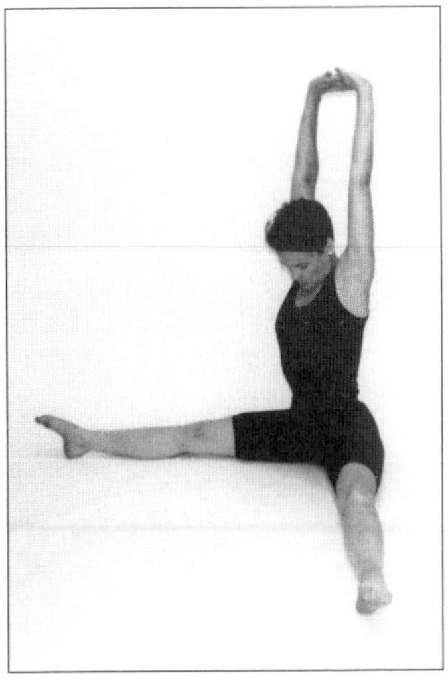

*Upaviṣṭhakoṇāsana sthiti*

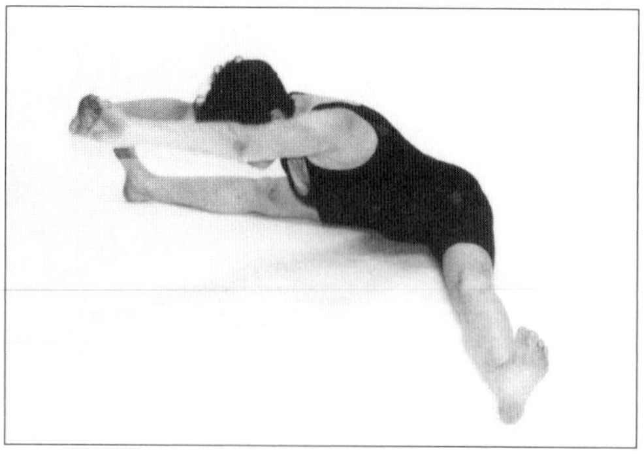

*Upaviṣṭhakoṇāsana*
(movement)

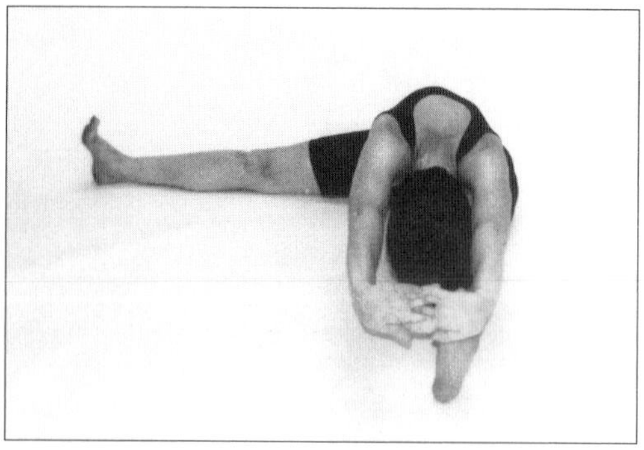

*Upaviṣṭhakoṇāsana (pārśva)*

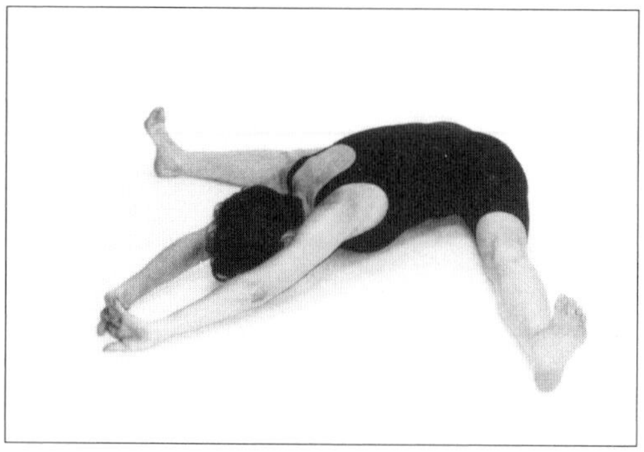

*Upaviṣṭhakoṇāsana*
(forward bend)

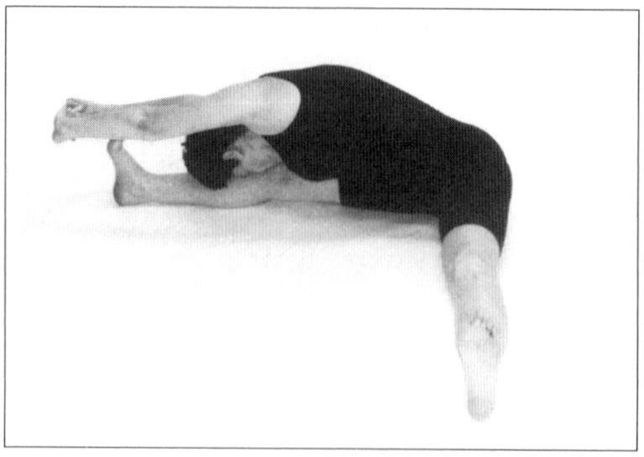

*Upaviṣṭhkoṇāsana* (*dakṣina-pārśva*, or right side)

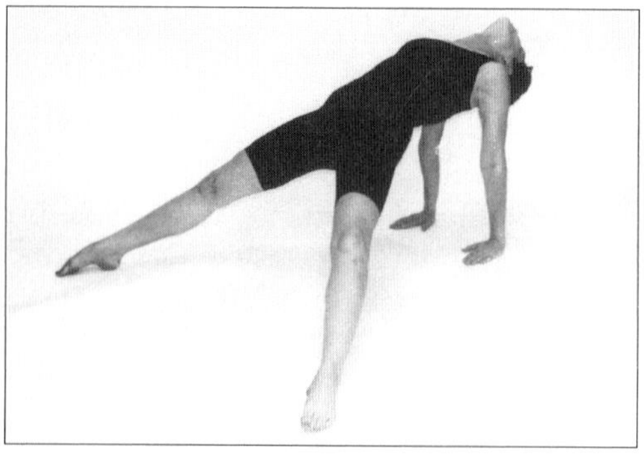

*Upaviṣṭhakoṇāsana (pratikriyā)*

# 12 *Padmāsana* and Other Postures for *Yoga Sādhana*

THE *HAṬHAYOGAPRADĪPIKĀ* OF SVĀTMĀRĀMA discusses *āsanas* first because they form the first stage of *haṭhayoga*. The text says that *āsanas* make one firm and free from diseases, and also make one feel extremely light and flexible. In his commentary *Jyotsnā* on the *Haṭhayogapradīpikā*, Brahmānanda says that *āsana* practice makes one firm because it weakens the *rajoguṇa (āsanena rajo hanti)* that cause fickleness (*vikṣepa* of the *citta*). Since *āsanas* eradicate diseases, they help the mind to concentrate. According to Patañjali, diseases *(vyādhi),* dullness *(sthyāna),* doubt *(samśaya),* inattention *(pramāda),* sloth *(ālasya),* worldliness *(avirati),* false notions *(bhrāntidarśana),* and instability *(anavsthita)* are the causes of the distraction of the mind, and as such are the obstacles for material or spiritual progress. Although it is impossible to explain clearly and thus realize the important truths that underlie the various *āsanas,* and until the human system is understood in all its intricacy and detail, suffice it to say that the various *āsanas* bring about many important results—physical, physiological, psychological, and spiritual. For instance, various nerve centers are activated in *āsana* practice, and these are effective in helping to control the irregularities of the body; what is more fascinating but no less true is the purification of the mental process that results—the mind becomes more and more attentive *(ekāgra).*

# *Padmāsana* and Variations

*Padmāsana* is one of the well-known *āsanas* and holds pride of place among sitting postures. It easily fits into Patañjali's dictum that an *āsana* be *sthira sukham āsanam,* that is, "steady and comfortable." *Padmāsana,* especially its important variation *baddhapadmāsana,* completely immobilizes the limbs and gives steadiness to the yogi's posture. The stretching experienced in all the stubborn joints—the neck, shoulders, elbows, wrists, lower back, hips, knees, ankles, and toes—makes it a complete posture. It gives one a firm foundation to sit for *prāṇāyāma, japa,* or study. No doubt it holds the fascination of many yoga aspirants.

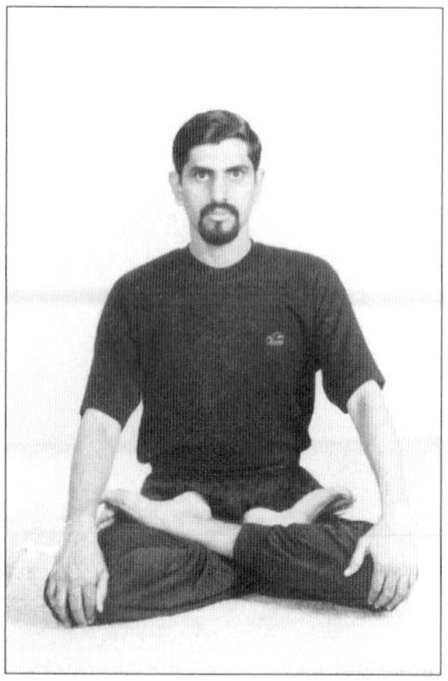

*Padmāsana*

According to Śrī Sureśvarācārya, the first *pīṭhādhipati* of Śrīngeri Śaṅkara Maṭh, *padmāsana,* along with *svastika, gomukha,* and *haṃsa āsanas,* are known as *brahmāsanas,* as is mentioned in the last *ullāsa* (chapter) in *Mānasollāsa,* an authentic and elaborate commentary on Śrī Śaṅkarabhagavatpāda's *Dakṣiṇāmūrthi Aṣṭakam.* The *narasiṃha, garuḍa, kūrma,* and *nāga āsanas* are known to be Vaiṣṇavite, while *vīra, mayūra, vajra,* and *siddha* are Rudra *āsanas. Yonyāsana* is known among Śākta groups, and *pascima-uttānāsana* is a Śaivite *āsana.*

The *vinyāsakrama* to reach *padmāsana* would require starting from *samasthiti* and proceeding to *daṇḍāsana,* the same *āsana* that is the intermediate stage in *paścimatānam. Daṇḍāsana* is the posture for all sitting *āsanas.* Sit up and stretch your legs, keeping your back straight. Exhale deeply, bend your right leg, and draw your right foot closer to your body with your hands, keeping it on top of your left thigh, in line with your groin. On the next exhalation, in similar fashion, bend your left knee and place your left foot on top of your right thigh. Now you have a very firm base upon which to sit and your lower back is relieved of the outward curve normally required to keep your body balanced. Now, with your palms fully covering their respective knees, stretch your arms, spine, and neck and place your chin on the center of your breastbone, making *jālandhara bandha.* Breathe normally, making a hissing noise through the partially closed glottis. This is *padmāsana.* After a few breaths, do the posture with your left knee bent first. Initially, there no doubt will be excruciating pain for some, but with deep exhalation, one should be able to slowly relax and repeat the movements. Those who are not used to squatting may have problems, especially in the early stages. Don't force the bending of your knees. Many people have left yoga after a vigorous attempt to do *padmāsana* in a hurry. But once the initial resistance is overcome, one will slowly start to experience the relaxing effects of *padmāsana*, which is undoubtedly a marvel among *yogāsanas*. One feels extremely secure and on a firm base, and the lower back enjoys freedom and a comfort unknown even on the most cozy of sofas. The body is erect but relaxed. The mind will naturally become relaxed and alert, unperturbed by the postural distractions. Those prone to rheumatism and stiffness in their knee joints will find benefits.

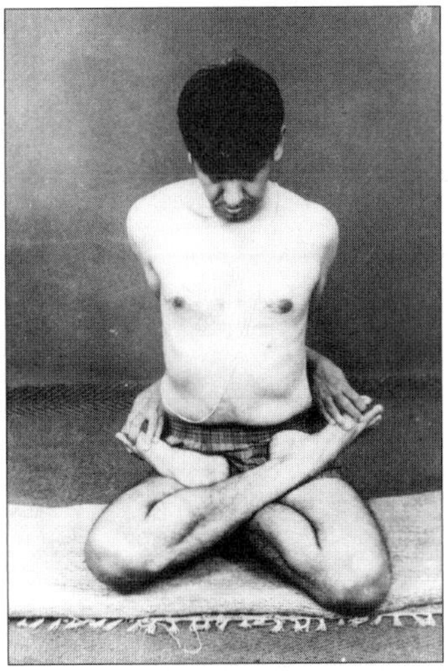

*Baddhapadmāsana*
(with *bandhas*)

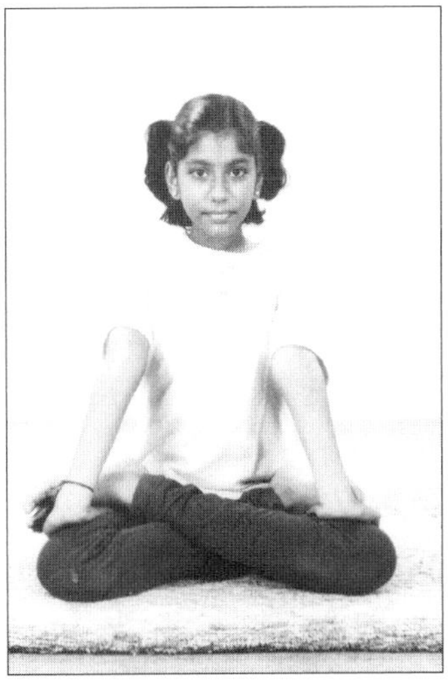

*Bhadrāsana*

After a few breaths, one may practice *mūla bandha* and *uddīyāna bandha*. Thus it is possible to practice *bandhatraya* (all three *bandhas*) in *padmāsana*. It is a good posture for *prāṇāyāma*, meditation, and *saṃyamas*. There are a number of variations in *padmāsana* that help to improve circulation and strength, and to develop the body proportionally.

The next variation is *bhadrāsana* (*bharadra* means "peace.") Sit in *padmāsana*. Inhale and raise your arms. On exhalation, lower your arms and keep your palms on their respective thighs with fingers pointing inward. Stretch your elbows, raise your trunk, and maintain *jālandhara bandha*. Do between six and twelve long inhalations and exhalations with the *bandhas*. This is very good for the wrists, shoulders, neck, and spine. Inhale and raise your arms overhead, interlock your fingers, and stretch your spine, shoulders, neck, elbows, and wrists. Keep your chin locked in *jālandhara bandha*. This is *parvatāsana* (*parvata* means "hill"). This posture helps

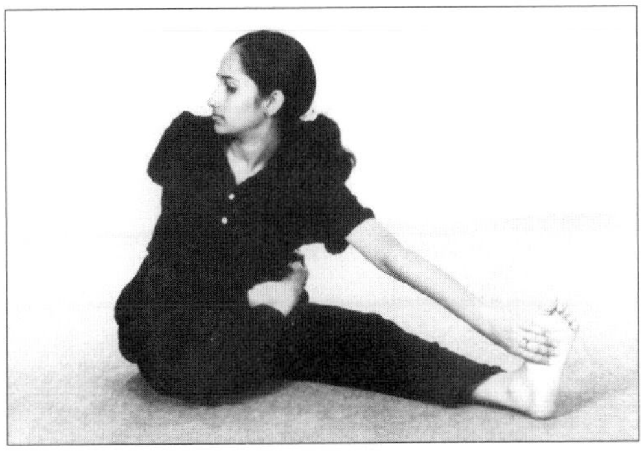

*Ardhamatsyendrāsana*
(in *ardhapadmāsana*)

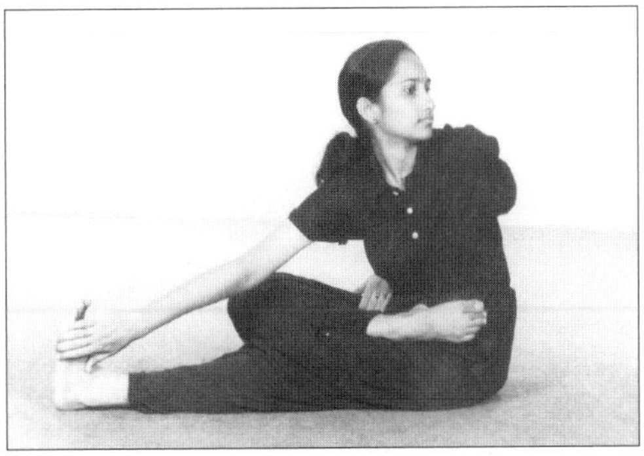

*Ardhamatsyendrāsana (vinyāsa)*

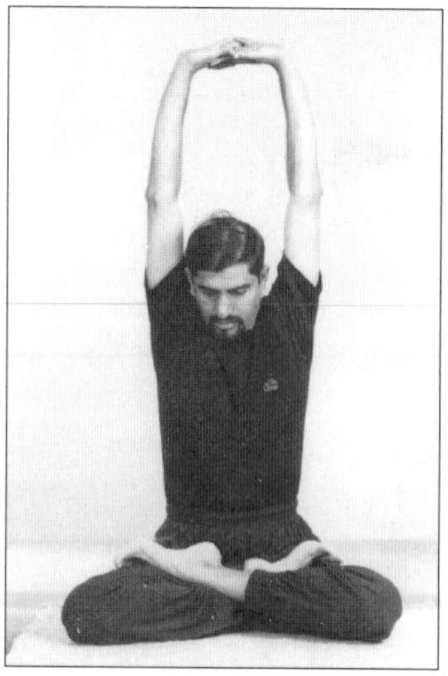

*Parvatāsana*

to develop the shoulders and makes the shoulder joints supple. Deep inhalation also helps to expand the chest and is especially useful for children, teenagers, and young men and women. It also helps to stretch the abdominal muscles, and it is beneficial to those suffering from respiratory ailments. After six to twelve breaths, exhale, bend at the elbows, lower your arms, and keep your palms behind the back of the neck, with your palms facing upward, your elbows pointing outward, and your shoulder blades touching each other. On inhalation, raise your arms, and on exhalation, lower them with good stretching of your neck and shoulder muscles. Repeat three to six times.

From *parvatāsana*, exhale deeply and bend forward, touching the floor with your forehead and keeping your arms stretched outward. This is particularly good for those who suffer from constipation and irregular or erratic peristalsis. It helps improve digestion and relieve flatulence. Yogis belonging to the *kuṇḍalinī* school of yoga credit it with the awakening of *kuṇḍalinī*. Stay for a few breaths and then return to *parvatāsana*. Another variation requires placing the top of the head on the floor instead of the forehead. From *parvatāsana*, exhale, and, rolling your shoulders back, keep your palms behind you, about one foot away from your buttocks, leaving about one foot between them. Inhale, press your palms and knees, raise your trunk, and stretch your neck backward. This acts as a counterpose to *yogamudrā*. The front portion of the torso is stretched, and the lower back also gets massaged. The wrists, elbows, arms, and neck get relieved of the slight pain encountered in such postures as *yogamudrā, parvatāsana,* and so on. After about six breaths, exhale and return to *padmāsana;* if raising the trunk is done while exhaling, this is *langhana kriyā*. From *pārvatāsana*, slowly exhale, round your back, raise your knees a bit, and completely lie down on your back, with arms stretched overhead and fin-

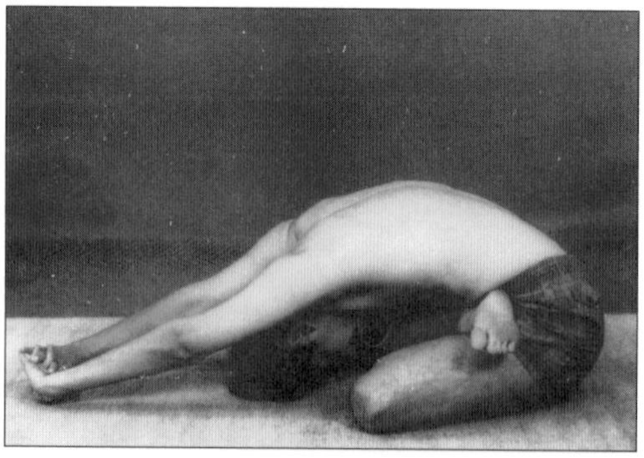

*Yogamudrā*

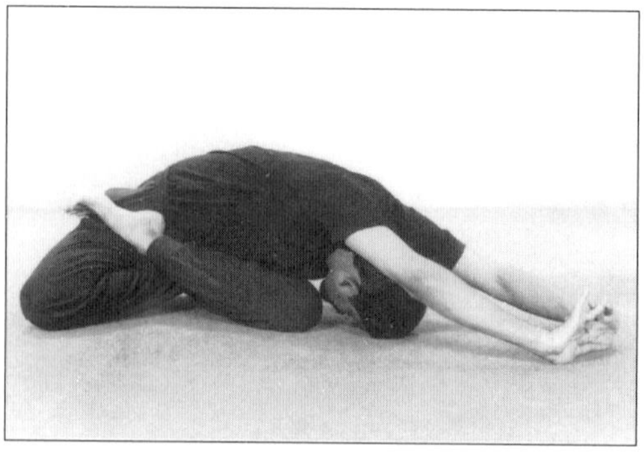

*Yogamudrā (pārśva)*

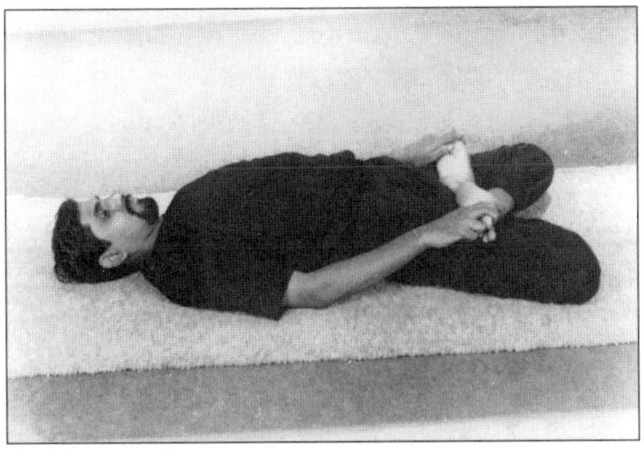

*Suptapadmāsana*

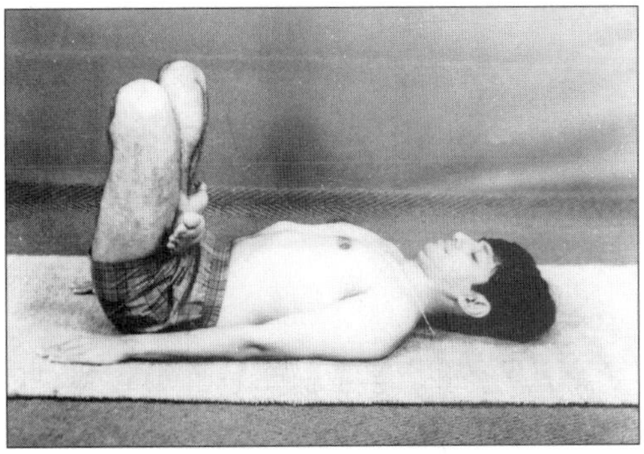

*Suptapadmāsana (vinyāsa)*

gers interlocked, and the *padma* portion (crossed legs) also on the floor. Stay for a few breaths, doing *mūla* and *uddīyāna bandhas* after exhalation. Exhale, lower your arms, and hold your toes. Try to stretch your spine and keep it on the floor; your neck should also be stretched so that your chin is not pointing upward but toward the chest. Close your eyes and do a few breaths. This is known as *suptapadmāsana* (*supta* means "lying down"). Now place your palms on the floor by the sides of your body, press your palms, and on exhaling raise the *padma* portion up to about ninety degrees and then, inhaling, return to *suptapadmāsana*. Repeat the movements six times. This helps to work on the lower hips and also helps to counter the ache one may develop owing to the stretching of the back in *suptapadmāsana*.

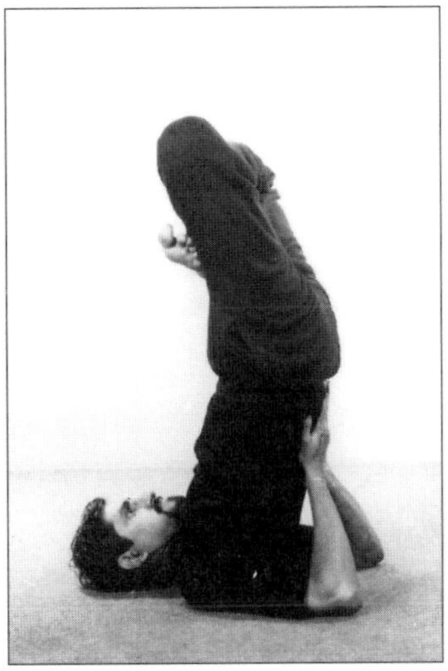

*Ūrdhvapadmāsana*

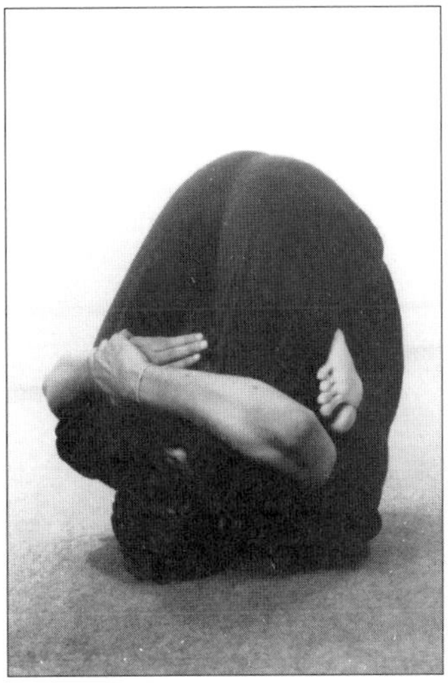

*Piṇḍāsana*

The posture *ūrdhvapadmāsana*, described in chapter 9, was included as a variation of *sarvāṅgāsana*. The same *āsana* can be done from *suptapadmāsana*. Exhale and raise your trunk as in *sarvāṅgāsana*, but instead of your legs being straight, they are in *padmāsana*. Stay for a few breaths. To proceed to *piṇḍāsana*, return to *parvatāsana* and sit in *padmāsana*. Extend your arms forward and place your palms on the floor. Now exhale, raise your hips, and stand on your knees with the support of your palms. Flex your elbows and lie facedown, so that your entire body, with legs in *padmāsana*, is on the ground. Now inhale, press your palms and knees, and raise

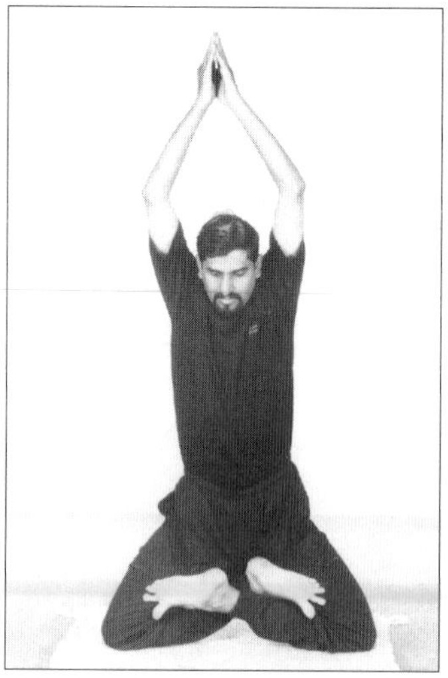

*Gorakṣāsana*

your trunk, stretching your arms, elbows, and shoulders. This is *adhomukhapadmāsana*. Stay for a few breaths. Then, pressing your palms and exhaling, slowly push your back and body so that you sit in *padmāsana,* and then stretch your upper body forward into *yogamudrā*. Inhale and raise your trunk back to *parvatāsana*.

*Padmāsana* and its variations can be practiced in a series and was recommended by our *ācārya* to attain *āsana siddhi* and to derive the maximum benefit of each variation. It saves time and ensures that one exercises all the parts of the body. This *vinyāsakrama* in *padmāsana* can be done as follows:

1. *padmāsana*
2. *parvatāsana*
3. *suptapadmāsana*
4. *ūrdhvapadmāsana*
5. *piṇḍāsana*
6. *parvatāsana*
7. *adhomukhapadmāsana*
8. *yogamudrā*
9. *ūrdhvamukhapadmāsana*
10. *parvatāsana*
11. *padmāsana*

*Adhomukhapadmāsana*

This series should be done a few times along with the recommended breathing. Then repeat it, changing the leg position. This group is exceptionally good for toning up all the usual stiff and stubborn joints, and makes knees, hips, and shoulders more flexible;

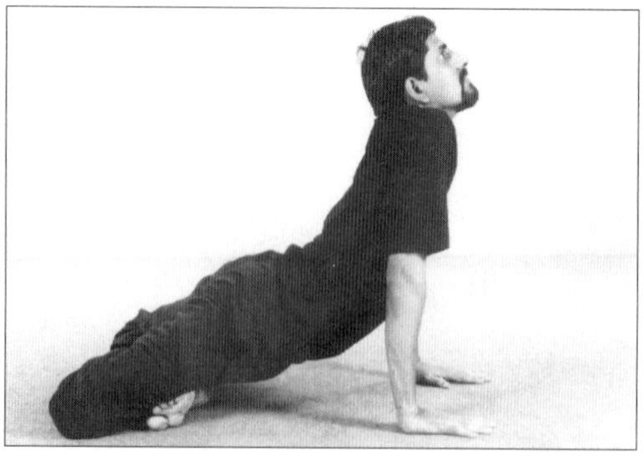

*Adhomukhapadmāsana (vinyāsa)*

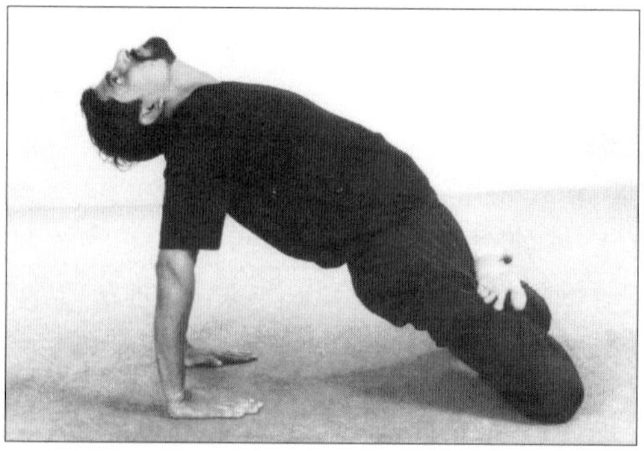

*Ūrdhvamukhapadmāsana*

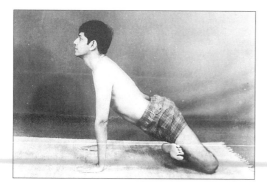

it also improves stamina, circulation, and general well-being. It is a compact and a very useful group to practice for young men and women. There are a number of other, more difficult variations. One of them is *baddhapadmāsana*. It is described as *padmāsanam* in the *Haṭhayogopradīpikā:*

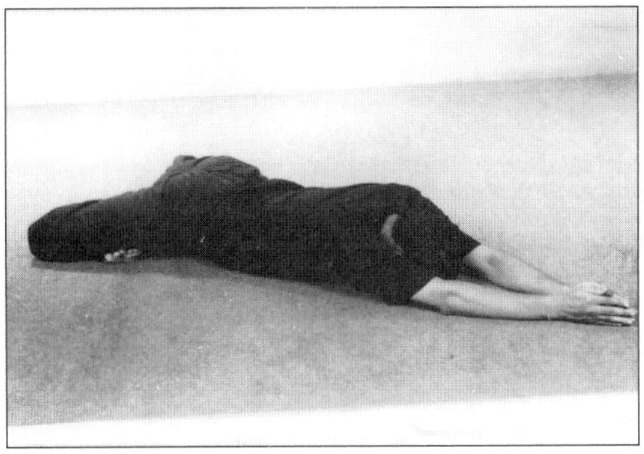

Adhomukhapadmāsana (vinyāsa)

*Vamorūpari dakṣinam*
*Caraṇam samsthāpya vāmam*
*tathā.*
*Dakṣinorūpari paścimenavidhinā*
*Dhṛtvā karābhyām dhṛḍham*
*Āṅguṣṭau hṛdaye nidhāya*
*Cibukam nāsagramālokayeth*
*Yetaṭḥ vyādhivināśakārī*
*Yamīnām padmāsanam procyate.*

"Place the right foot on the left thigh and the left foot on the right thigh, cross the hands behind the back [your own back, of course!], and firmly take hold of the toes [the right toe with the right hand and the left toe with the left hand]. Place the chin on the breastbone and gaze at the tip of the nose *(nāsāgra)*. This is called *padmāsanam*. It destroys diseases for the self-restrained yogis *(yamis)*."

*Baddhapadmāsana* requires subtle control of the deep muscles of the shoulders and legs. It is a very deep-cleansing exercise that is exceptionally beneficial. If one can stay in the posture, one can do long inhalations and exhalations. As noted by Svātmārāma, and also by authorities like my *ācārya*, it removes all diseases emanating from the stomach and abdominal region. Pregnant women should not practice this *āsana*. *Padmāsana*, as mentioned before, is not merely an exquisite physical posture, but also is believed to hold the key for proper meditation and the arousal of *kuṇḍalinī*. As the *Haṭhayogapradīpikā* puts it:

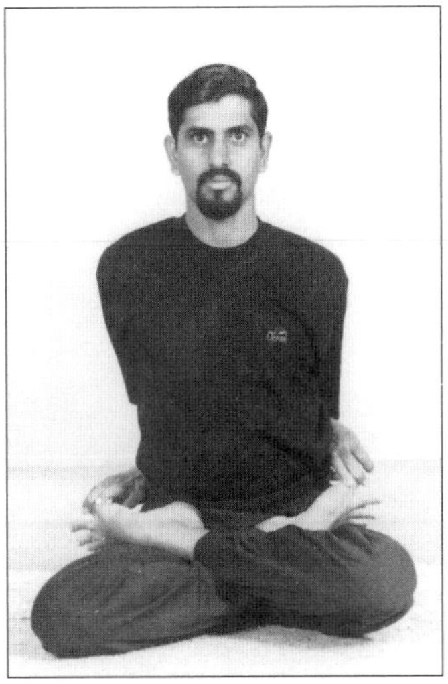

Baddhapadmāsana

> Staying well in *padmāsanam*, with the palms placed on the lap, fix the chin on the chest, and, contemplating (Brahman or *iṣṭa devatā*) in the mind *(citta)*, repeatedly raise the *apāna* upward (by contracting the anus, which is *mūla bandha*), and bring the inhaled *prāṇa* downward (after inhalation). By this a man obtains unequaled knowledge through the power of *kuṇḍalinī* (which is roused by this process).

*Yogamudrā (vinyāsa)*

It should be noted that as a further extension of the practice suggested earlier, the *mūla bandha* started after *bāhya-kumbhaka* is also maintained by some on inhalation. And by means of *mūla bandha* and *jālandhara bandha,* both the passage of the down-going *apāna* and the up-going *prāṇa* are sealed, so to speak. Then by forcing the *prāṇa* downward and the *apāna* upward, the union of *apāna* and *prāṇa* is achieved. This is also referred to in the Bhagavad Gītā. By the union of *prāṇa* and *apāna*, the *jāṭharāgni* (gastric activity) is aroused, and the mythical *kuṇḍalinī,* awakened by the heat of the gastric fire, straightens out from its coiled position and moves upward in the *suṣumṇā.* The *prāṇa* and *apāna* are forced through the *suṣumṇā,* and the union of these two takes place, which is the ultimate goal of *haṭhayoga.* Suffice it to say that *padmāsana* is an excellent posture for physical, physiological, and psychological well-being as well as for mystical and spiritual experiences.

After a strenuous stint in the various *padmāsana* variations, one may wish to enjoy the relaxation obtained by such exercises. *Śanmukhīmudrā* helps in directing the attention inward. It is also known as *yonimudrā.* There are some schools that-state that it is also known as *sāmbhavīmudrā.*

Sit in *padmāsana* or another convenient posture like *siddhāsana—vajrāsana* may also be chosen—but *padmāsana* appears to be the best. Keep your back erect and head level, without the *jālandhara bandha.* Raise your arms, keeping your elbows at shoulder level. Close your ears with your thumbs and place your forefingers and middle fingers over your closed eyelids, the forefinger above and the middle finger below the position of the eyeballs. You should not press the eyes hard, but maintain a very mild pressure so that it is barely felt. Your ring fingers should partially close your nostrils and your little fingers are kept at the side of your closed mouth. The attention is directed toward the middle of the eyebrows. One may follow the breath. Stay for about five minutes. This is a very relaxing procedure and may be adopted after a strenuous day's work, or even before starting or after *prāṇāyāma.* Since the senses are under control, it helps to calm the mind, especially when practiced in a noiseless, clean place devoid of unpleasant odors and other distractions. It is a good exercise for *pratyāhāra,* or cleansing the senses by withdrawing them and directing them inward. In fact, it is considered one of the methods of *pratyāhāra.*

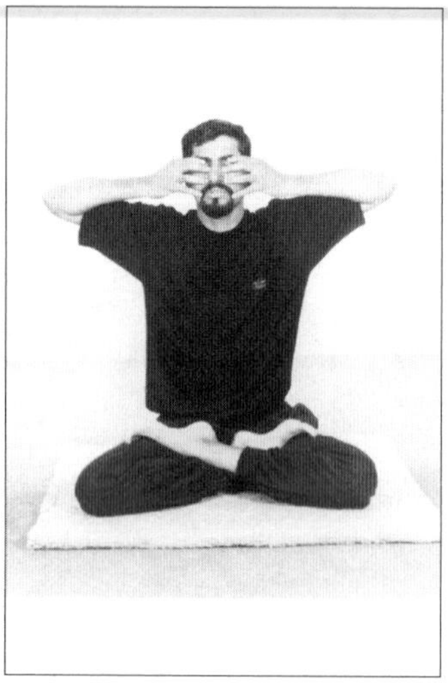

*Śanmukhīmudrā* in *padmāsana*

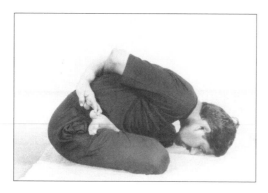

Whether it is *śīrṣāsana*, *sarvāṅgāsana*, or sitting postures such as *padmāsana*, after considerable practice the body adjusts to the different positions and a certain delightful feeling starts flowing. It manifests as a slow rhythmic breathing and indicates perfection in the posture *(āsana siddhi)*. The beneficial effects mentioned by *ācāryas* and ancient yoga texts then start accruing. The capacity to stay comfortably and steadily in a posture should be acquired, for then *prāṇāyāma* and *dhyāna* become easier, and beneficial. For the purpose of more intimate practices like *prāṇāyāma* and the *antaraṅga sādhana*, such as meditation on one's *iṣṭa devatā*, certain specific sitting *āsanas* are normally practiced.

*Padmāsana* with its *vinyāsas* has been described. A few more important sitting—or, as they are more commonly known among modern yoga practitioners, "meditative"—postures will now be taken up. The first, *siddhāsana*, like *padmāsana*, is equally well known and practiced. Texts like the *Gheraṇḍa Saṃhitā*, the Śiva Saṃhitā, the *Haṭhayogapradīpikā*, and others refer to *siddhāsana* as an important one. There are, however, slight variations in the practice of this *āsana*, and many texts refer to them as well.

Start with *samasthiti*. Inhale, raising your arms overhead; exhale, and do *utkaṭāsana*. Then, keeping your palms by the side of your buttocks, squat, and, inhaling, stretch your legs straight, keeping your knees and ankles together. This is the starting point of all sitting postures and is known as *daṇḍāsana*.

On the exhale, spread your left leg and flex the knee, keeping the heel on the *yoniṣṭhāna*. Stretch your ankle, keeping your toes pointing outward and your heel along the groin and thigh. On the next exhalation, in a similar fashion, bend your right knee and keep your right ankle on top of your outstretched left ankle, so that your right heel is on top of your generative organs and pressing against the pubis. Your right lateral malleolus should be between your left medial malleolus and heel. Then, keeping your back straight, you should close your eyes and direct your attention toward the middle of the eyebrows. The Śiva Saṃhitā recommends *pavanābhyāsa*, or the practice of *prāṇāyāma*, in this posture, and according to it, Lord Śiva's instruction to Pārvati is that there is no posture more potentially beneficial than this one. Since one has to practice *prāṇāyāma* and meditation in *siddhāsana*, naturally the *mūla*, *uḍḍīyāna*, and *jālandhara bandhas* can all be practiced in this posture. *Mūla bandha* is helped by the pressure on the *yoniṣṭhāna*, which is actually the perineum. In his commentary on *Haṭhayogapradīpikā*, Brahmānanda refers to *yoniṣṭhāna* as *gudhaupasthayohmadhyam*, "the place between the rectum and the generative organs," in which place is the perineum. This posture is comparatively easy for some who may have difficulty with *padmāsana*, and since there is pressure on the



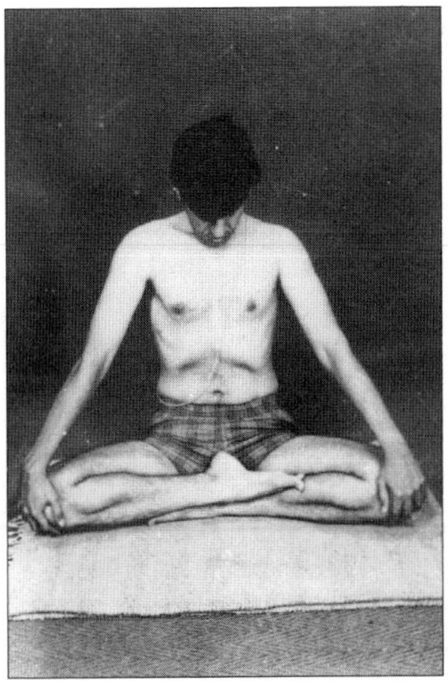

*Siddhāsana* with three *bandhas*

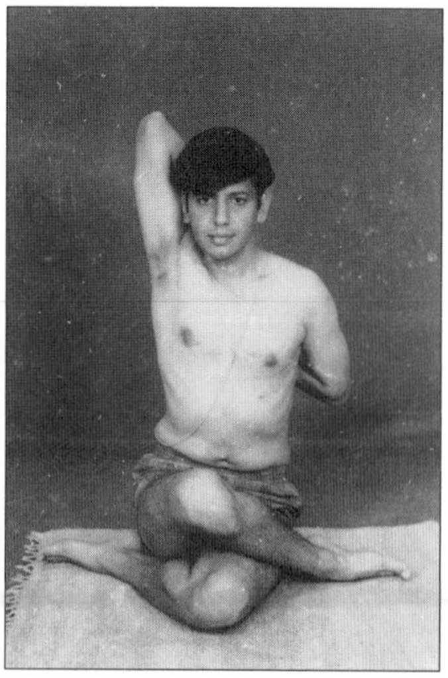
Gomukhāsana

pubic region and rectum, it evidently works on *kuṇḍalinī*. More specifically, *siddhāsana* helps in the early stages of hemorrhoids and improves circulation in the knees, lower back, and abdomen. With practice, the stubborn sacroiliac joint becomes more flexible. After some time, it is refreshingly relaxing.

Another sitting posture is *gomukhāsana*, or cow-faced posture. Start with the initial sitting position. Exhale and place your left outstretched ankle by the side of your left buttock. On the next exhalation, keep your right ankle by the side of your left buttock. Then, keeping your palms on your heels and slowly pressing, raise your buttocks and adjust the position of your knees so that one is exactly over the other. Stay for a few breaths and repeat on the other side. The disposition of the limbs resembles the face of a cow *(gomukhasya akriti).* The two knees with the gap in between resemble the mouth, the shin, the side of the face; and the feet, the ears. The chin is kept in *jālandhara bandha.* As a variation, raise one arm over your head and, bending your elbow, lower your forearm onto your back between the shoulders. Your other arm is lowered, elbow bent, forearm raised up. Clasp the fingers of the downward hand with those of the other hand. Repeat on the other side. You may stay for a few breaths. People who have disproportionately heavy thighs and buttocks may attempt to practice *gomukhāsana* and derive great advantage. The normally dormant group of muscles in the lower back and buttocks, such as the gluteus and iliac are well stretched and get a good blood supply. One attains a certain measure of sphincteric control with this posture as well. Men should practice it carefully, especially while crossing the legs (in the initial stages) ,to avoid any pressure on the scrotum.

How many *āsanas* are there? There are different answers even among the ancient yoga exponents. According to the *Gheraṇḍa Saṃhitā,* there are as many *āsanas* as there are animal species, and the author proceeds to state that, according to Lord Śiva, there are eighty-four thousand *āsanas,* of which, according to him, eighty-four are the best and thirty-two the most beneficial.

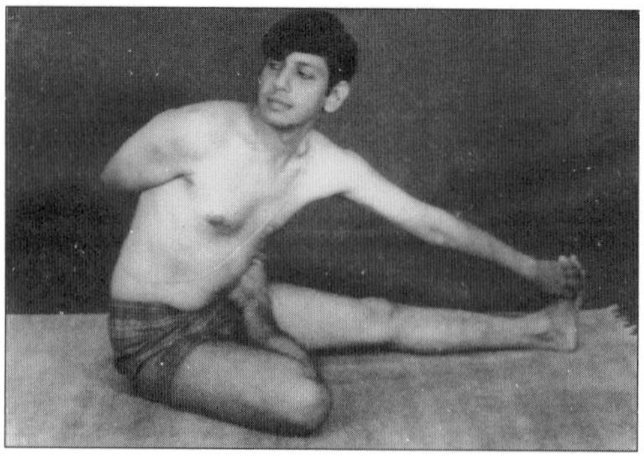
Ardhapadmāsana (vinyāsa)

In addition to *āsanas* that resemble various species of animals, there are *āsanas* that resemble other things such as a lotus (*padma),* mountain *(parvata),* and a stick (*daṇḍa*), as well as a desk *(dvipāda pitha),* a table *(catuṣpādapīṭham),* and so on. Further, there are *āsanas* whose names derive purely from the positions of the limbs and organs or the effect they have on the system, such as *jaṭharaparivṛtti* (activating the stomach) and *paścima-uttāna* (posterior stretching). Then there are the classical *āsanas* based on the names of the *ṛṣis* who are supposed to have discovered and perhaps used them for *tapas.* Examples include *bharadvājāsana, vasiṣṭh-āsana, dūrvāsāsana, kapilāsana, buddhāsana,* and *viśvā-mitrāsana.* Then there are *āsanas* named after the *avatāras* of the *trimūrtis* and other gods. These include, for example, *trivikramāsana, skand-āsana, bhairavāsana, vīrab-hadrāsana, yoganarasiṃhāsana,* and *naṭarājāsana.* Additionally, if the various *vinyāsas* are considered, one can appreciate the amount and scope of the research the ancients have done in the domain of the physical and how they brought this understanding to perfection. One group of *ṛṣis* practiced and developed yoga as an art. Just as a sculptor takes an otherwise formless stone and converts it into a beautiful work of art, the yogi used his own body and made it a beautiful, well-sculpted, perfect, live object. Approaching yoga, even on only a physical level, can be highly satisfying, matching any other art in its content, complexity, and divinity.

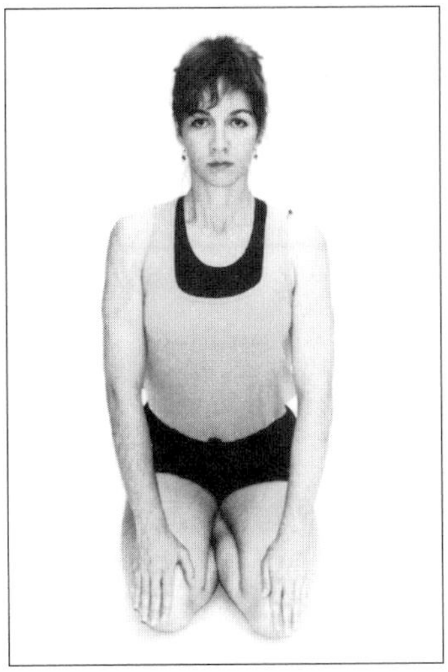

*Siṃhāsana* (position)

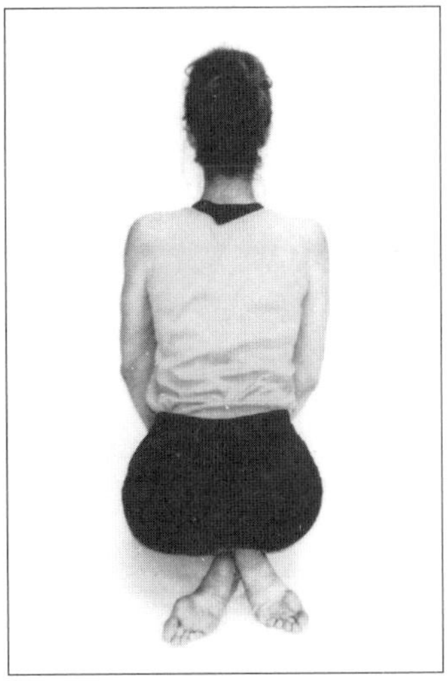

*Siṃhāsana* (rear view)

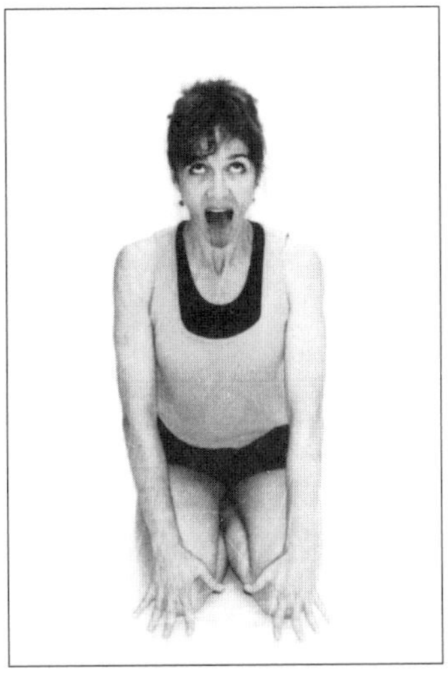

*Siṃhāsana*

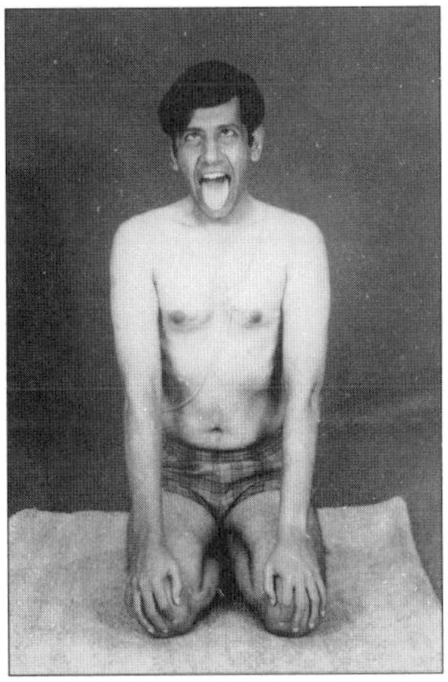

*Siṃhāsana* (with *dṛṣṭi* and no *bandhas*)

*Siṃhāsana* is another important sitting posture, derived from observing a lion waiting for its prey and with its tongue hanging out. Start by sitting erect and keeping your legs stretched in front. Exhale, and put each of your heels below the opposite thigh, that is, your left heel below the right thigh and your right heel below the

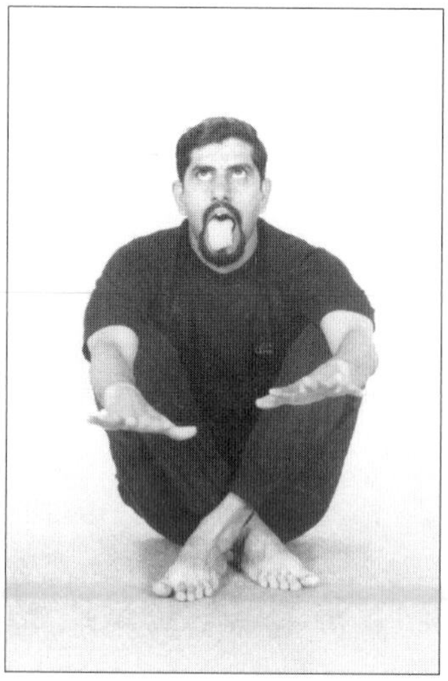

*Narasiṃhāsana*

left, just to the side of the scrotum. You should actually be sitting on your heels, with your ankles stretched and your shins on the floor. Keep your palms on their respective knees, with your fingers stretched and slightly apart. Open your mouth, stretching your jaw, and hang your tongue out as much as possible—exposing the throat, as it were. With open eyes, squint slightly and look at the top of your nose *(nāsāgra).* Breathe through your mouth for a while. According to Svātmārāma, this posture will also be helpful in mastering the three *bandhas.* This is true because in postures in which one is seated with buttocks on the ground, the anal muscles are not free to move; whereas in this case, since one sits elevated, as it were, on the heels, the *mūla bandha* is easier to do. One incidental advantage of this posture is that it helps in ventilating the oral and throat regions that harbor bacteria. One of the causes of bad breath is that the throat region is generally not kept clean. While *dantaśuddhi* (cleaning the teeth) keeps out bad breath, this aeration of the throat region will help oral hygiene to a greater extent. It should also be noted that from the rectum up to the tip of the tongue, the entire alimentary system is pulled up, as it were, providing a good tonic effect on the whole digestive system. Certain schools refer to this *āsana* as *yoganarasiṃhāsana.* Other variations of *siṃhāsana* are to stay in *adhomukhapadmāsana,* stretch the tongue out, and direct the visual attention to the *nāsāgra.* It resembles a lion ready to pounce on its prey.

The *ṛṣi* Bharadvāja is well known and said to be the father of Dronācārya. There are many others who belong to the great sage's *gotra* (lineage). The Bharadvāja group of *āsanas* basically require the twisting of the trunk in one direction and the neck and head in the opposite direction, giving a tremendous toning effect to the spine because of the torsion. The well-known posture named for this sage is a sitting one. Start with *daṇḍāsana.* Exhaling, flex your left knee and keep your ankle close and alongside your left thigh with your stretched ankles on the floor, just as in *vīrāsana.* Exhaling, bend your right knee and place your right ankle on your left thigh, high up. Sit straight with both buttocks on the floor. Now slowly exhale, hold the big toe of your right foot with the fingers of your right hand from behind. Inhale and raise your left hand; exhale and bend forward. Inhale again, raise your trunk to the erect sitting position, and, on exhaling, keep your left palm fully on the floor between your knee and buttocks, fingers turned inward and below the thigh, then turn your head to the left and look over your left shoulder. Close your eyes and do long inhalations and exhalations, stretching and twisting the spine a little more on each exhalation. Repeat on the other side. This is *bharadvājāsana.* Another variation would require sitting in *parvatāsana.* Exhaling, twist to one side keeping your interlocked palms on the floor near your thigh between your knee and buttock.

Exhale and turn your head over to the other side. This *āsana* combines the advantages of *vīrāsana* and *padmāsana* and helps to twist the spine, thus making it supple. The cervical and lumbar regions and the small back muscles are all stretched.

## *Mudrās*

*Mudrās* involve contracting a group of muscles, which also include the *bandhas*. We have already discussed some *mudrās* such as *tatākamudrā, śaṇmukhīmudrā,* and *yogamudrā,* and also *mūla, jālandhara,* and *uddīyāna*, the three famous *bandhas*. The *mudrās* should also be practiced and, with *prāṇāyāma*, are very important in *haṭhayoga*. Sage Gheraṇḍa refers to twenty-five such *mudrās*. For one of them he says, *Akuncayeth gudhadhvāram prakaśayeth punafpunaḥ sa bhavet aśvinīmudrā śaktiprabodhakārinī:* "Contracting and dilating the anal aperture—as a horse *(aśvinī)* does—in any posture in which it is convenient is called *aśvinīmudrā*. This is said to give one energy."

Many of the *āsanas, bandhas,* and *mudrās* stress the importance of keeping the muscles and *nāḍīs* of the lower part *(mūla)* of the body in good tone. According to yogic theory, many important *nāḍīs* are situated in the anal and pelvic region, and hence it is repeatedly stressed that one keep that area in good shape. Further, it is the area of the sex glands (prostate, uterus, ovaries) as well, and good muscle tone is especially essential to proper functioning. Without these *āsanas, bandhas,* and *mudrās*, these areas are never exercised. People equate yoga and other forms of physical exercise and say that yoga is as good or as bad as other games, sports, or exercises. One has to appreciate the extent to which minute muscles and *nāḍīs* are attended to in yoga, which requires enormous concentration and self-control. The yoga of our ancestors attempted to perfect the human physical system, so that whatever is best in the physical realm was achieved and experienced in full measure. *Aśvinīmudrā* can be practiced as

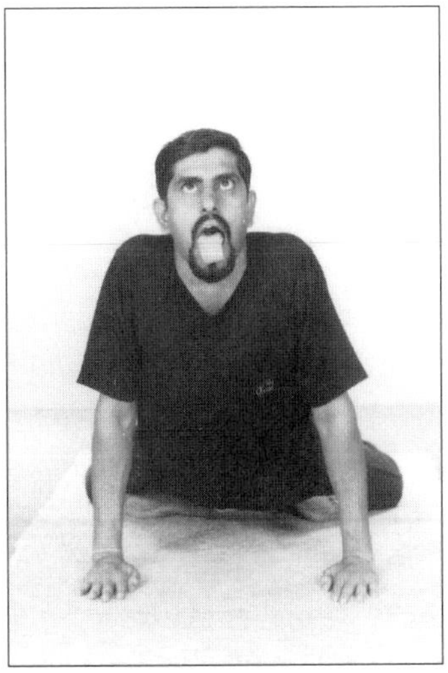

*Siṃhāsana (vinyāsa)*

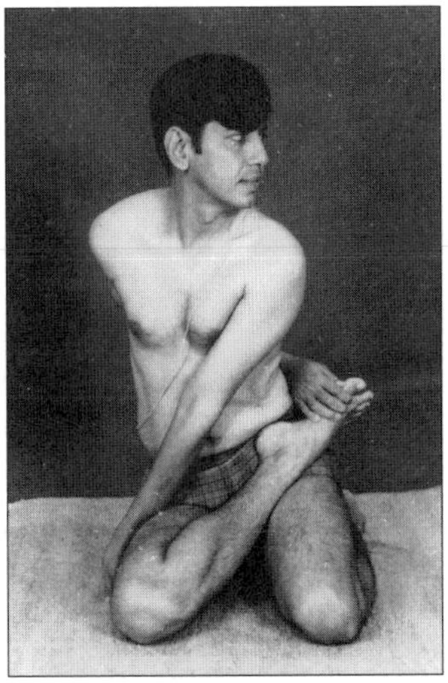

*Bharadvajāsana*

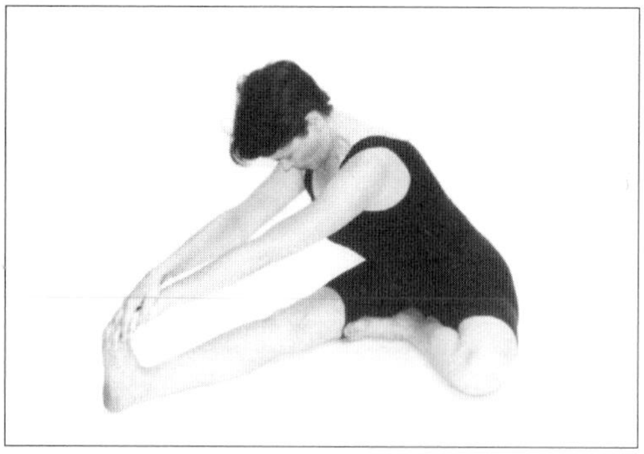

*Mahāmudrā*

a prelude to achieving perfection in *mūla bandha*. It can be learned while in certain *āsanas* such as *sarvāṅgāsana* and *śīrṣāsana*, among others.

*Mahāmudrā* is referred to in almost all the yoga texts, including the Śiva Saṃhitā, the *Gheraṇḍa Saṃhitā*, the *Haṭhayogapradīpikā*, the Dhyānabind Upaniṣad of Kṛṣṇa Yajur Veda, and the Yoga Cudamani Upaniṣad of the Sāma Veda. According to our *ācārya*, this *mudrā* should be included in one's daily practice of yoga.

Start with your legs outstretched. Press your perineum *(yoni)* with the left heel; your knee should be bent and pushed away to the side at about ninety degrees to your body. The sole of your left foot should be flush with your right thigh. Pressing the perineum, exhale and, keeping your back straight, hold the big toe of your right foot with both hands. Lock your chin for *jālandhara bandha* and practice the other *bandhas* on exhalation. Repeat for a few breaths. Change legs and repeat on the other side. According to the *Haṭhayogapradīpikā*, *mahāmudrā* helps overcome such maladies as tuberculosis, leprosy, constipation, abdominal diseases, and indigestion. Specifically, it helps tone up the pelvic organs. It is especially important for gynecological problems such as prolapse and incontinence.

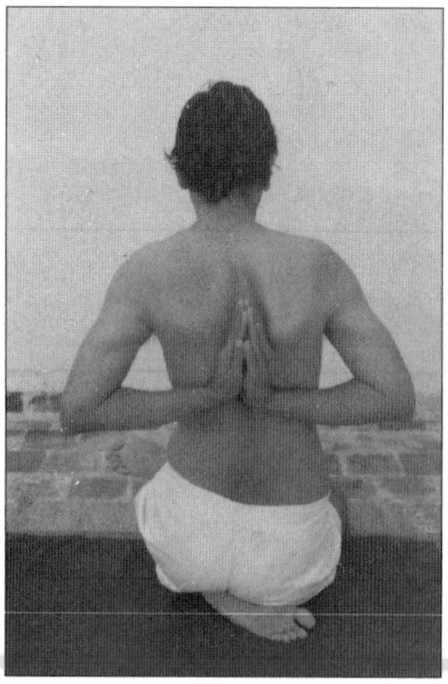

*Mahā bandha* with *pṛṣṭanjali*

Next is *mahā bandha*. Start with your legs outstretched. Exhale, bend your left knee, and sit on your heel, the heel pressing and closing the anus. On the next exhalation, keep your right foot on your left thigh, as in *padmāsana*. Keep your palms on your knees and practice the *mūla, uddīyāna,* and *jālandhara bandhas.* This is a good posture for the practice of *prāṇāyāma* with the *bandhas.* As in *siṃhāsana*, the arms are free, and *mūla bandha* becomes more effective with the pressure of the heel. Repeat on the other side. The arm position in a saluting gesture on the back can be attempted in many other postures, such as *padmāsana*, though it is not specific to *mahā bandha*. If *āsanas* are practiced with *bandhas, mudrās, vinyāsas,* proper breathing, and *prāṇāyāma*, it is better to do so under proper guidance. This has been the traditional approach for study of the *śāstras* in India.

In the Darśana Upaniṣad, which belongs to the Sāma Veda, the last *āsana* referred to is *sukhāsana*. It is recommended for those who cannot do difficult *āsanas* but who are interested in other yogic practices such as *prāṇāyāma: Yena kena prakārena, Sukham dhairyam ca jayate, Tat Sukhāsanam Ithyuktam, Asaktastat Samāśrayeth*

("In whatever way [posture] one attains comfort and steadiness, this is called *sukhāsanam.* That should be adopted by the infirm for practice of *prāṇāyāma.*"

## *Vajrāsana*

Of the many sitting postures, *vajrāsana* is comparatively easy to do and combines grace and poise. It is a good posture for *prāṇāyāma* and meditation and, when performed with synchronous breathing and movements *(vinyāsas),* it works on different joints and muscles and also helps to relax them.

Use a thick ($^1/_8$") carpet folded in two; the seat should be neither too hard nor too soft. Start from *samasthiti.* Inhale, raise your arms overhead, interlock your fingers, and turn them outward. Exhale, raise your heels, bend your knees, and come down, landing on your knees and sitting on your heels. Exhale, lower your arms, and place your palms on your bent knees. Sit, bending your legs, with knees, shins, and ankles together and stretched toes pointing outward so that you sit on your heels with your shins on the floor. Keep your palms on your knees and stretch your back. Stretch the back of your neck and place your chin a couple of inches below your neck. Throw your shoulders back a little so that the shoulder blades come closer together and form a canal along the spinal column. This is *vajrāsana.* The chin lock, *jālandhara bandha,* helps partially close the glottis and thus helps control the breathing.

Now let us see further movements and variations *(vinyāsas)* of *vajrāsana.* Interlock the fingers of both hands and turn them out. Inhaling, raise your body and your

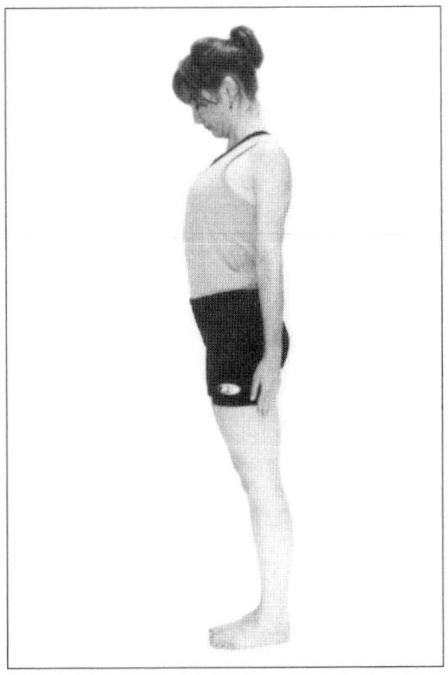

*Samasthiti*

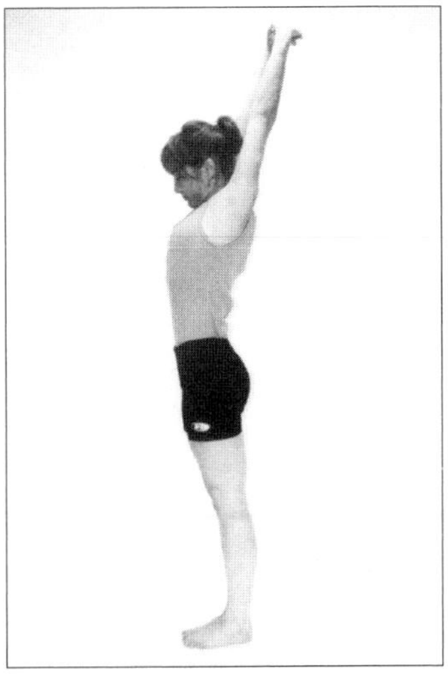

*Paḍāsana*

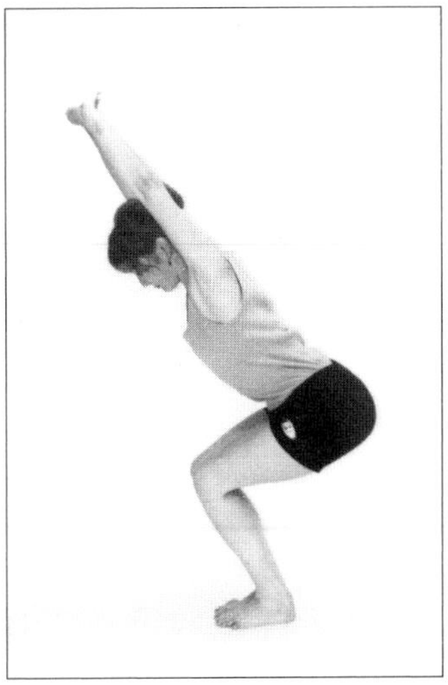

*Ardha-utkaṭāsana*

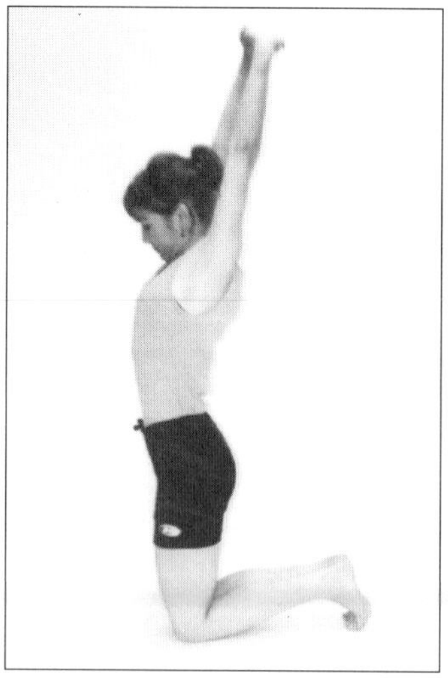

*Vajrāsana* (preparation)

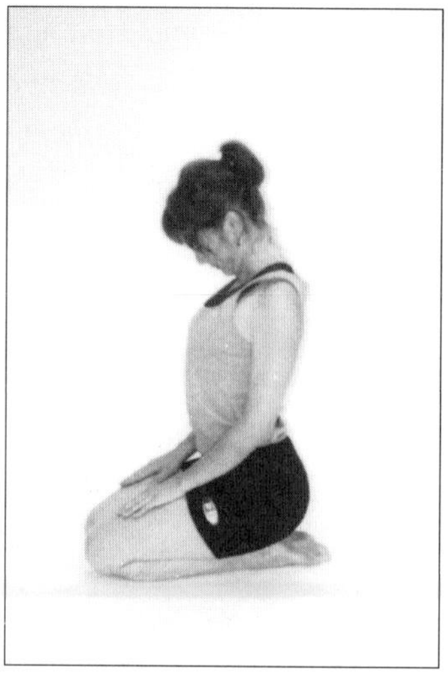

*Vajrāsana*

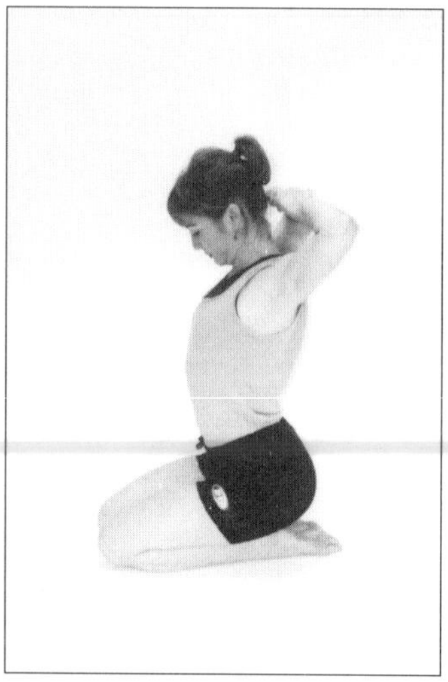

*Vajrāsana (vinyāsa)*

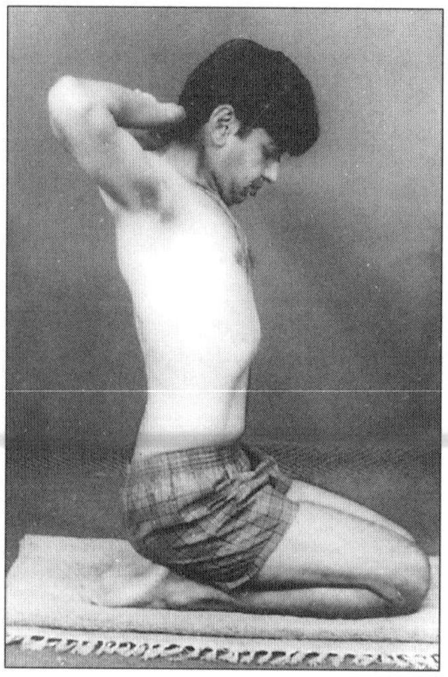

*Vajrāsana* with three *bandhas*

arms overhead. While you inhale, the chin lock will produce a hissing sound in the throat with the partial closing of the glottis. The period of inhalation and the movement of the trunk and arms should synchronize. On completion of the inhalation, you will be on your knees and the front portion of your legs. Stay for two or three seconds, holding the breath in. As you exhale, return to the original seated position. Now seated in *vajrāsana*, raise your arms on inhalation. Stay for a few seconds. On exhalation, flex at the elbows, lowering your hands to the back of your neck. Repeat three times. The next *vinyāsa* requires sitting on your heels, but bending forward so that your face touches the floor; your arms are still stretched outward. This movement—which is to be done on exhalation—should be avoided by pregnant women.

Now let us consider a counterpose for this forward movement. Exhaling, lean slightly back and keep your palms on the floor about one foot behind your legs and about one foot apart. Inhale, press your palms and the entire portion of your legs touching the floor, as well as your ankles and knees, and raise your trunk, stretching your neck and throwing your head backward. Exhale and return to the original position. Repeat about three times. Those who are obese may do the above movement of raising the trunk on exhalation, which is then called *langhana kriyā*. Return to the original position on inhalation. Pregnant women may do this movement. Those with high blood pressure need not drop the head back. An advanced *vajrāsana* variation would require the practitioner to spread the ankles about eighteen inches apart and sit between the ankles and heels, instead of on them as earlier; this variation is known as *vīrāsana*. *Vīrāsana* has many *vinyāsas*, including *paryaṅkāsana* (couch posture), variations of *bharadvājāsana*, and a host of others.

Now inhale, raise your arms, interlock your fingers and turn them outward, and raise your trunk, sitting on the shins. Exhale, and on the next inhalation arch your back and push your hips forward, and with cupped hands, bend further down and hold your heels from above. This is called *uṣṭrāsana*, or camel posture. You can stay for a few breaths, arching your back and pushing your hips forward on each inhalation. Then, as you inhale, arch your back further and, pushing your hips, place your head between your heels, as you press your heels with your palms. Then, as you inhale, stretch both arms forward and hold your knees. This

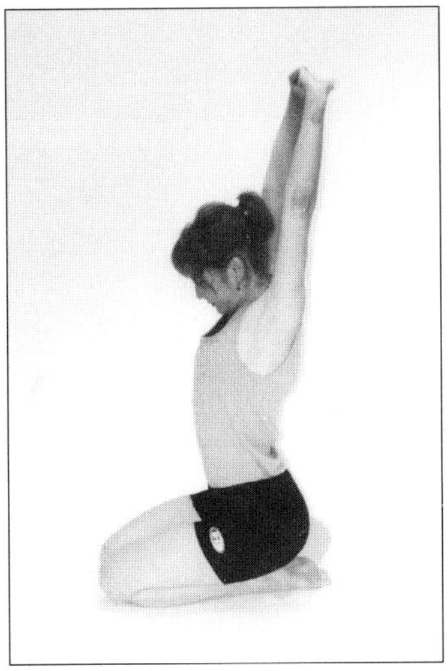

*Vajrāsana*

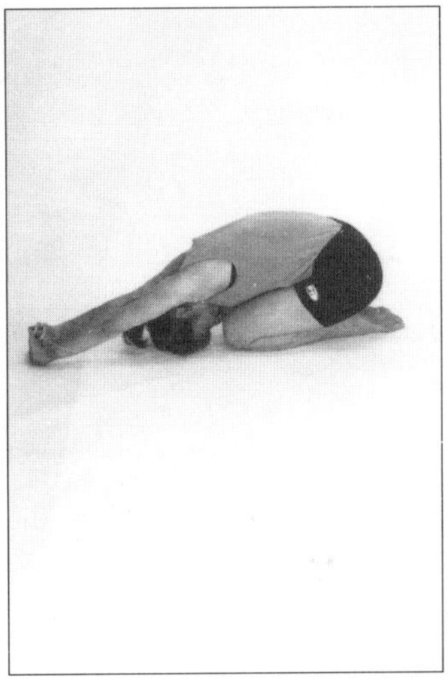

*Vajrāsana* (forward bend)

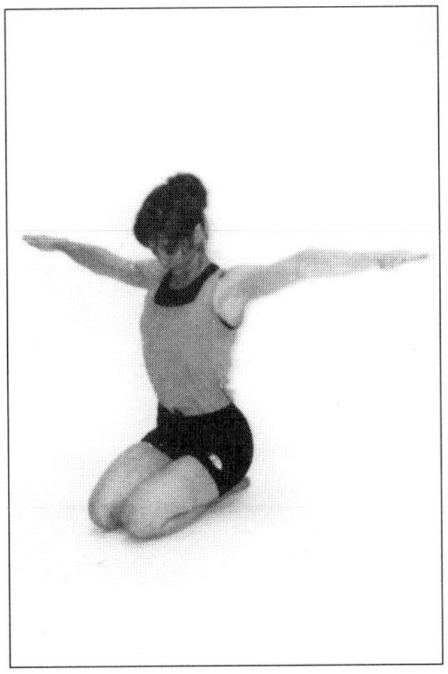

*Vajrāsana (vinyāsa)*

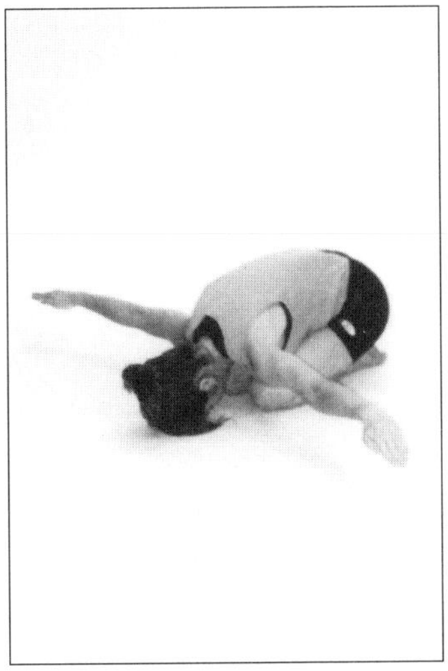

*Vajrāsana* (forward bend *vinyāsa*)

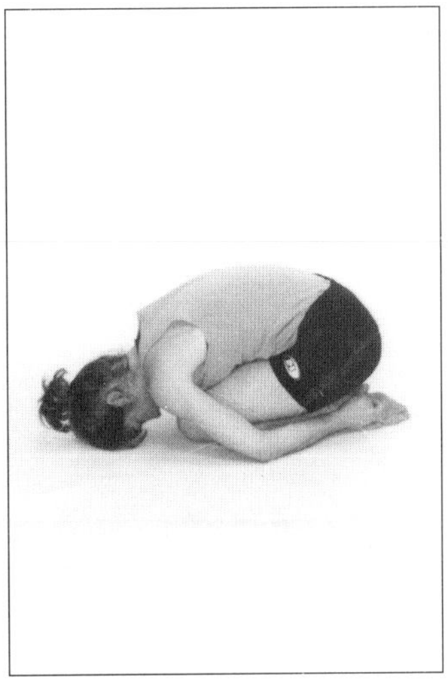

Another *vinyāsa*

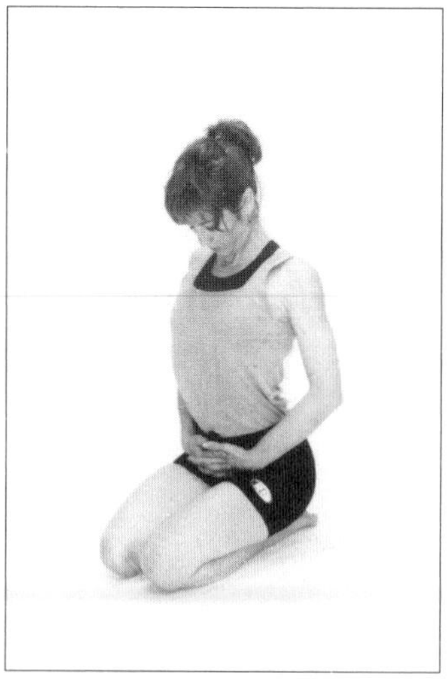

*Vajrāsana (vinyāsa)*

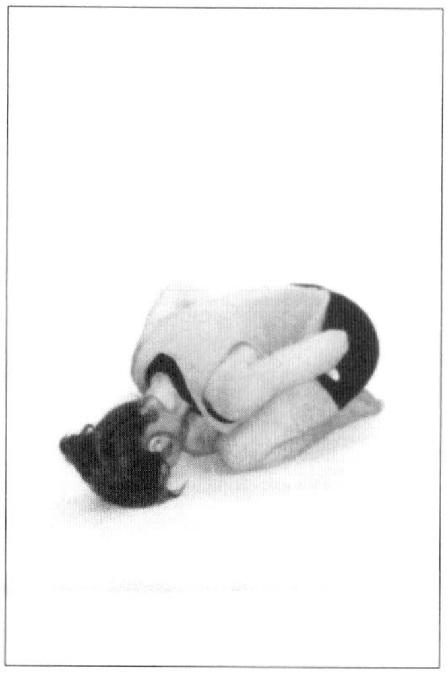

Forward bend with stomach lock

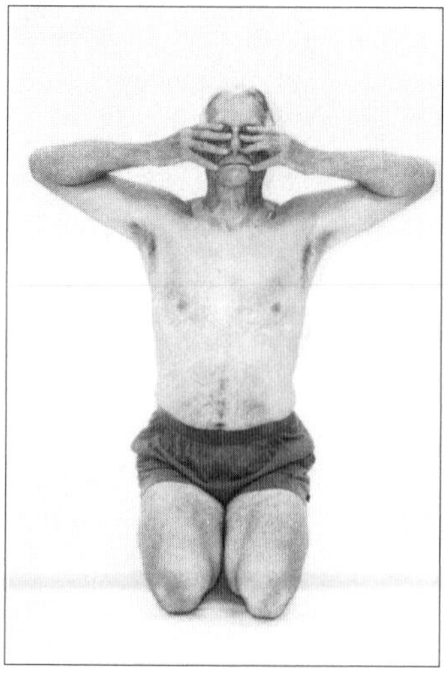

*Śaṇmukhīmudrā*

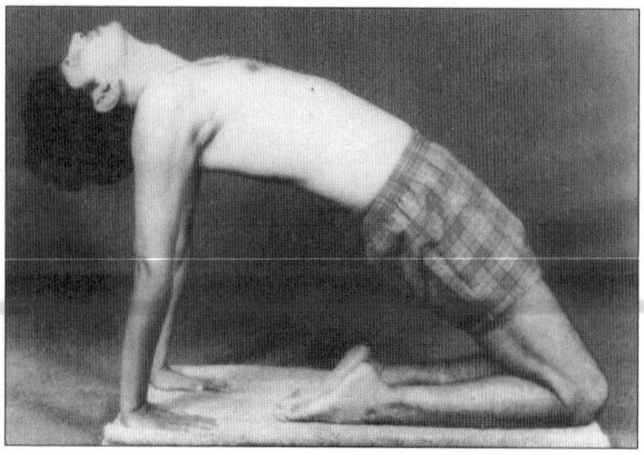

*Vajrāsana pratikriyā*

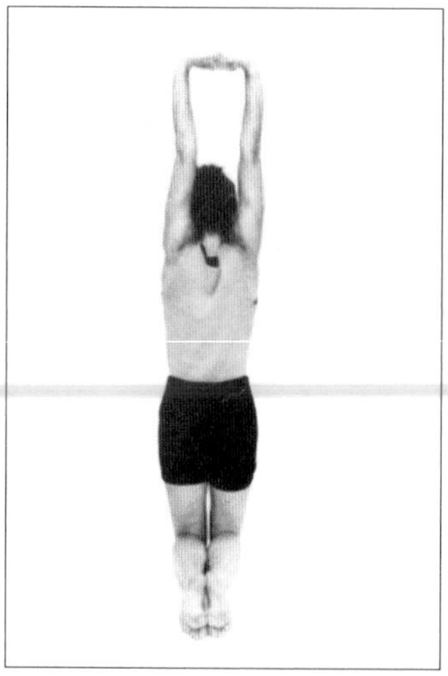

*Vīrāsana* (preparation)

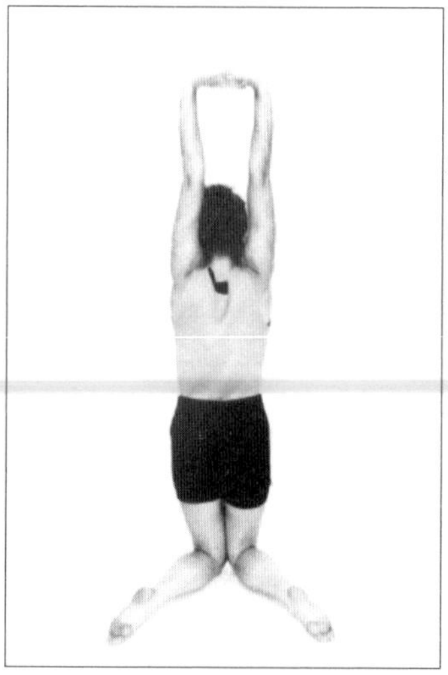

*Vīrāsana* (preparation of legs)

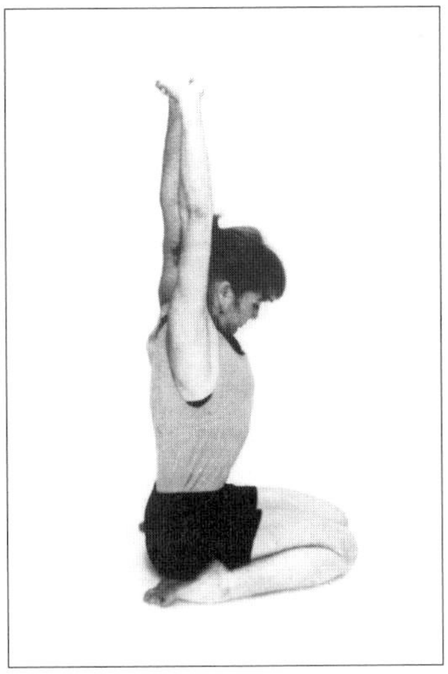

*Vīrāsana*

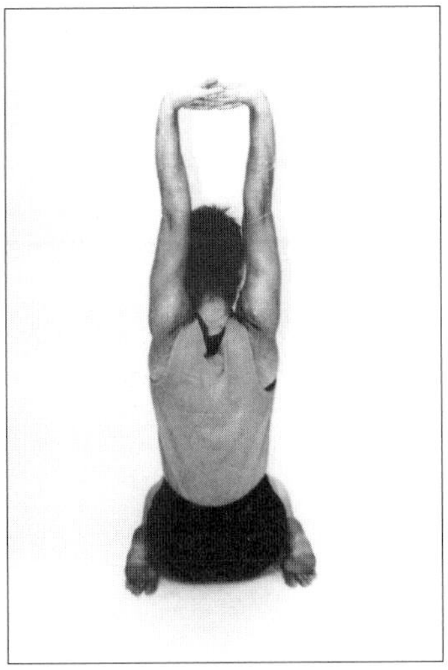

*Vīrāsana* (rear view)

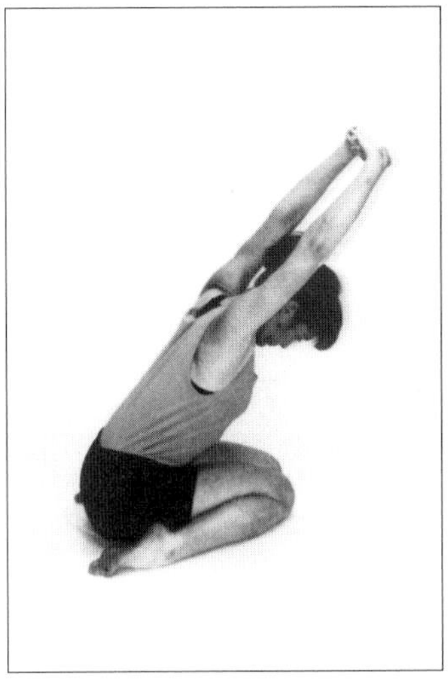

*Vīrāsana*
(forward bend, preparation)

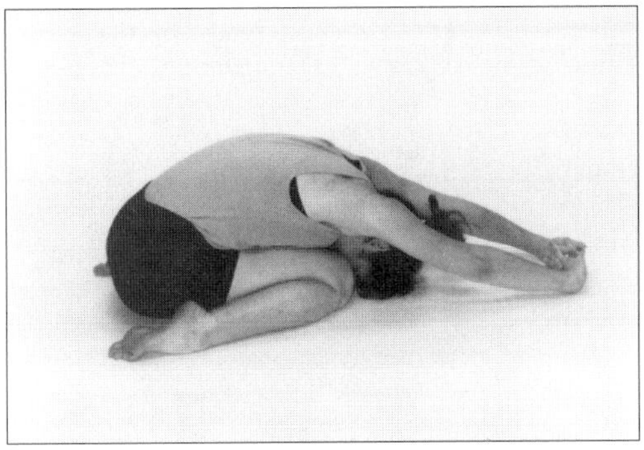

*Vīrāsana*
(forward bend)

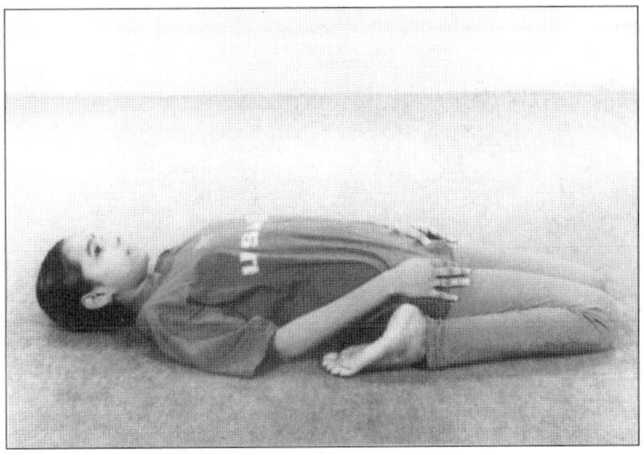

*Paryaṅkāsana*

posture is called *kapotāsana,* or pigeon posture, as the *āsana* resembles the exaggerated forward curvature of a pigeon's chest. It makes the spine supple and is believed to raise *kuṇḍalinī.*

*Vajrāsana* is very relaxing. Because of the stretching of the ankles and the front portion of the knees, it gives relief to those who are prone to rheumatism or who suffer from gout. Asthmatics have been found to respond well, especially to forward and back bending. Pregnant women will find that the trunk raising helps relieve the persistent lower-back pain and also strengthens the perineal muscles. It should be noted

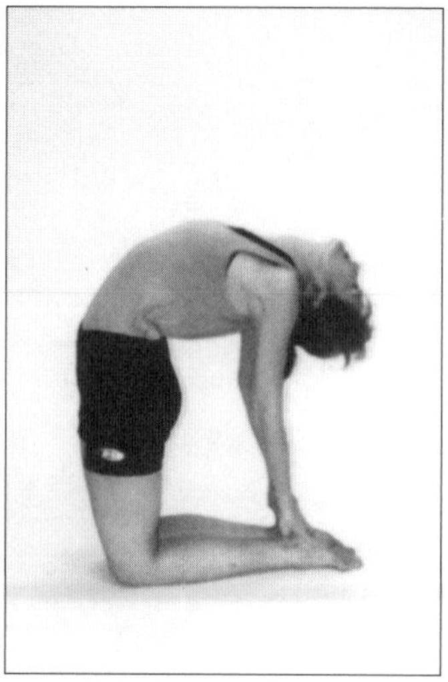

Uṣṭrāsana

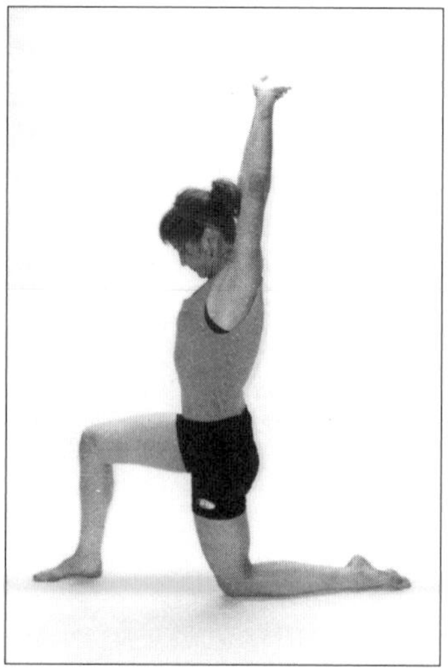

*Uṣṭrāsana (vinyāsa)* preparation

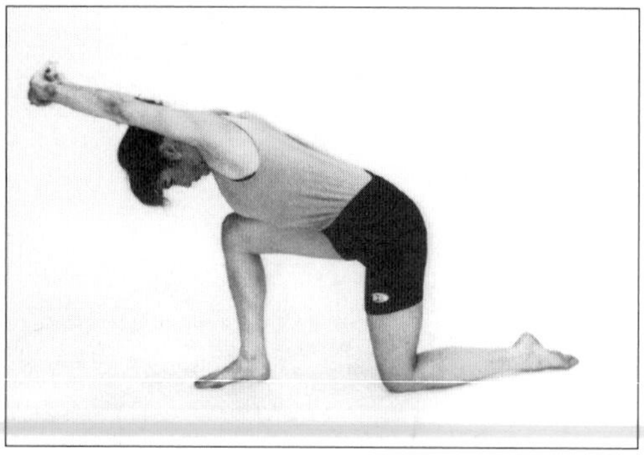

Preparation for forward bend

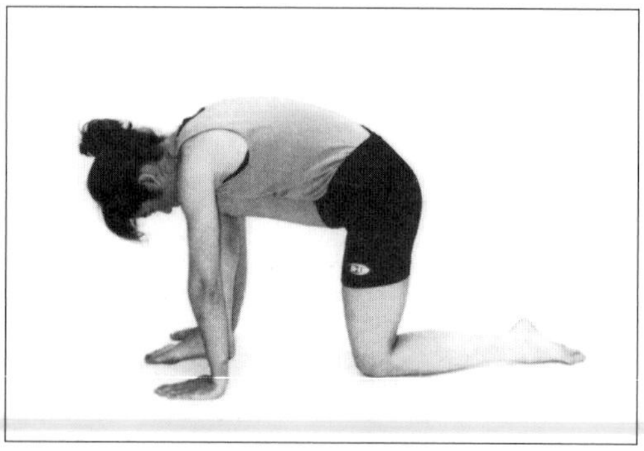

Forward bend

that the postures and movements are done with a breathing pattern. Breath is the link between body and mind. With proper breathing in *āsanas*, according to our *ācārya's paddhati*, one develops good mind-body coordination and control.

## Balancing Postures

Apart from the many groups of *āsanas* discussed so far, some requiring good balance merit attention. These postures help to develop one's sense of balance, correct disproportions in the body, and give the *abhyāsī* a tremendous sense of self-confidence. Children love to do many of them. Some of them resemble gymnastic movements, but in yoga, as always, the movements should be done with corresponding breathing patterns. Among the balancing postures there are those that require balancing on one foot, on one hand and one foot, or on both hands. Balancing on the hands is usually called *utpluti,* and this can be tried in almost all of the sitting postures. Balancing *āsanas* also include inverted postures. These require strong arms *(sthairya)* as well as suppleness of the limbs and joints *(aṅgalāghava).* Starting with *tāḍāsana*, many balancing postures are possible that depend upon the position of one of the legs, (the other foot is kept on the floor). Standing in *tāḍāsana*, exhale, stretch your right leg forward, and hold the big toe with the fingers of your right hand. Keep your left hand on your hip. Keep both knees

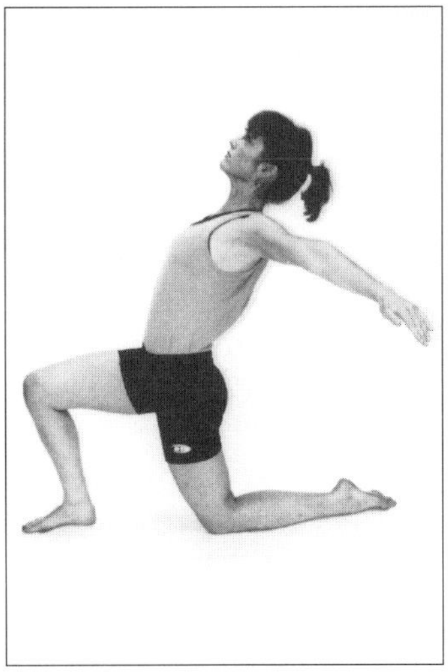

*Uṣṭrāsana (pūrva)* preparation

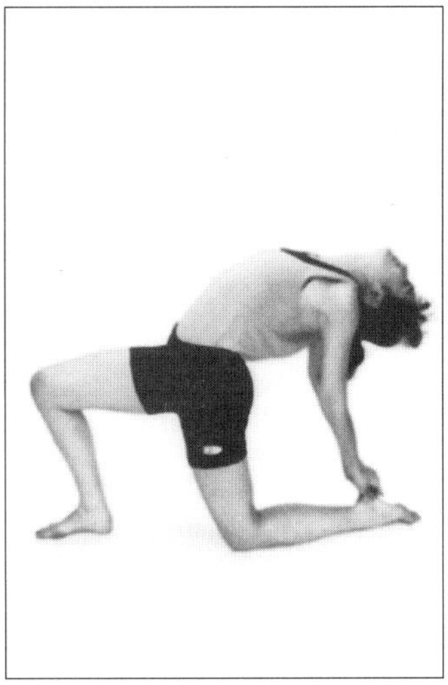

*Uṣṭrāsana* (advanced)

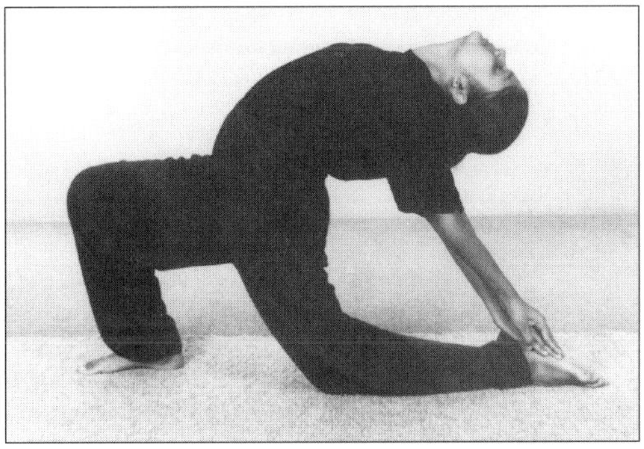

*Uṣṭrāsana* (full stretch)

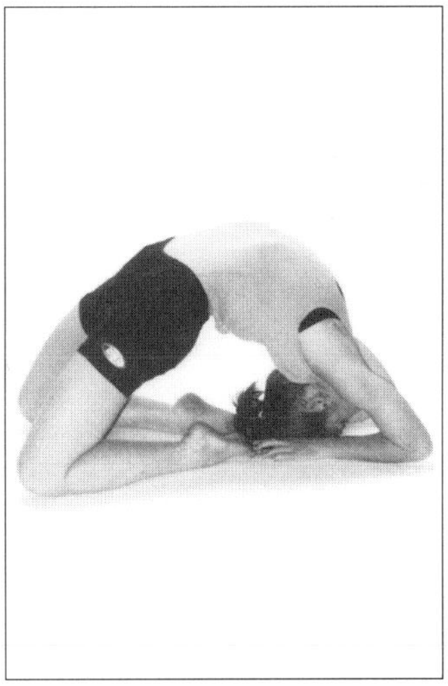

*Kapotāsana*

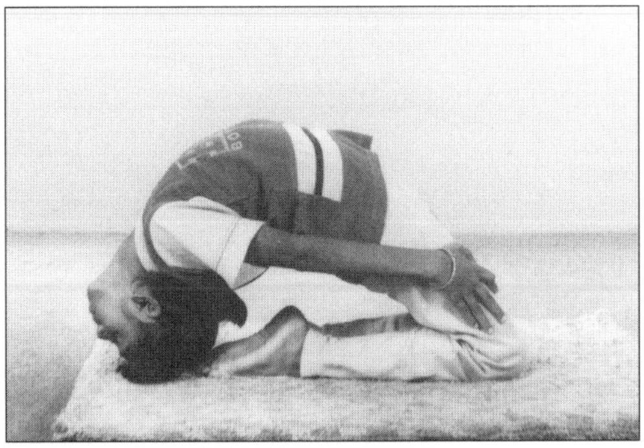

*Kapotāsana (nirālamba)*

stretched and maintain balance for a few breaths. Now stretch your other arm and hold your right foot. Exhale and raise it still further. The final position requires you to stretch your spine and bend forward on exhalation, so as to keep your forehead, nose, or chin on your right knee. After some practice, you may stay in the posture for a few breaths, maintaining your balance, of course. These one-legged *āsanas* can also be considered part of the group of standing postures. It is possible that one may lose one's balance in the initial stages, while raising the leg. In this case, one may bend the knee, hold the big toe with the fingers, and keep the other hand on the hip and stretch the knee. Alternately, one may keep the leg stretched and keep the heel on a raised platform or table and then raise the leg off the table. This gives strength to the hip and the leg muscles and gives one steadiness and poise. This posture is known as *utthitapādāṅguṣṭhāsana.*

There is yet another interesting way of attaining this posture, but it requires the *yogābhyāsī* to have supple joints and a better sense of balance. From *tāḍāsana*, proceed to *utkaṭāsana.* Staying in that posture, exhale, keep your left hand on your hip and stretch your right leg, and hold your big toe with the fingers of your right hand. Now inhale, rise up, and keep your right leg stretched, but without flexing your right knee.

Another balancing posture is *ardhabaddhapadma-uttānāsana.* Starting from *tāḍāsana*, exhale, bend your right leg, and place your foot at the top of your left thigh. Inhale, raise your right arm, and then, exhaling, from behind hold the big toe of your right foot with the fingers of your right hand. Stay for a few breaths. Exhale, bend forward, and, keeping your left palm on the floor by the side of your left foot, place your forehead on your stretched knee. The added requirement in this posture is that one has to stand on one foot and do the movements without falling. This posture helps in strengthening the shoulders; it also opens up the chest and thus facilitates free breathing. The pressure of the heel on the abdomen helps abdominal and pelvic organs and muscles.

There are many other postures that require balancing on one foot. *Garuḍāsana* requires keeping one leg encircling the other, straight leg right from the groin. Keeping one foot on the inside of the thigh with the corresponding knee bent and at a right angle to the straight leg is called *vṛkṣāsana,* or tree pose, especially when the arms are also raised overhead and the palms kept together. Keeping the right leg in *padmāsana*, on exhalation bend the left knee so that the right knee is kept on the floor, still maintaining balance. In this position, the left foot and the right knee are on the ground. This is called *vātāyanāsana.* All these require considerable concentration but bestow grace, poise, and stability to the *abhyāsī.* Other *āsanas,* such as *naṭarājāsana,* are more complicated ones in the same group of postures. *Āsanas* requiring one to balance on one foot and one palm help to stretch and tone up the side muscles *(pārśva).* They are also helpful in strengthening the arms and giving greater flexibility to the hip joints. Another group of *āsanas*, beginning with *vasiṣṭhāsana*, requires balancing as well.

Proceed from *caturaṅga-daṇḍāsana*, explained in chapter 7. Start with *tāḍāsana*. Exhaling, proceed to *utkaṭāsana*. Then, on the next exhalation, place your palms to the sides of your feet. Then, holding the breath, jump back to *caturaṅgadaṇḍāsana*. On the next exhalation, raise your hips in *adhomukhaśvān-āsana*, but slowly tilt your body to one side, with your right palm and the outside of your right leg on the floor. Keep your left arm by your body. On the next exhalation, press your right palm and arch your body further so that both feet are on the floor. Inhale, raise your left arm, and look up. This is *vasiṣṭhāsana*. This *āsana*, attributed to the great sage Vasiṣṭha, apart from strengthening the hips, helps the lumbar region, the rather stubborn coccyx, and the entire cervical region. Stay for a few breaths. There are interesting variations possible in this posture. For one, exhale, remaining in *vasiṣṭhāsana;* then bend your left knee, hold your big toe with the fingers of your left hand, and stretch it up. Bend your left knee on exhalation and keep it on the top of the right thigh. Exhale, balancing on your palm and leg, and hold the big toe of your left foot with the fingers of your left hand from behind. Inhale, press your palm and foot and raise your hips and trunk, and look up. This is *kaśyap-āsana*, an important and difficult variation of the simpler *vasiṣṭhāsana*. The shoulders and especially the sacral region are benefited. There are a number of variations on this kind of balancing that include *viśvāmitrāsana* and *kapiñjalāsana*. These also require balancing on one hand and one leg.

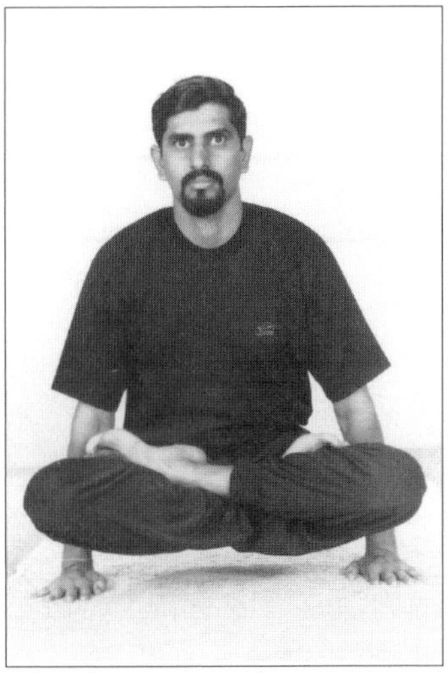

*Tolāṅgulāsana*

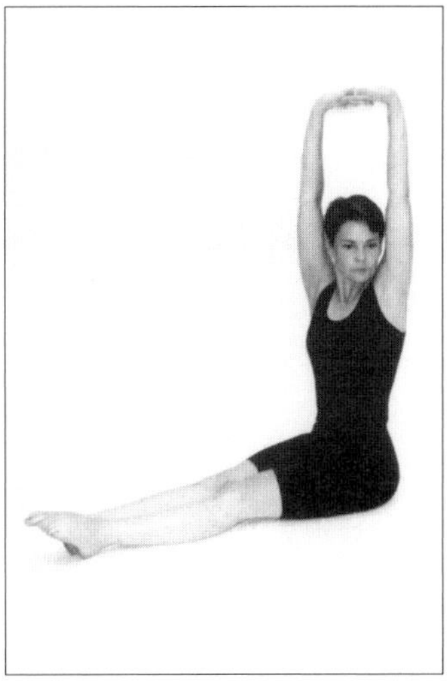

*Vasiṣṭhāsana* (preparation)

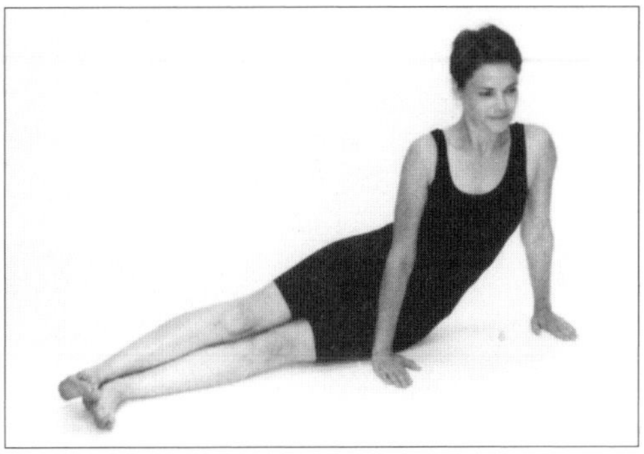

*Vasiṣṭhāsana* (preparation)

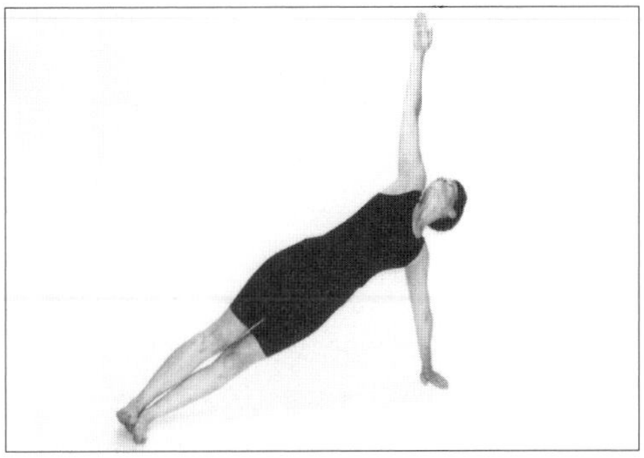

*Vasiṣṭhāsana*

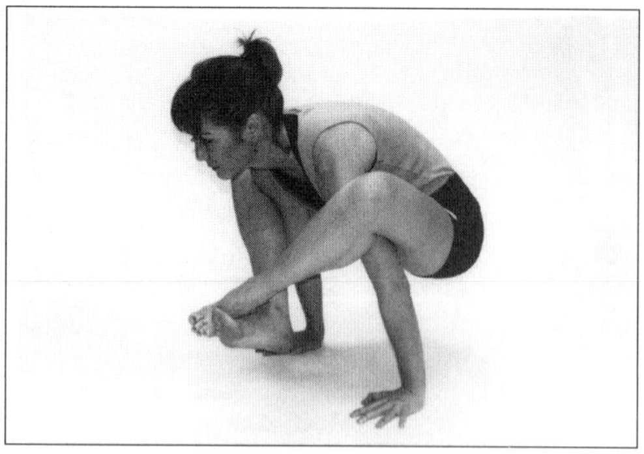

*Bhujapīḍāsana*

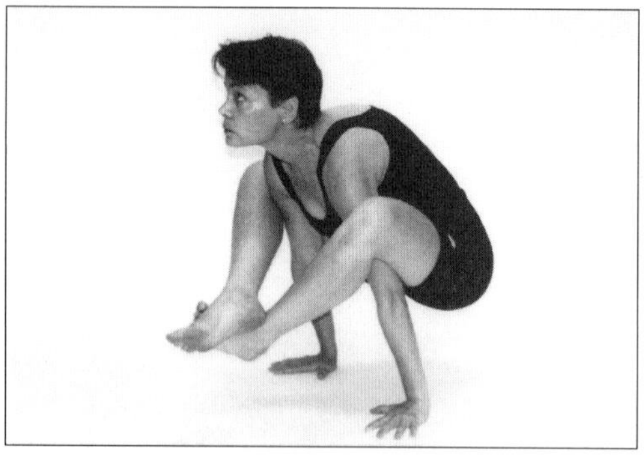

*Bhujapīḍāsana (vinyāsa)*

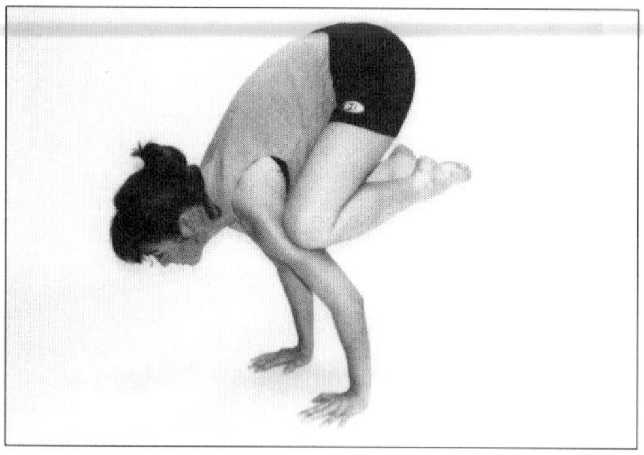

*Bhujapīḍāsana (vinyāsa)*

Balancing on both hands is fascinating to anyone interested in physical culture. Gymnasts and others make use of this with telling effect. To yogis doing this on the floor, the variations are far too many. As noted previously, in almost any sitting posture the palms may be placed on the floor and the body raised up, which is called *utpluti*. Perhaps the most common *utpluti* is raising the body while in *padmāsana*. Sit in *padmāsana*. Exhale, place your palms on the floor, hold your breath, and raise the body by about four *aṅgula* (finger widths), which is known as *tolāṅgulāsana*. Swinging to and fro, which children enjoy, is called *lolāsana*. While balancing on the palms, one may twist the body to one side beyond the base and by the side of one arm, which is known as *pārśva-uttānakukkutāsana*. There are of course different starting points for these *āsanas*; one may start from *śīrṣāsana* or *ūrdhvapadmāsana* and proceed to the balancing postures. *Utpluti* may also be attempted in *paścimatānāsana*, *siṃhāsana*, *vajrāsana*, and so on.

In raising the body, there are a number of variations. Many can be done, interestingly enough, from *śīrṣāsana* when one presses and balances the weight of the body with the hands, thus enabling the head to be lifted. One interesting but simple posture is *bhujapīḍāsana*. Place your palms with your feet on the floor. Press your palms, spread your knees, and raise your feet, balancing on your palms. There are further variations. This simple balancing posture helps strengthen the wrists, and one tends to feel lighter over the course of time. *Upaviṣṭhakoṇāsana*, done with the legs spread more than 90 degrees (from *daṇḍāsana*), gives rise to several *vinyāsas*, all of which help to make the hip joint supple and strengthen the pelvic and lower-back muscles.

# 13 Yogic Breathing Exercises and Their Health Benefits

HAVING DESCRIBED SOME IMPORTANT GROUPS of *āsanas*, such as *padmāsana*, *sarvāṅgāsana*, and *trikoṇāsana*, it is perhaps time (although a few more useful and well-known *āsana* groups will be taken up later) to discuss in more detail the next step in yoga, *prāṇāyāma*. Patañjali places *prāṇāyāma* next to *āsana*, but authors of *haṭhayoga* texts, even as they follow the same outline, recommend other purifying practices before the *kumbhaka*, or breath-holding, *prāṇāyamas* are taken up. Six such practices, known as *sat-kriyās*, are mentioned by Svātmārāma in his *Haṭhayogapradīpikā*. These are not obligatory exercises, even according to *haṭhayogis*, but are recommended for those who are obese and phlegmatic and are not for those whose *vāta*, *pitta*, and *kapha* are perfectly balanced.

The six practices are *dhouti* (stomach wash), *vasti* (colon wash), *neti* (nasal wash), *trātakam* (gazing), *nauli* (stomach churn), and *kapālabhāti* (skull polishing). Of these the first three, which use water, cloth, or other external agencies, were not recommended or encouraged in the system in which I was trained. *Trātaka*, which is a good exercise for the eyes, *nauli*, which is for the lower abdomen, and *kapālabhāti*, which is primarily for the respiratory system, are, however, frequently used by many *abhyāsīs*. None of these three practices introduces external aids into the system, and none is as displeasing as the first three *kriyās*. *Kapālabhāti* is most beneficial in preparing one for *prāṇāyāma;* it purifies the *prāṇamayakośa* just as *āsanas* purify the *annamayakośa*. *Kapālabhāti* is made up of two words, *kapāla*, meaning "skull" and implying the entire head, and *bhāti*, "that which makes it shine." Thus one who practices *kapālabhāti* feels rejuvenation in the head and gradually finds his face attaining some luster. These cleansing procedures help to rid the system of all the *doṣas*, and *prāṇāyāma siddhi* accrues without undue effort.

## *Kapālabhāti*

Even though *kapālabhāti* is not a *prāṇāyāma* in the orthodox system, it works thoroughly on the respiratory equipment. Hence, just as for *prāṇāyāma*, one should choose a place to practice that is free from noise and other atmospheric pollutants such as dust, dirt, and unpleasant odors. A good workout in *āsana* practice, which should be well planned to include movement of all the parts and joints of the body, should come first. A good workout includes a judicious combination of *āsanas* and their *vinyāsas* and a little rest. Then one should sit comfortably in *padmāsana* or another sitting posture. It has been found that *padmāsana* is among the best for *kapālabhāti*. Since the exercise is a highly dynamic one, it is better to choose a posture that can be maintained in the midst of vigorous activity involving the abdominal muscles. *Padmāsana*, with its interlocking of the legs, provides a firm base and enables one to keep the lower extremities under good control. For those who have trouble getting into correct *padmāsana*, another sitting posture like *vajrāsana* or *vīrāsana* may be chosen.

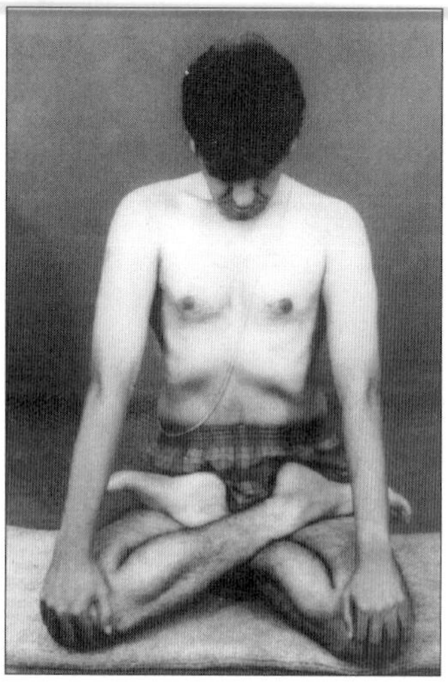

*Kapālabhāti* in *padmāsana*

Sit in *padmāsana*. Place your palms on your knees. Slightly bend your head forward as in *jālandhara bandha*, but do not constrict the glottis. After a few normal breaths, inhale and exhale quickly in succession about twenty-four times (or less, depending upon one's capacity). The breathing should be of the abdominal or diaphragmatic type and should be done through the nose. The abdominal muscles can contract quite vigorously and rapidly. With each stroke the viscera are drawn in and pressed, and the diaphragm is pushed up. As soon as the vigorous exhalation is over, the abdominal muscles relax and the abdominal viscera come down to their original position. Simultaneously, the diaphragm also comes down, creating a partial vacuum in the chest cavity, and the external air enters the lungs automatically. The active part of *kapālabhāti* is the expulsion of air, and one's inhalations are almost imperceptible. Then immediately following the first round, begin a second one by contracting the abdominal muscles and rapidly inhaling and expelling air. Again, twenty-four repetitions is a good beginning number.

*Kapālabhāti* is primarily an exercise of the viscera and diaphragm. It may be noted in practice that even though this is a breathing exercise, the movement of the chest wall is negligible. The intercostal muscles, in fact, are kept mildly contracted throughout and the slight inhalation is made possible only by the mobility of the diaphragm. This can easily be verified in practice, and, in fact, could be used as a check to see if one is doing it correctly. The inhalation *(pūraka)* is done silently and without effort, as distinct from the deep breathing involving deliberate expansion of the chest and the stretching of intercostal muscles. The expiration *(recaka)* is done with considerable effort at contracting and drawing in the abdominal muscles. Necessarily, therefore, when the air is forced out through the nostrils, a noise is produced resembling that of a bellows. In the *Haṭhayogapradīpikā,* Svātmārāma himself indicates this fact: *Bhastravat lohakārasya recapūram sasambhrame. Kapālabhātīṛk-hyāta kaphadosa vināśinī* ("Practice exhalation and inhalation rapidly [repeatedly like a blacksmith's bellows.] It is called *kapālabhāti,* which destroys *doṣa* of *kapha* [respiratory or phlegmatic]"). Since the *pūraka* is slow and imperceptibly soft, the exercise appears to be just a series of vigorous exhalations.

The depth of exhalation is more than normal, but it is not as much as in deep breathing or *prāṇāyāma.* The volume of air expelled is reasonably high, but is much less for women and those with emphysema.

There are four aspects to be looked into in *kapālabhāti:*

1. *The intensity of exhalation* refers to the force of expulsion and is primarily a function of the strength of the abdominal muscles, provided the respiratory system can withstand the intensity.
2. *The speed* is the time taken for completing one exhalation and inhalation. Intensity and speed are complementary, and their particular combination should be found by trial and error by each *abhyāsī.* Speed at the cost of intensity should be avoided, but so should proceeding too slowly. In the initial stages of practice, some may experience bouts of coughing or develop cramps in the stomach. In fact, in any group that starts this exercise, one finds that at least one-fourth of its members start coughing violently after a few attempts. Progress is slow and halting at the outset. In addition, those with excessive phlegm in their respiratory systems, which may be expelled during the practice, will have necessarily to stop in the middle. Certain asthmatics who have not been prepared well by preliminary *yogāsanas* may experience a bout of coughing, which may even precipitate bronchial constriction. It should be noted, however, that *kapālabhāti,* introduced at the proper time, is for an asthmatic highly

beneficial and is actually one of the important aids in treating asthma.

3. *The frequency* or number of times one does *kapālabhāti* at one stretch varies from person to person. In the initial stages one may not be able to do it more than ten or twenty-four times; with practice, though, a few hundred times becomes possible. Gasping for breath in the initial stages restricts the frequency. But later on, as one is more relaxed and develops one's second wind (improved stamina), one may continue until one feels a pleasant exhaustion or fatigue. When one's abdominal muscles are strong enough, and with increased practice, not only the abdominal muscles but also the pelvic and rectal muscles come into play. It is not necessary to practice *mūla bandha* to facilitate expulsion, but some find it useful to contract the rectal muscles. For the majority, use of the pelvic diaphragm and rectum becomes almost automatic. There are a few who prefer *mahā bandha* for doing *kapālabhāti,* since the gluteal muscles are raised and the rectum is pressed by the heel, thus facilitating a more conscious involvement of these muscles. Those with a weak abdominal wall should not attempt this without clearance from a doctor or therapist. One should consider the possibility of inducing a hernia.

   The intensity, speed, and frequency for a round of *kapālabhāti* should be determined by the practitioner and improved upon gradually. There should be no violent jerking of either the chest, shoulders, or head. Some attempt to constrict the nostrils to produce a distinctive sound, but the expelled air is allowed to escape freely through the glottis (no constriction there, please) and passes smoothly (though the nasal passage) to the end of the nostrils anyway. When the nostrils are not constricted, they themselves open out a bit to facilitate the passage of expelled air. Hence it is neither necessary nor desirable to try to control either of the nostrils or to indulge in facial contortions to regulate the passage of the air. Anyone who "makes faces" while doing *kapālabhāti* is not doing a good job of it. The air should be allowed smooth passage on its way out. Of course it does produce some friction at the lower ends of the nostrils, but it does not create any problems. One should be careful not to constrict the upper portion of the nose, so that there is no friction in the delicate parts of the mucous membranes lining the nasal passages. Those suffering from acute rhinitis or sinusitis should not do *kapālabhāti* during the period of acute nasal blockage; if *kapālabhāti* is done regularly, however, nasal blockage itself most likely will be prevented. The normal speed of doing *kapālabhāti* is about two per second. One may start at half that pace in the beginning. Eighty to 120 per minute is quite satisfactory.

4. *The number of times per sitting,* that is, a round of *kapālabhāti,* should be followed by *prāṇāyāma*, but mere long inhalation and exhalation should suf-

fice between rounds of *kapālabhāti*. This may be done for a minute or so before the next round is started. It will be good to do about three rounds per sitting, interspersed with a few rounds of long inhalation and exhalation. Those who have learned some *prāṇāyāma*, such as *ujjāyī* or *nāḍī śodhana*, may practice these after *kapālabhāti*, but more on those later.

*Kapālabhāti* should be attempted only with guidance from a teacher. Those suffering from hernia, acute rhinitis, or earache should not attempt this practice. Asthmatics should do it only under supervision. They will observe that a cough develops toward the end of each round; the phlegm should be spat out. In most cases the cough subsides, but if it continues, after a few days' practice it will abate. It is said that passage of air over the mucous membrane of the air passages could act as an inhibitory stimulus. In *kapālabhāti* the ratio of time for expiration to inspiration is about one to three. Since during inhalation the sympathetic nervous system is stimulated, which in turn is beneficial, it could be of considerable use to an asthmatic. Further, because of vigorous expulsion owing to the upward movement of the diaphragm, the residual air is thrown out. In early stages of emphysema, it helps very much in restoring the lungs to normal functioning.

The congestion in the bronchi and bronchioles is decreased gradually; the mucus is forced from the bronchial walls and is coughed out. After some time, there should be very little mucus to excite, thereby decreasing the possibility of precipitating a spasm. Furthermore, the powerful expiratory blasts of air through the entire respiratory passage act as a powerful inhibitory stimulus to the cough centers. Hence cough and the associated spasms of the bronchi diminish. Even for a generalized cough, it could be very useful; and since it improves blood circulation to the head and face, one gets a healthier look.

Perhaps equally important is the fact that the abdominal organs get thoroughly massaged through this practice. The liver, spleen, pancreas, kidneys and adrenals, and stomach and intestines get massaged and hence have improved vascularity. When combined in a group with such *āsanas* as *sarvāṅgāsana* and *paścimatānam*, it helps to alter the shape of the belly from its usual and unseemly half S shape to one more trim. Those suffering from irritable colon, constipation, certain types of early-stage diabetes due to a sluggish pancreas, flatulence, or dyspepsia will find it beneficial. Pregnant women and those suffering from menorrhagia or fibroids in the uterus are advised not to practice *kapālabhāti*. Those with an acute pulmonary or cardiac condition are also advised to be extremely cautious in attempting *kapālabhāti*.

For those interested in the esoteric aspects of *haṭhayoga*, *kapālabhāti* is said to arouse *kuṇḍalinī śakti*. The forcible movements of the abdominal muscles, when done properly and intensively, press the viscera and the various plexuses of the autonomic nervous system and stimulate them to activity, and hence, one could conjecture, brings about the arousal of *kuṇḍalinī śakti*. Apart from the respiratory system, the digestive and other pelvic organs as well as the heart also get massaged. The pericardium is attached to the upper surface of the diaphragm. Therefore, during each forcible exhalation, the thrust by the diaphragm massages the heart. Needless to say, it is absolutely essential that *kapālabhāti* be practiced on an empty stomach. Though it involves a simple technique, it has a salutary effect on the overall circulation of the body. The vibrations set in motion by *kapālabhāti* reverberate throughout all the cells of the body.

## *Prāṇāyāma* and Breathing

The simple, involuntary physiological function of breathing lends itself to a variety of *prāṇāyāmas* that have different benefits depending on a number of parameters. These variables may be broadly classed as follows: (1) the site in the respiratory passage at which the flow of breath is regulated; (2) whether or not the breath is held; (3) the ratios of the duration of inhalation, holding of the breath, and exhalation; (4) whether or not mantras are used; (5) whether or not *bandhas* are used; (6) whether inhalation and exhalation are continuous or discrete; (7) whether inhalation and exhalation are active or passive; (8) specific or nonspecific visual attention; (9) whether or not breath holding is accompanied by breathing; (10) the number of rounds of *prāṇāyāma* per sequence; (11) the number of sequences per sitting; (12) the frequency of doing *prāṇāyāma* per day; (13) hybrid *prāṇayamas;* (14) whether performed with or without *utghāta;* (15) the stages of *prāṇāyāma siddhi* as revealed by physiological and psychological transformations.

In inspiration, the air passes through the nostrils, pharynx, larynx, trachea, bronchi, and bronchioles and into the lungs. The reverse order occurs in expiration. The larynx, trachea, bronchi, and bronchioles form one continuous tube. At its lower end the trachea divides into two bronchi, one for each lung. The bronchi consist of a framework of rings of cartilage united by fibrous and muscular tissue, and the bronchioles branch off and divide further, narrowing to about half a millimeter in diameter. Their walls are formed of a fibrous elastic membrane with fibers of muscle. These muscles are controlled by two sets of nerves; one is called the vagus, which contracts the muscles when stimulated, and the other, the sympathetic, which relaxes the muscles on stimulation. In certain types of *prāṇāyāma,* the effort is to stimulate either of these nervous responses. During active inhalation, the muscles of the chest wall cause the volume of the chest to increase, which in turn causes a vacuum between the lungs and the chest wall; and the lungs, being elastic, immediately fill this vacuum. So the airspace inside the lungs also increases, and the pressure differential between the external air and the lungs causes the atmospheric air *(bāhya-vāyu)* to rush in and fill up the lungs, which also causes the diaphragm to become parallel to the floor, thanks to the expanding lungs. Expiration being normally passive, the reverse process takes place; the muscles contracted during inhalation now relax, and the elastic lung tissues also return to their nonstretched state. It could be observed that in the case of an asthmatic, since the bronchial tubes are constricted, the passive action of exhalation is not sufficient to expel the contaminated air; but inhalation is easy because of the activity of the powerful intercostal muscles.

The variety of *prāṇāyamas* have been designed by yogis so that all the aspects of respiration are completely free and perfect. By controlling the various aspects of breathing, one is able to control the nervous stimuli as well as what are otherwise involuntary functions.

## *Ujjāyī Prāṇāyāma*

Those who have practiced *āsanas* according to our *ācārya's paddhati* will find that *ujjāyī* is quite easy to practice. Since all the movements in the various *vinyāsas* are done with controlled breathing, and since the control is attained only in the throat at the glottis, *ujjāyī* is almost invariably done in *āsana* practice. In fact, *ujjāyī* is given pride of place by many *haṭhayogis. Ujjāyī prāṇāyāma* has many variations. But its primary function is controlling inhalation and exhalation at the site of the glottis, between the larynx and the trachea. The principle underlying *ujjāyī* is that we learn to control the bronchial muscles through the vagus nerve. We know that a nerve carries an impulse to its muscles and causes it to contract. In *ujjāyī* we voluntarily send impulses through the vagus nerve to the intricate muscles of the larynx near the vocal cords and learn to breathe well under such conditions. The hissing sound is produced because of the proximity of the vocal cords to each other. The air passage is regulated by the partial closing of the glottis. The glottis is a valve-membrane that closes completely when one swallows and is completely open the rest of the time. In *ujjāyī,* the partial closing of the glottis helps to regulate the breath, and the hissing sound that is a by-product is also indicative of the correctness of one's practice of *ujjāyī prāṇāyāma.*

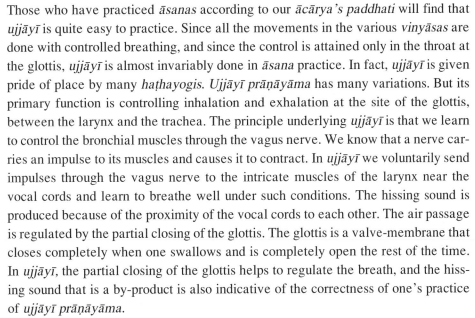

The normal way to practice *ujjāyī* is to seat oneself in a comfortable, steady posture. It can also be done standing, for example, in *tāḍāsana* or *samasthiti.* In the beginning, *ujjāyī* can be practiced without *kumbhaka,* or retention of breath. For many beginners, it may be done in an easy posture like *vajrāsana*, with long inhalation and exhalation and a hissing sound in the throat, between six and twelve times. It may be done immediately after doing the various *vinyāsas* in *vajrāsana.* Later on, breath holding, or *antaḥ-kumbhaka,* may be attempted. Its benefit to those with respiratory ailments is considerable, as is mentioned in the yoga texts and as borne out by experience. Asthmatics benefit a great deal from *ujjāyī.* As noted above, in normal breathing, exhalation is a passive process. This being the case, one can see why it is especially difficult for air to be expelled when the bronchi and bronchioles are contracted, as with asthma. On the other hand, since inhalation in the course of normal breathing is an active process, the air is forced through the constricted tubes, and there is less difficulty with inhalation in one with asthma. In bronchial asthma, the muscles of the tubes undergo paroxysmal contractions that may last from a few minutes to some hours, and in certain cases, days. When the spasms last for a number of days, this is called "status asthma" and requires drastic treatment.

For such a person, when expiration becomes difficult, the lungs are not completely deflated before another short, jerky, or spasmodic inhalation takes place. The lungs, as a result of the trapped air, become more and more distended, and the movement of the chest walls becomes more restricted. When the lungs get permanently distended as a result of many neglected attacks, the condition is known as emphysema, and yogic treatment in such a case is not as effective. With emphysema, the shoulders are held high and the whole chest is permanently increased in size. Such a barrel-shaped chest loses its usual suppleness and elasticity. The alveoli of the lungs are blown up into large chambers as a result of the destruction of the septa that separate them. Naturally, the disappearance of septa, which support blood vessels, means a drastic reduction in oxygen exchange and the consequent loss of vital capacity. The suffering of an asthmatic *prāṇa avasthā* (painful state) is dreadful. The face becomes pale and anxious, the fingertips cyanotic. Experimentally, when we stimulate the vagus we produce a condition exactly similar to bronchial asthma. In asthma, the mucous membranes of the bronchi and the bronchioles form a thick secretion: The bronchial muscles are in spasm, and the small bronchioles practically close, which makes breathing the hardest job.

*Ujjāyī*—some scholars say its meaning is "to produce sound"—is done with the glottis partially closed. The space between the two vocal cords varies with the sound we produce. In *ujjāyī* the vocal cords are brought nearer to each other than in normal breathing. Therefore, when the air rushes in or out through the narrow slit, the well-known hissing sound, resembling that of a cobra, is produced. This exercise is perhaps the first that is taught in our *ācārya's* system, as all *vinyāsas* are done with controlled breathing. But it is very easy to do when one observes closely and does it in a relaxed fashion. The sounds produced are somewhat similar to asthmatic breathing. The muscles, which control the movements of the vocal cords, are activated by branches of the vagus nerve, which innervate the muscles of the bronchioles.

The principle underlying *ujjāyī* (which increases secretions of the pituitary and relaxes bronchiole muscles) is that one learns to control these bronchial muscles through the vagus nerves. In an asthmatic paroxysm, the bronchial muscles contract and the patient is helpless. In *ujjāyī* one reverses the process; one voluntarily causes contraction of these muscles in order to regulate breathing. It may be found that with a little practice, one gradually controls these muscles and that the muscles no more control the patient. *Ujjāyī* can be practiced standing or sitting, in an office, or even in other places. It is thus not difficult to practice, and may be done one hundred times a day. Slowly one may increase the duration of each round so that it takes between half a minute and a minute to complete one round, thereby enabling the *abhyāsī* to gain good control over the respiratory muscles. It has also been found that the lungs' vital capacity increases anywhere between two hundred and three hundred cubic centimeters. The effect of *ujjāyī* is enhanced when retention of breath is introduced between inhalation and exhalation. As mentioned in yoga texts, the duration of the breath retention, in the final stages, should be four times that of inhalation. The effects of *ujjāyī* practice are described below.

The heart is enclosed in a sac, the pericardium, the lower part of which is attached to the center of the upper surface of the diaphragm. On either side of the heart is a lung, each of which is enclosed by a sac. This sac is composed of two thin but strong membranes. Inside them, the pressure is negative, which allows the elastic lung to stretch a little. When we inspire, the negative pressure increases, and thus venous blood rushes up to the right atrium. The only thing separating the pericardium and blood vessels from the pleural cavity is this membrane, the pleura. Therefore, when pressure in the pleural cavity is decreased, the pressure in the right atrium and the two venae cavae, which take venous blood to the right atrium, also decreases significantly. The pressure in the veins elsewhere, in the neck or abdomen, for instance, is much higher. Therefore the venous blood automatically rushes into the right atrium. Thus one may say that inspiration acts as a second pump to the heart, a kind of respiratory pump. During inspiration the diaphragm presses against the abdominal viscera, and therefore the pressure on the abdominal cavity is also increased, which again forces the blood in the abdominal veins to rush into the right atrium. The arteries in the chest, however, are not affected, since their walls are thick and strong. Moreover, their blood pressure is higher compared to that of the veins.

When the pericardium distends as a result of this low chest pressure, the right ventricle, which is much thinner than the left ventricle, is also distended. Hence, more blood rushes from the right atrium into the right ventricle and then to the lungs for oxygenation.

Breath retention, or *kumbhaka,* following inspiration *(antaḥ-kumbhaka)* is given importance in all forms of *prāṇāyāma.* In *antaḥ-kumbhaka,* increased negative pressure in the thorax is maintained throughout the period of retention. The increased flow of venous blood into the heart necessarily continues for a much longer period. This is the special physiological significance of *antaḥ-kumbhaka.* Increased blood flow into the heart implies that with every systole of the heart, an increased volume of blood will be sent out, and there will be no stagnation in the venous return. Blood pressure rises during *kumbhaka* to a considerable degree, to about twenty milligrams for a healthy person, hence the practice is forbidden to those with high blood pressure. In fact, it may be maintained that *ujjāyī* inhalation and *antaḥ-kumbhaka* are energizing processes, which is a plausible explanation for holding the breath four times longer than the time taken for inhalation. The *prāṇāyāma* procedure described by our *ṛṣis* is both physiologically and psychologically energizing. Conversely, long exhalation and a longer pause, or *bāhya-kumbhaka,* following exhalation will be beneficial to those suffering from high blood pressure or mental agitation. More research should be done along these lines. Patañjali refers to long exhalation and suspension of breath after exhalation as helpful for calming the mind (1.34): *"pracchardhana vidhāraṇābhyāṃ vā prāṇasya."*

There is yet another important aspect to *kumbhaka:* The respiratory centers that involuntarily send impulses for inhalation and exhalation are brought under one's voluntary control. When *antaḥ-kumbhaka* is done after a robust inhalation, the inspiratory center is greatly stimulated and the expiratory center is inhibited, that is, the automatic impulses are stopped. Conversely, when we perform *bāhya-kumbhaka* at the end of a deep exhalation, aided by *mūla bandha* and *uddīyāna bandha,* the inspiratory center is inhibited and the expiratory center is greatly stimulated. By doing this practice regularly many times a day (up to 320 times a day is mentioned in *haṭhayoga* texts), one may learn to stimulate or inhibit either the inspiratory or expiratory centers at will.

In normal inspiration, impulses go through the vagus nerve to the respiratory centers, causing inhibition of the inspiratory center and stimulation of the expiratory center (also known as the Hering-Breuer reflex). With *antaḥ-kumbhaka,* however, these impulses are made inoperative so that the respiratory centers do not respond to the stimulation of the vagus nerve. In other words, deliberate control over the respiratory center is established. Thus repeated practice of *kumbhaka* strengthens the control, the *saṃskāra,* of respiration. Furthermore, when we retain breath after inhalation, that part of the larynx immediately below the two vocal cords is distended by air under pressure. This area is asthmagenic, or sensitive, and thus there is an immediate tendency to cough (which can be observed in many who begin learning *prāṇāyāma*). But since we deliberately stop the cough, we gain control of the respiratory centers. In *prāṇāyāmic* exercises, the will plays a great part by sending impulses through the cerebrum to the respiratory centers. Those who suffer from asthma breathe abnormally, which in turn strengthens the abnormal breathing *saṃskāras. Ujjāyī prāṇāyāma* helps to correct this situation and to establish a healthy and more normal breathing practice by fine-tuning the respiratory apparatus and its control.

The normal practice of *ujjāyī* is as follows:

1. Sit in a comfortable *āsana*, such as *vajrāsana* or *padmāsana*.
2. Exhale deeply.
3. Lock the chin, so that the vocal cords are brought closer together, and inhale by expanding the chest.
4. After complete inhalation, pause for a moment and exhale with a hissing sound in the throat.
5. Pause for a moment after exhalation, and then inhale through throat, again making a hissing sound. Follow the breath mentally.

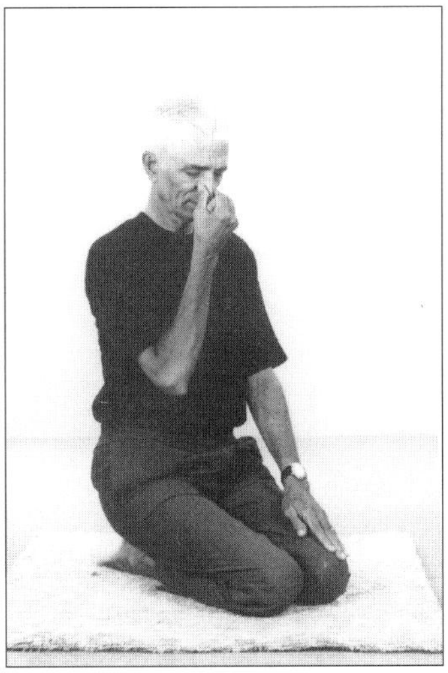

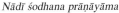

*Nādī śodhana prāṇāyāma*

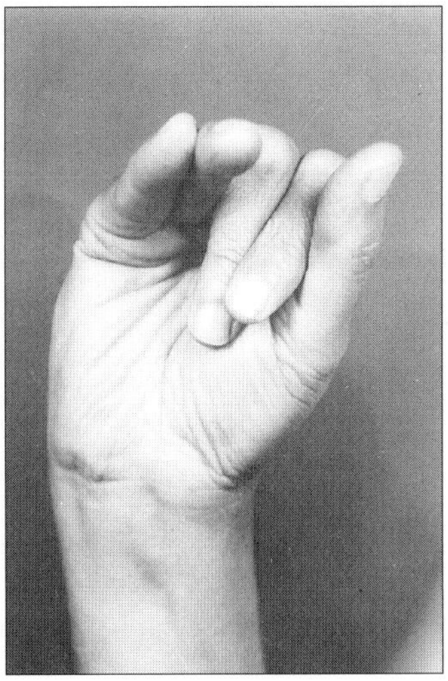

*Mṛgī mudrā*

*Ujjāyī* is easy to do when practicing *āsanas* and *vinyāsas*, and it is extremely beneficial. Yoga texts describe in detail a variety of *ujjāyī prāṇayamas* and their benefits. Vyāsa says, *Tapo na paramprāṇāyāmath,* "There is no *tapas* or purifying activity superior to *prāṇāyāma*." It burns always all defilements—mental and physical—and enables the intellect to shine forth.

## *Prāṇāyāma* and Mantras

Nārada describes the use of mantras in *prāṇāyāma:*

*Prāṇo vayūśśarīrastha*
*āyāmastasya nigrahaḥ!*
*prāṇāyāma iti proktā*
*dvividhaf procyate hi saha.*
*agrbhasca sagarbhasca*
*dvitīyastu tayorvaraḥ!*
*apidhyānam vinā agarbhaḥ*
*sagarbhastat samancitaḥ.*

*"Prāṇa* refers to the *vāyu* (force) in the body. *Āyāma* means to completely control it (to bring under voluntary control). Such control of the life force, known as *prāṇāyāma,* is of two kinds, *agarbha* and *sagarbha,* the latter of which is superior. *Agarbha* entails practicing breath control without *dhyāna,* and *sagarbha* entails practicing with an object for contemplation."

In chapters 7 through 12, sequences of *āsanas* with their related breathing patterns, *pratikriyās,* and benefits have been presented. These are quite sufficient to provide many *yogābhyāsīs* the means to exercise various joints and muscles and maintain reasonably good health. A few somewhat more difficult *āsana* groups remain to be discussed. But it is time to describe the next important aspect of *bahiraṅga sādhana* (external practice), which is *prāṇāyāma.*

Breathing, to which very little attention is paid by many of us in day-to-day life (except if we suffer from asthma or some other respiratory ailment), has been discussed in great detail by our ancient yogis and sages. In fact, many have proclaimed that *prāṇāyāma* alone could be the key to attainment of *samādhi.* The choice of *prāṇa* alone as the object of contemplation comes naturally to many people. Unlike other types of meditation, the advantage of *prāṇāyāma* is that one need not have an external object or an abstract idea as a guide for contemplation. The yogis have found that by exercising control over *prāṇa,* one can control the mind and thus transcend it. *Prāṇa* exercises are treated in depth in Vedic, Tantric, and also *haṭha* disciplines.

The practice of *āsana* and *prāṇāyāma* is an important prelude to *antaraṅgasādhanapūjā, upāsāna, japa,* and *dhyāna. Āsanajaya,* or mastery of a posture, is a prerequisite for the practice of *prāṇāyāma.* By definition, *āsana* means to remain in a steady and comfortable position, but that position or posture should be a yogic posture. But this does not mean that one needs to have mastered all the *āsanas* to practice *prāṇāyāma.* In fact, it is rare to find someone who can do all the postures. But the method of *yogāsana* practice that includes use of breathing with the various *vinyāsas* and *pratikriyās* ensures that one's circulation and respiration are improved and that one feels deep relaxation before starting *prāṇāyāma.* The practice of *yogāsana* with *vinyāsa,* as propounded by our *ācārya* and based on such authorities as Patañjali, the *Yoga Kuranṭam,* and the *Vṛddha Śātātapam,* is scientific and comprehensive, and hence gives the maximum benefit to the *abhyāsī* by improving physiological functioning. The mind is trained and attuned to follow the breath and consequently attain the capacity for *ekāgra,* which is essential for *antaraṅgasādhana* and all other mental and spiritual attainments.

While defining *prāṇāyāma,* Patañjali also stresses the mastery of at least one *āsana* before proceeding to do *prāṇāyāma:*

*"Tasmin sati śvāsa praśvāsyoḥ gati vicchedaḥ prāṇāyamaḥ,"* "remaining in a posture [which is comfortable and steady] and controlling the inward and outward movement of breath is *prāṇāyāma.*" In his commentary, Vyāsa is more specific. He

says, "*Āsana jaye sati,*" which means "Having mastered a particular posture, one should start on *prāṇāyāma.*" As described in chapter 7, there are four distinct stages to yogic breathing. Expelling the air completely from the lungs *(kauṣṭasya vāyu)* is one, called *praśvāsa,* or *recaka: kauṣṭasya vāyoh nissaranam praśvāsah.* Another is inhalation, or *pūraka,* which is drawing in the atmospheric air and completely filling up the lungs: *Bāhyavāyoḥ ācamanam śvāsaḥ.*

The other part of breathing, *kumbhaka,* the act of preventing the activity of both inhalation and exhalation, is of two kinds. One is holding the breath after complete inhalation, and the other is to hold the breath out, as it were, after complete exhalation. The four stages are:

1. *Pūraka,* or *abhyantara vṛtti,* complete inhalation;
2. *antaḥ-kumbhaka,* or *stambha vṛtti,* holding the breath in after inhalation;
3. *recaka,* or *bāhya vṛtti,* complete exhalation;
4. *bāhya-kumbhaka,* or holding the breath out after exhalation.

The time of day, the duration of the breath holding, the depth to which one feels the effects of the breathing, the frequency, the method of controlling the passage of air, the various ratios of inhalation to holding and exhalation, the uniformity and fineness of the breath, and the use of mantra or not are the various parameters of *prāṇāyāma.* All of these together make for a formidable number of *prāṇāyāma* types. Hence the guidance of a teacher is required to study and practice *prāṇāyāma.*

The respiratory function is both voluntary and involuntary. Normally, our breathing is shallow and involuntary. In *prāṇāyāma* a deliberate attempt is made to bring the breath under greater voluntary control, thereby bringing many other involuntary conditions of the body and the mind under voluntary control. The *yogābhyāsī* can achieve certain extraordinary powers over his or her own physiological functions. According to a well-known Indian neurosurgeon, it appears that the basic factor in yoga is the control of respiration. Respiratory function can be more easily influenced than any other vital functions, and the yogi uses it as the first step in gaining control of the nervous system. When cortical higher brain control is achieved over one basic function, it is possible to achieve control over others, such as vasomotor functions. It is therefore possible to dilate bronchial tubes in an asthmatic, reduce blood pressure or increase it, and reduce the heart rate, all with the help of *prāṇāyāma.* Neurological brain disorders such as epilepsy, as well as skin allergies and other conditions, also respond to *prāṇa* control.

A number of bodily functions classified as autonomous are not so for an adept yogi. He or she is able to control by will many functions that are controlled in ordinary human beings by subcortical areas—which areas are normally beyond voluntary control. The mechanism involved could be neurological and chemical. Once regular control of respiration is achieved, there is perhaps a reciprocal biochemical steady state that is achieved that helps in the maintenance of this control. When one establishes full control over this lower vital and emotional function by the exercise of one's cortex (will), this is achieved by the reciprocal connections among the cortex, the reticular system, and the various centers in the brain. Constant yogic practice of both *prāṇāyāma* and meditation quite likely leads to an enlargement in the scope of the function of the reticular system and the cortex. It is quite possible that in the real yogi the reticular system and the cortex are both functionally altered and structurally proliferated. Patañjali seems to suggest that such a mutation of brain cells is possible. The *citta pariṇāma,* or degree of alteration in the arrangement of brain cells, is inherent in every individual, and practice is the only cause of such a mutation. It is an activity of the mind on the mind to transcend the mind. Like a farmer *(kṣetrika)* who diverts the flow of water in a field, the yogi has only to channel his neurological energies along certain paths. There is no external cause *(nimittamaprayojakam)* for such cortical and neurological changes. And the key to such changes appears to be the control of breath, or *prāṇāyāma.*

*Prāṇāyāma* is of two kinds, *samantraka,* or *sagarbha,* which is practicing *prāṇāyāma* with mantras, and *amantraka,* or *agarbha,* which is practicing without them. What mantras should be used in *prāṇāyāma*? The practice of *prāṇāyāma* with mantras is well known to Hindus. Many authorities have stated how *prāṇāyāma* should be done with the *gāyatrī, praṇava,* and *bījaksara* mantras. These days, while the mantra part is maintained by many who observe *sandhyā* and other religious rites, the actual practice of *prāṇāyāma* is completely left out; most people merely touch the nose, or worse yet, only suggest taking the hand toward the nose. The oft-quoted definition of *samantraka prāṇāyāma* is given in the Manu Smṛti: *Savyahrtikām sapranavām gāyatrīm śirasā saḥ, trifpatet āyatapraṇaḥ prāṇāyamāssa ucyate,* "Controlling the breath and meditating *(japa)* three times on *gāyatrī* with *vyāhṛtis, siras,* and the *praṇava* is known as *prāṇāyāma.*" According to the the *Yoga Yājñavalkya, prāṇāyāma* involves doing *japa* of *gāyatrī* preceded by *praṇava* and associated *vyāhṛtis* and followed by *śiras.* Elaborating on this, the *Vighneśvara* says that one has to control the *vāyu* in the face and nostrils. The *Yājñyavalkya* gives a more detailed account of *samantraka prāṇāyāma;* the mantras are *bhūḥ, bhūvaḥ, suvaḥ, mahaḥ, janaḥ, tapaḥ,* and *satyam* along with *omkara;* then *tatsavituḥ,* followed by the *śiras "omāpaḥ"* (the *śiras* mantra is found in the Taittirīya Upaniṣad). When one does this three times, it is known as *prāṇāyāma.*

Details of the actual methods of *prāṇāyāma* are found in such yoga texts as the *Yoga Yājñavalkya,* the Śiva Saṃhitā, the *Gheraṇḍa Saṃhitā, and* the *Haṭhayogapradīpikā,* and in the Amṛtanada, Kṣurikā, Triśikhibrāhmaṇa, Darśana, Dhyānabindu, Nādabindu, Yogakuṇḍali, Yogacuḍāmaṇī, Yogatattva, Yogaśikha, Varāha, and Śaṇḍilya Upaniṣads, various Purāṇas, and of course the Gītā.

To what extent should one draw in external air is a question often asked. The answer is to draw the air in completely so that all the *nāḍīs* are "filled up." This kind of drawing in is known as *pūraka*. Holding the inhaled *vāyu* in different parts of the body, as it were, by means of the various *bandhas* and after deep inhalations is referred to by Patañjali (2.50) in his mention of *deśa paridṛṣṭi*, or the "place" where the breath is held. When the inhaled breath forces circulation from the roots of the hair and the ends of nails and is held *(nirodha)*, this is the best, according to the *ṛṣi* Atri, because a chain of changes is created in the body: Through *prāṇa nirodha*, *vāyu* is generated, from *vāyu*, *agni*, and from *agni*, *jala (vāta sāram, vāhni sāram, vāri sāram)*. With these three, one becomes completely purified. Then, one should exhale gradually through the nostril, so that it is never forced or abrupt. The body should be kept steady. Such a practitioner is known as yogi of the highest order.

*Prāṇāyāma* should be done with *dhyāna*. This practice, however, requires a teacher. The better-known method of *dhyāna* is mentioned by Vyāsa, who says that when doing *pūraka*, one should meditate upon the four-faced Brahma whose complexion is red and whose position is in the navel region *(nābhi cakram)*; during *antaḥ-kumbhaka*, one should meditate on the form of Lord Viṣṇu, whose complexion is that of a blue lotus; and while doing *recaka*, one should meditate on the white-complexioned form of Lord Śiva in the region of the forehead. He further explains the form of Śiva:

*Lalāṭastha śivam śvetam recakenabhicintayet.*
*Sādhum sphatikasaṅkāśam nirmalam pāpanāśanam*
*śaṅkaram trayambakam śvetam*
*Dhyāyan mucyate bandhanāt.*

"Śiva is like a spotless *sphaṭika* (jewel). He removes all defilements. He is peaceful, three-eyed, and white. One who meditates on him thus in *recaka* is released from all sins." When one practices *prāṇāyāma* with *gāyatrī*, the more popular method is to do *recaka* with the mind closely following the breath. While doing *kumbhaka* one should say the *prāṇāyāma* mantra silently, which mantra is *gāyatrī* with *praṇava*, *vyāhṛtis*, and *śiras*. The exhalation should be done with the mind closely following the breath. In the *Smṛti Ratnākara*, it says that *japa* should be done while practicing *kumbhaka:*

*Dakṣine recakam kuryat krāmenapūritodaraḥ* |
*Kumbhakena japam kuryāt prāṇāyamasya lakṣanam* | |

Here the method of doing *prāṇāyāma* is clearly described. It involves drawing in the air through the left nostril, doing *japa* during the *kumbhaka* phase, and then exhaling through the right nostril. It should be understood that the next inhalation is through the right nostril and the next exhalation through the left.

What should be the duration of the inhalation, holding the breath, and exhalation? Patañjali provides an answer in sūtra 2.50—*kāla paridṛṣṭi*; that is, *prāṇāyāma* should conform to some measure of time. Here again there are many variations, but there are many authors who suggest that the duration of *kumbhaka* should be four times as long as *pūraka* and twice as long as *recaka*. Many of the Upaniṣads that refer to yoga, as well as other yoga texts, give specific instructions concerning the duration. For instance, in the Triśikhibrāhmaṇa Upaniṣad, we find:

> *Idayā vāyumpūrya brahman ṣodaśamātrayā*
> *Pūritam kumbhayet pascāt catur ṣaṣṭyāttu mātrayā*
> *Dvāṭṛsanmātrayā samyak recayet pīngalāmalam.*

Here the recommended duration for the inhalation is 16 *matras* (units); holding the breath, 64 *matras;* and exhalation, 32 *matras*. Following the method mentioned in *Smṛti Ratnākara*, *japa* should be done during the holding of the breath. *Matra* merely means a measure, here a measure of time. For *japa*, taking one *matra* to mean one syllable is valid. Thus the *prāṇāyāma* mantra is made up of 64 syllables—21 for the *vyāhṛtis*, 24 + 1 for the *gāyatrī* portion with *praṇava*, and 18 for the *śiras* position. In practice, it takes about twenty seconds for the mantra. Thus it works out to be five seconds for *pūraka*, twenty for *kumbhaka*, and ten for *recaka*. If one practices the *bandhas* after exhalation, it will take nearly forty seconds for each breath.

*Prāṇāyāma* with *gāyatrī* is an activating process. *Gāyatrī* is an energizing or invigorating *(pracodayāt)* mantra. There is also a method of using the *praṇava* in *prāṇāyāma*. One meditates on the *a* during inhalation, on the *u* while holding the breath, and on the *m* upon exhalation. The goal is to merge the mind with the unmanifest *praṇava* in *bāhya-kumbhaka*. This is naturally for "out of this world" yogis, so one has to practice *prāṇāyāma* according to his *āśrama*, or station in life.

Gheraṇḍa describes *sagarbha prāṇāyāma* and the repetition of *bīja* mantra:

> Seated in a comfortable *sukhāsana*, facing east or north, let the *abhyāsī* meditate on Brahma, full of *rajas* and of a blood red color, in the form of the letter OM. Let him inhale by the left nostril, repeating OM sixteen times. Then before he begins retention after completing inhalation, let him perform *uddīyāna bandha* [this requires considerable control and one should attempt it only under the immediate guidance of a guru]. Then let him retain the breath by repeating OM sixty-four times, contemplating Lord Hari, full of the *sattvic* quality. Then let him exhale through *piṇgalā* [right nostril] by repeating OM thirty-two times, contemplating Lord Śiva,

> full of the *tamas* quality. Then, again, inhale through the right nostril, retain by [the breath] *kumbhaka* and exhale through *iḍā* [left nostril], as in the above method, changing nostrils alternately. Let him practice thus, alternating the nostrils again and again. When inhalation is completed, close both nostrils, the right one by the thumb [of the right hand] and the left one by the ring finger and the little finger, never using the index and middle fingers. The nostrils are to be closed as long as the breath is held in *kumbhaka*.

There are some who (not initiated in *gāyatrī* or *praṇava*) make use of one- or two-syllable Tantric mantras to practice *sagarbha prāṇāyāma*. Patañjali also refers to the number of breaths or rounds to be performed in *prāṇāyāma* by the term *sāṃkhya paridṛṣṭi* (2.50). Here again, different authors give different numbers. Svātmārāma and other *haṭhayogis* recommend 80 per sitting and four sittings, making 320 *prāṇāyamas* per day. This number should be taken as the upper limit, however, and the instructions specify a gradual increase to that amount.

> *Prātarmadhyandine sāyamardharātre ca kumbhakān!*
> *Śanaivasītiparyantam caturvāram samabhyaset!*

In this stanza from the Triśikhibrāhmaṇa Upaniṣad, it could be observed that eighty rounds per sitting in the morning, noon, evening, and midnight is suggested. By the expression *śanaiva* one should understand "gradually," and *asītiparyantam* would mean "up to eighty rounds." The sage Bharadvāja suggests that one should practice *prāṇāyāma* with *japa* during *kumbhaka* ten times before proceeding to *gāyatrī japa*. It should be noted that *sagarbha prāṇāyāma* requires that one first master a yogic posture before one develops the capacity to do *kumbhaka* for the length of time required to complete the mantra and to do it without a break for the required number of rounds. Such ability may be obtained by a variety of *prāṇāyāma* and *kumbhaka* practices referred to in *haṭhayoga* texts. The ultimate benefit of *prāṇāyāma* is *samādhi* itself, according to certain schools. In the Gītā this process is referred to as the merger of *prāṇa* and *apāna*, which is achieved by a very long *(dīrgha)* and fine *(sūkṣma) prāṇāyāma*.

As for the benefits of *sagarbha prāṇāyāma*, according to Manu, if it is done with *vyāhṛtis, praṇava,* and *śiras* three times, this is the greatest *tapas* for a *brāhmana* (Vedic scholar). Just as a metal is cleaned in a smelter, the *indriyas* lose their impurities through *prāṇāyāma*. If one does this practice sixteen times a day, in a month even the dreaded *brahmahatti doṣa* (the sin of harming or killing a Vedic scholar) is destroyed. According to Sounkata, if one practices three times with great concentration, all *doṣas* vanish instantaneously. With twelve breath controls, the *citta* becomes clear. Doing *prāṇāyāma* twenty-four times is the greatest *tapas. Prāṇāyāma* done with ten *praṇava* (seven with the *vyāhṛtis,* one with *gāyatrī,* one at the beginning of *śiras,* and one at the end) and fourteen times for a month releases one from *brahmahatti doṣa* and all other minor condemnable deeds *(upapātaka),* according to *yama.* Vyāsa simply states that the *prāṇāyāma* mantra of *japa* makes one absolutely fearless. And the *Yoga Yājñyavalkya* relates the seven *vyāhṛtis* to the seven worlds or seven levels of consciousness. With that, the yogi gains the capacity to communicate with all the higher worlds.

Patañjali, the authority on yoga, says: *Tataḥ kṣīyate prakāśa āvaraṇam,* with *prāṇāyāma* "the clouding of the mind is reduced and the intellect shines in its true splendor" (2.52). Further, *Dhāraṇāsu ca yogyatā manasaḥ,* "As a natural consequence, such a mind, and only such a mind, becomes fit for *dhāraṇā,*" or the first step of *antaraṅga sādhana* (2.53).

The uniqueness of our *ācārya's* system is that it attempts to include all the various systems of yoga and the gradual combination of the different *aṅgas* so that there are no abrupt changes. Thus in the practice of *āsanas,* the introduction of breathing practices helps to prepare the breathing apparatus for subsequent *prāṇāyāma.* Practicing *āsanas* with breath control, a certain mental discipline is achieved, so that when one starts *prāṇāyāma,* the mind also cooperates in following the breath, and thus in *kumbhaka* one may use Vedic mantras, *bījaksara,* or other Tantric mantras. With the requirement of the *adhyayana* (chanting) according to one's *śākha* (branch of the Veda), and the study of yogic texts such as Yoga *darśana, haṭhayoga* texts, and Upaniṣads with the foundation of *savinyāsa āsana* practice, one may hope to experience the greatness and thoroughness of our ancient system of yoga. There are schools of yoga that insist on *prāṇāyāma* alone as the key to yoga, as they declare that control of *prāṇa (prāṇanirodha)* inevitably brings control of mind *(citta nirodha).* In the classic *Yoga Vāśiṣtha,* the *ṛṣi* Vāśiṣṭha explains the relationship between mind and breath and extols the efficacy of *prāṇāyāma* in controlling the mind.

> Dear Rāma, the body is like a vehicle. The Lord has created the mind and *prāṇa* for the functioning of the body. When *prāṇa* rejects the body, the mechanism of the body also ceases. And when the mind works, *prāṇa* moves; it acts. The relation between *prāṇa* and *manas,* which are extremely close *(anyonya)* to the body, is like a driver and his chariot. The way the *prāṇa vāyu* acts, in the same way *manas* reacts. So the highest achievement of mind control is to be obtained by the concentrated effort of mastery over *prāṇa.* The regulation of *prāṇa* brings in its wake all worldly achievements *(rājyādi)* as well as others and leads to the highest spiritual attainment, that is, to total independence of the indwelling

consciousness from the gross, subtle, and causal bodies that are operated by *prāṇa* force. Hence, study the science of breath.

In previous sections, a few *prāṇāyamas* and the general benefits of *prāṇāyāma* were discussed. There are a few more *kumbhakas* mentioned in the yoga texts that are also now in vogue:

*Brahmadayopi tridaśāḥ*
*pavanābhyāsa tatparāḥ* ।
*abhūvam antakobhāyat*
*tasmāt pavanamabhyaset* ।।

"The gods, including *caturmukha* Brahma, practice the highest activity, *prāṇāyāma*, because of the fear of death. Therefore practice *prāṇāyāma* always." It is also said that as long as the breath is restrained in one's own body, the mind is calm and steady, and also that when the vision *(dṛṣṭi)* is directed toward *bhrūmadhya*, why should there be fear of death? The *nāḍīs* are purified by a properly regulated course of *prāṇāyāma*. The sage Brahmānanda, in his *Jyotsnā*, or commentary, on the *Haṭhayogapradīpikā*, details the routine to be followed by a full-time *yogābhyāsī*. It becomes important when one finds time heavy on one's shoulders after discharging one's necessary responsibilities and the mind yearns desperately for spiritual quest and rest.

## *Prāṇāyāma* Practice

Let us detail the routine of a *yogābhyāsī* for achieving the goal of *prāṇāyāma* practice. The *yogābhyāsī* should wake up a couple of hours before dawn *(uṣatkāla)*—or at least early in the morning *(prataḥkāla)*. He should contemplate his guru in his mind and his dear deity *(iṣṭa devatā)* in his heart. Then he should clean his teeth *(dantaśuddhi)*, complete his other morning ablutions *(suddhi)*, take a bath, and apply *bhasmadhāranam* (for a Saivite) or *punḍradhāranam* (for a Vaiṣṇavite), as the case may be. Then he should choose a clean place in a pleasant room *(ramya maṭha)*. He then should seat himself in a comfortable yogic posture on a soft *(mṛdu)* spread. He should then again meditate intently on Īśvara before proceeding to state his resolve *(saṅkalpa)*, mentioning the place and time (*deśa* and *kāla*) for the particular yogic activity.

*Adyetyādi śriparameśvara prasāda pūrvakam* ।
*samādhi tatphala siddhyartam āsanapurvakam prāṇāyamadhīn kariṣye* ।।

"With the grace of Lord Parameśvara, I now start the practice of yoga with *āsanas*, and other *aṅgas* such as *prāṇāyāma* for attaining *samādhi* and other yoga benefits thereof." Since Nāgārāja is referred to as the deity of yoga, one should utter a suitable prayer and proceed with the practice of *āsanas*.

During the practice of *āsanas*, when one naturally becomes fatigued one should assume *śavāsana*. If one feels refreshed thereafter, one may continue with *āsanas;* if one still does not feel up to the mark, one should not proceed with further practice. Instead one should practice a *viparītakaraṇī* (somewhat between *ūrdhva-prasāritapādāsana* and *sarvāṅgāsana*) where the back of the neck is stretched, facilitating the chin lock in later *kumbhaka*. The next step will be to do *ācamana* and begin that division of yoga called *prāṇāyāma*. Think then of the great yogis *(yogīndra)* for inspiration and proceed to do *prāṇāyāma* as detailed by Lord Śiva in the Kurma Purāṇa. Start with mentally saluting the great yogis and their *śiṣyas* (disciples) and Lord Vināyaka. With a calm mind one should contemplate the Lord (Śiva). Then, sitting in *siddhāsana* or *baddhapadmāsana,* one should practice *prāṇāyāma,* accompanied by the great *bandhas* at the appropriate stages. To start with, one should do ten breath controls, then increase it daily by five. This should be done until one is in a position to do eighty *kumbhakas* in one sitting, without any difficulty and with a positive sense of well-being *(susamāhita)*.

The first *prāṇāyāma* should be *nāḍī śodhana* with the use of alternate nostrils. It is referred to as *anuloma* and *viloma* by some (they are, however, differently interpreted by various schools). A *kumbhaka* called *sūryabheda* with the requisite *bandhas* should then be practiced. It should be followed up with *ujjāyī, śitkārī, śītalī, bhastrikā,* or any other *prāṇāyāma*. This should be followed by certain *mudrās*, (especially *mahāmudrā*) as taught by one's teacher. The posture is *padmāsana*, and the higher yoga practices such as *nādānucintanam,* which are enabled by *śaṇmukhīmudrā*, should be attempted.

Thereafter one should mentally surrender all the benefits of such practice to the Lord (Īśvarapraṇidhānam). After practice is over one should bathe in hot water *(uṣnena vāriṇā)*. Then one should perform one's daily duties *(nitya karma)*. The above-mentioned yoga practice should be repeated at noon. After some rest, one should have *patya* (that *sattvic* food mentioned in yogic and Āyurvedic texts), lunch, but never those prohibited items. One should, immediately after lunch, take cardamom *(yelam),* cloves, or *karpura*, if desired, betel leaves *(tāmbula)* without lime, if he practices intensely the praiseworthy *prāṇāyāma*. The *yogābhyāsī* should not indulge in frivolous small talk. After lunch, he should listen to the Purāṇas, practice *nāmasaṅkīrtanam* of Īśvara, but preferably research *(avalokana)* authentic texts of liberation *(mokṣaśāstra)* such as Yoga, Sāṃkhya, Vedānta, and so on. At dusk, he should perform the *sāyam sandhyā*, but preceded by over an hour of *yogābhyāsa,* as mentioned earlier.

The different types of *kumbhakas* require some elucidation. The Yogaśikha Upaniṣad says:

> *Atha abhyaset sūryabhedam*
> *ujjāyīm cāpi śītalam*
> *bhastram cān sahita nāma*
> *syāt catuṣtayakumbhakaḥ*
> *bandhatrayeṇa samyukte*
> *kevalaprāptikaraḥ.*

"There are four types of *kumbhakas* to be practiced, *sūryabhedam, ujjāyī, śītalam,* and *bhastram,* which are known as *sahita-kumbhakas.* One should practice them,and *kevala-kumbhaka,* facilitated by the three *bandhas.*"

*Nāḍī śodhana prāṇāyāma* is an extremely popular *prāṇāyāma* referred to in Vedic texts. *Sūryabheda-kumbhaka* requires a proper *āsana.* Then the inhalation is done slowly and deeply through the right nostril. According to *haṭhayoga,* such inhalation and subsequent *kumbhaka* should induce *prāṇic* effect up to the hair follicles and the fingertips. Thereafter one should exhale slowly through the left nostril. The procedures are repeated a fixed number of times. *Sūryabheda* helps to relieve heaviness in the head and sinuses *(kapāla doṣa),* the four types of *vāta doṣa,* and other diseases caused by microorganisms *(krimi doṣa).* Repeated practice, according to the *Haṭhayogapradīpikā* and the *Yogakuṇḍalī,* is a superior yoga practice. According to the Yogaśikha, it also helps in cases of many abdominal *(udare bahuroghaṇām)* disorders. In general, *sūryabheda* is believed to "heat up" the system. Hence those with low blood pressure and lethargy may benefit from it. Some schools say that *candrabheda,* which just reverses the process of *sūryabheda,* can help those with hypertension.

Yet another *prāṇāyāma,* called *śītalī,* is also quite popular, and the procedure is as follows:

1. Sit in a comfortable *āsana.*
2. Curl the tongue into a roll, protrude it, and inhale through the wet tongue, slowly stretching the neck and dropping the head back in the process.
3. At the end of inhalation, release the curl, fold the tongue, and touch the top of the upper palate, touching if possible the uvula. This is called *jihva bandha.*
4. Then stretch the back of the neck, drop the chin to about three inches below the neck pit, forming *kaṇṭha bandha.*
5. After *kumbhaka,* exhale through alternate nostrils.
6. Repeat wetting the tongue (before inhalation)—the "air-conditioning" *prāṇāyāma.*

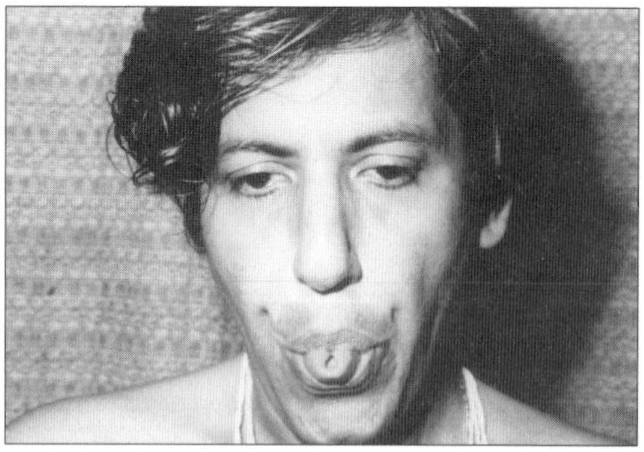

*Śītali* position

Done on hot days, this practice helps remove fatigue. According to the Yogaśikha Upaniṣad, it helps to correct *pitta doṣa* and suppress hunger and thirst. The *Haṭhayogapradīpikā* and Kuṇḍalī Upaniṣad attribute to *śītalī* other benefits, such as the eradication of diseases of the spleen *(plīha)*, abdomen *(gulma)*, fever, and bodily toxins *(viṣān)*.

*Bhastrikā* is like *kapālabhāti*, except that there is an additional constriction of the glottis so that the resounding effect is felt in the throat, nostrils, and even in the skull. The effects are similar to *kapālabhāti*, but are more pronounced for a potential asthmatic, working as a preventive but not necessarily as a cure.

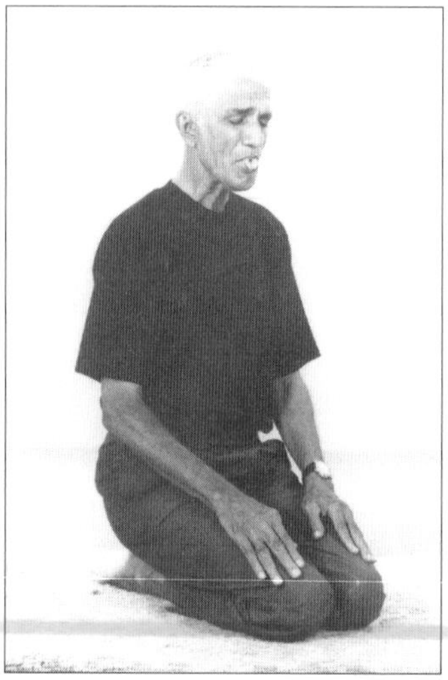

*Śītali prāṇāyāma*

Summarizing the effects, it may be mentioned that *sūryabheda* is heat generating. It is energizing and contraindicated for those with hypertension. *Bhastrikā*, *kapālabhāti*, and *nāḍī śodhana* maintain equitable heat (or temperature), whereas *śītalī*, *sītkanī*, and perhaps *candrabheda* have cooling effects. For those who follow Āyurveda, *sūryabheda* controls excess of wind *(vāta doṣa)*, *ujjāyī* controls phlegm *(kapha doṣa)*; *śītalī* controls bile *(pitta doṣa)*; and *bhastrika*, *kapālabhāti*, and *nāḍī śodhana* work to harmonize.

It is interesting to note that the various terms in yoga, such as *āsana*, *prāṇāyāma*, and *bandhas*, have been given entirely different connotations by certain Vedāntins. The Tejabindu Upaniṣad has the following to say about *prāṇāyāma:*

> *Cittādi sarvabhavāsu*
> *brahmatvenaiva bhāvanam*
> *nirodheḥ sarvavṛttīnām*
> *prāṇāyāmāssa ucyate*
> *niṣedanam prapancasya*
> *recakakhyatha samśritaḥ*
> *brahmaivāsmi iti ya vṛttiḥ*
> *pūrako vayuctyate.*

"To renounce involvement in *prapañca*, or the manifest universe, is called *recaka*, or exhalation; making the mind full with the realization that 'I' am identical with Brahman is called *pūraka* or inhalation." And further,

*Tatastadvṛttinaiscalyam*
*kumbhakam prānasamyamaḥ*
*ayancāpi prabhuddhanam*
*ajñānam ghrāṇapīdanam.*

"That mental state of 'I am Brahman' permanently maintained is called *kumbhakam (kevala).* This is how *prāṇāyāma* is to be understood by the wise. Mere holding of the nostrils is ignorance." The above stanzas also appear in one of the classic works of Śrī Śaṅkarācārya, the *Aparokṣānubhūti.*

# 14 Yoga for Women

THERE IS NO DOUBT THAT WOMEN HAVE BEEN practicing yoga since the olden days. In fact, there are yogic practices meant specifically for women. In his *Yoga Rahasya,* the sage Nāthamuni considers the special conditions of women and prescribes yoga practices that can be done during pregnancy for the proper development of the fetus *(garbha vṛddhi).* He also recommends specific prenatal exercises, as well as *āsanas* that work to tone up the "delivery apparatus" and help in normal birthing. A third group of exercises consists of those that are useful in family planning *(mitā santāna)* and for contraception *(garbha nirodha).* Readers may wonder whether these have been medically tested; it should be noted that for them to be effective, women need to have practiced these *āsanas* from early childhood, prior to puberty, since many *āsanas* are not at all possible to perform at the time they are needed—unlike taking a pill or undergoing instant surgery. All of them, however, are logical, and those interested should take them up at a young age to see the efficacy of the system.

Concerning those yogic practices that are prescribed for the healthy development of the fetus, Nāthamuni offers the following *śloka.*

> *Pūrvatāna dvipāt baddhakoṇa padmacatuṣtayam*
> *śīrṣa, sarvāṇga, pavanāyāmaiḥ, garbho vivardhate.*

This passage says that fetal development is helped by (1) *pūrvatānāsana,* or anterior-stretching posture; (2) *dvipāda pīṭham,* or desk pose; (3) *baddhakoṇāsana;* and

(4) *padmāsana,* or lotus pose. In addition, *sarvāṅgāsana* and *śīrṣāsana* are suggested. Together, these *āsanas* make up a daily routine that will facilitate proper fetal development. In describing these *āsanas,* the approach is *cikitsākrama* (therapeutic), and thus the classic *vinyāsakrama* may not be applicable in toto.

*Pūrvatānāsana,* or anterior-stretching pose, was mentioned in chapter 11 as a counterpose for *paścimatānāsana.* Briefly, one should sit erect with feet together and stretched forward. This is called *daṇḍāsana,* or stick pose. Then inhale, raise both arms overhead, and stretch and interlock your fingers. Next, exhale, and keep your palms on the ground about one foot behind your back. Then, keeping your back straight, press your palms, exhale, and raise your trunk, dropping your head back and pushing up your chest and pelvis. This is *pūrvatānāsana.* Inhale and return to starting position. Do this cycle about six times, or stay in the posture for three to six breaths. It is a very good stretching movement involving the front of the ankles, shins, knees, thighs, and especially the pelvis, abdomen, neck, shoulders, and arms. The chest is opened up. It also helps to tone up the breasts by improving vascularity and could help later in proper lactation. A milder variation of it is called *catuṣpādapīṭham,* which could also be attempted.

For *dvipāda pīṭham,* or desk pose, lie down on your back on a soft carpet. Support your neck and head with a small soft pillow. Exhale, bending your legs at the knees, drawing and placing your feet close to the buttocks. Do a few modulated breaths with the chin lock, or *jālandhara bandha.* If possible, hold your ankles with your hands; if not, keep your palms pressed on the floor. Inhale, press the back of your head, neck, and feet, and raise your trunk slowly as high as you can, arching and stretching your spine. Stay for a few seconds, pushing your hips (and stretching your lower back in the process). Exhale, slowly lowering your body. Repeat three to six times. This is *dvipada pīṭham.* The trunk raising may be done on exhalation, if one tends to obesity during pregnancy. This is a comparatively easy but very effective *āsana.* It is especially useful in relieving the lower-back pain so common among pregnant women.

*Baddhakoṇāsana* should be practiced daily by women. From *daṇḍāsana,* exhale, bend, and push one knee outward so that the thigh is at about ninety degrees. Keep your heel pressed against the perineum and bend your other knee also, so that both feet are together and your heels are pressed against the perineum. Keep your palms on your toes. Stay for a few minutes, doing normal inhalation and exhalation. This is *baddhakoṇāsana.*

It should be noted that unless one has been practicing this *āsana* from childhood, the hips will have become too rigid to do this *āsana* properly. This is the one *āsana* in which one stretches the pelvic muscles and the perineum as well, so that the normal development of the fetus is facilitated by the elastic pelvic muscles. Furthermore, it also helps in toning up those muscles that can help at the time of delivery. It is one

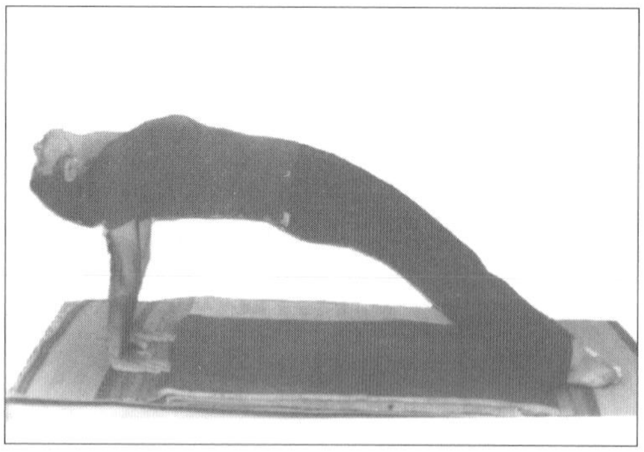

*Pūrvatānāsana*

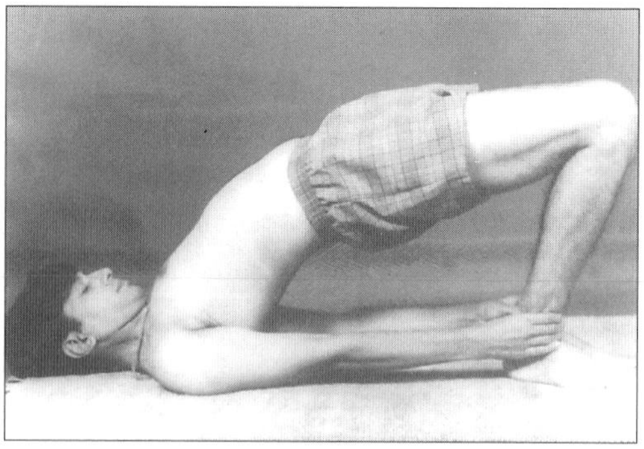

*Dvipādapīṭham*

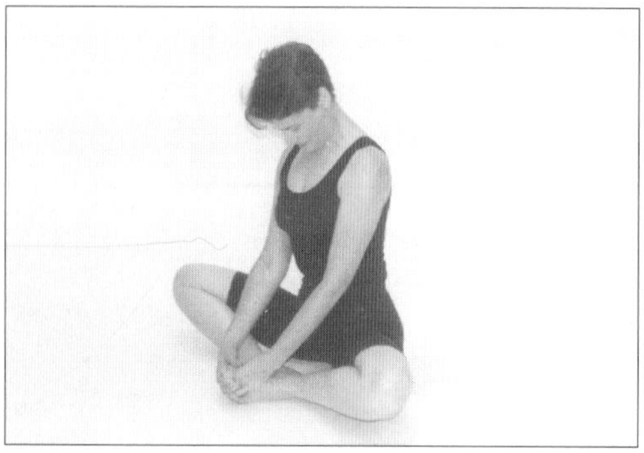

*Baddhakoṇāsana*

of the few *āsanas* recommended for practice during menstruation.

*Padmāsana*, or lotus posture, is the fourth *āsana* that Nāthamuni suggests. One of the best-known *āsanas*, it holds pride of place among the sitting postures. Sit in *daṇḍāsana*, exhale deeply, bend your right leg, and draw your right foot close to your body with your hands and place it on top of your left thigh, in line with the groin. On the next exhalation, in a similar fashion, bend your left knee and place your left foot on top of your right thigh. Now you have a

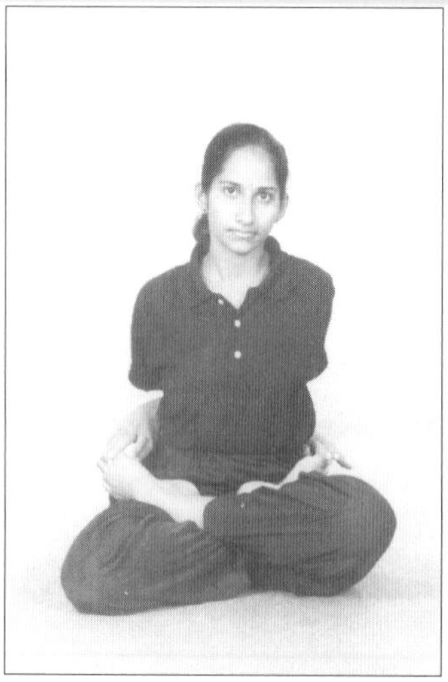

*Padmāsana (baddha)*

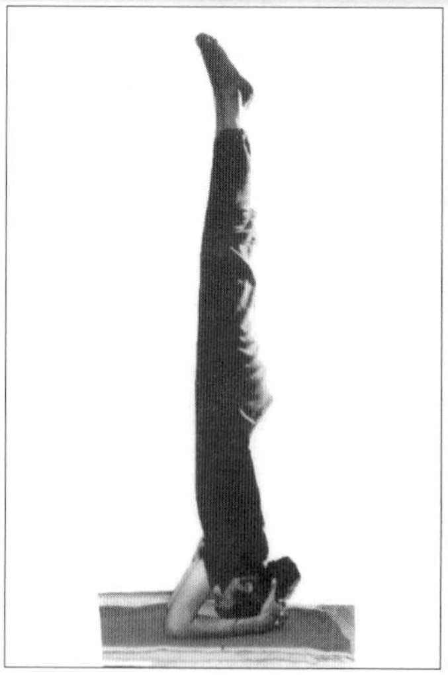

*Śīrṣāsana*

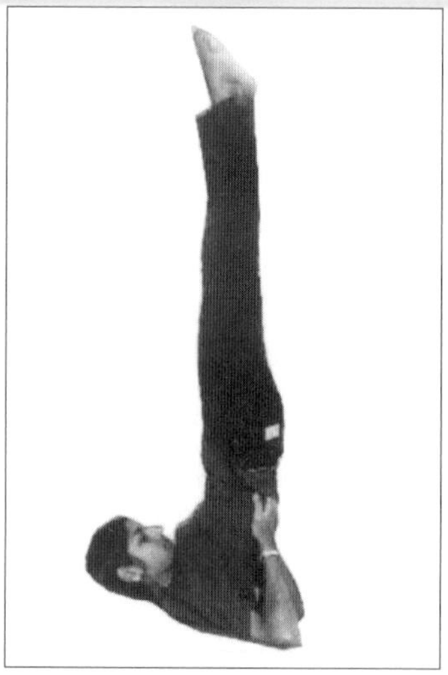

*Sarvāṇgāsana*

very firm base to sit on and the lower back is relieved of the strain of the outward curve normally found in squatting. Keep your palms on your knees, lock your chin, and do normal breathing, with the mind following the breath. This is *padmāsana*. In this position, one feels extremely secure and on a firm base, and the lower back enjoys freedom and comfort. The body should be erect. Naturally the mind will be relaxed and alert, unperturbed by postural distractions. This posture is recommended for both *prāṇāyāma* and some relaxation procedures like *śaṇmukhīmudrā*.

In addition to these four, Nāthamuni recommends two inverted postures, *śīrṣāsana* and *sarvāṅgāsana*. The techniques of doing both *sarvāṅgāsana* and *śīrṣāsana* have been explained in chapter 9.

According to yogic theory, diseases are caused by the displacement of vital internal organs and muscles, and yogic practice works to normalize the body. This kind of correction is accomplished by *śīrṣāsana* and *sarvāṅgāsana*. There are many benefits attributed to the practice of these *āsanas*. They have a tonic effect on the ovaries and pelvis through the removal of congestion. *Śirṣāsana* has a sedative effect. Pregnant women tend to get circulatory problems in their lower extremities, and *śīrṣāsana* helps to restore circulation. *Sarvāṅgāsana* has the advantage of working on the thyroid and helps to tone it. A sluggish thyroid affects the fetus. Even here, Nāthamuni cautions that inverted postures should be performed only up to the sixth month of pregnancy. In addition to these *āsanas*, an appropriate *prāṇāyāma* while pregnant is *nāḍī śodhana*. *Kumbhaka*, or retention of breath, should be very limited. One's diet should be *sattvic* and nourishing.

It should be clear that one cannot start to learn yoga after pregnancy. One should have been practicing yoga regularly prior to becoming pregnant. One should avoid all forward-bending movements; *prāṇāyāma* should not be preceded by *kapālabhāti* or *bhastrikā;* and *uddīyāna bandha* should also be avoided. For the purposes of relaxation, *śavāsana* and *śaṇmukhīmudrā* can be practiced after *prāṇāyāma*. Apart from the *āsanas* already explained, there are certain others that—if practiced from the early prenatal period—will facilitate normal delivery.

The purpose of this chapter on the possible applications of yoga therapy is mainly to indicate the potential of yoga and to appraise the depth of insight the yogis had on human anatomy and physiology and the wide range of yoga's therapeutic applications. This information should not, however, be taken as a workbook for direct application "off the shelf," as it were. It is important to emphasize that in all cases, a guru or a teacher is essential for the practice of yoga. It is all the more so in the case of the therapeutic applications of yoga.

Before discussing the mechanics of some other yoga practices, let us consider what natural childbirth, or *sukhaprasava*, could mean. Medical doctors say that when the cortex of the brain functions properly, our emotions cease to have an upsetting effect upon us. If one considers the effect of fatigue, a phenomenon we live with increasingly, it can be said that emotion or agitation occurs when there is no restraining influence. One can feel the devil working havoc when one is weak with fever. It is said that the necessary restraint comes from the cerebral cortex, which has the power to stop the disturbance originating in the subconscious centers of the brain. Hence it follows that agitation will occur when the cortex is disturbed. With less agitation, one's muscles can act normally, facilitating easy childbirth. Thus the goal of yoga practice, according to *sampradāya* (tradition), is both to provide the necessary strength to the uterus and the secondary muscles that work in unison during labor and to produce a serene mind that has the capacity to prevent disturbing emotions from appearing. Yoga attempts to provide both physical strength and mental control. With yoga, the expectant mother is able to direct childbirth, rather than meekly submitting to it, in which case the whole process becomes painfully chaotic. Of course, there are conditions like cephalopelvic disproportion and other mechanical, obstructive causes that may not allow for natural childbirth. But cases of cervical dystocia that may be related to psychological conditions or intrinsic neuromuscular disturbances may benefit greatly by these practices. Thus doing *yogāsanas* with proper modulated breathing and the specific *prāṇāyāmas* mentioned by Nāthamuni can help *(a)* create a relaxed and confident mind, able to "manage" labor properly; *(b)* strengthen the "delivery apparatus" so that it is relaxed and tuned to function properly; and *(c)* produce a sedative effect on the mother. These practices also help to provide the proper oxygenation so very necessary to the mother and the fetus during the birthing process.

The yoga practices that are helpful in facilitating normal delivery are given by Nāthamuni in the following verses.

*Ādhyam jaṭharabhāgasya*
*vivṛtiḥ koṇa pancakam*
*Śītalī nāḍīkā śuddhiḥ*
*dvipāt pītañca vajrakam*
*daṇḍāsanam pūrvatānam*
*sukhaprasava hetawaḥ.*

The suggested *āsanas* are:

1. *Jaṭharparivṛtti,* the abdominal stretch;
2. five *koṇāsanas*: *(a) utthitatrikoṇāsana (b) ūrdhvakoṇāsana,* done in either *śīrṣāsana* or *sarvāṅgāsana,* but only up to the sixth month of pregnacy; *(c) upaviṣṭhakoṇāsana,* sitting triangle pose; *(d) suptakoṇāsana, koṇāsana* done lying down; and *(e) baddhakoṇāsana,* an extension of *upaviṣṭhakoṇāsana;*

3. *dvipāda pīṭham,* desk pose;
4. *vajrāsana;*
5. *daṇḍāsana,* stick posture;
6. *pūrvatānāsana,* anterior-stretching pose.

The suggested *prāṇāyāmas* are *śītalī,* for cooling the system, and *nāḍīśuddhi,* for purifying the *nāḍīs.*

There are many variations of *jaṭharaparivṛtti.* The simplest and the most appropriate one is described here. Lie down, faceup, on a soft carpet. Keep your legs together and arms alongside your body. After a few breaths, and when you feel relaxed owing to steady breathing, preferably controlled in the throat, inhale, stretch your arms, and swing them to shoulder level. On the next exhalation, slightly raise your head, turn it to the left, and place the left side of your face on the floor. After a couple of breaths, on exhalation, press your arms and upper body, and, anchoring your hip, slowly swing your legs, one by one, to the right side, stretching the left side along its whole length. Close your eyes and do six to twelve inhalations, with very little holding of the breath in between. One may stay up to five minutes in this stretching pose. Then inhale and return to the starting position. Repeat on the other side. *Jaṭharaparivṛtti* is helpful in stretching the abdominal and pelvic muscles. The long modulated breathing helps the relaxed stretching and enhances muscular strength.

*Trikoṇāsana,* or triangle pose, is a posture that should be done carefully. Only those who have good balance and who have been regularly practicing yoga should continue this posture during pregnancy. Start with *samasthiti.* Exhale and spread your legs about three to four feet, depending upon your height. Take a few normal breaths and get a feel for the posture. Inhale and raise your arms to shoulder level. Then exhale, turn your head and neck to the left so that you look over your left shoulder, and, bending your hip, exhale as you lower your trunk on the right side, as much as possible without undue strain. Hold your knee, shin, or ankle or place your palm on the floor by the side of your right foot, depending upon your ability to stretch. Inhale and return to the starting position. Repeat a few times or stay in *utthitatrikoṇāsana* for a few breaths. Then repeat on the other side. One may do this *āsana* up to the sixth month. A long exhalation coupled with smooth movement will help produce a good stretch of the sides, especially the hip. If one is even slightly unwell, feeling weak, or giddy, this exercise should be skipped. It may be preferable to do this posture lying down, as *jaṭharaparivṛtti.*

*Upaviṣṭhakoṇāsana* is done sitting. Start with *daṇḍāsana.* Exhale and spread both legs as much as possible, stretching the groin area and thighs. Then inhale, raise your arms overhead, and do a few breaths. Next, exhale slightly, push your pelvis forward, and hold your toes, keeping your chin locked. This may be possible

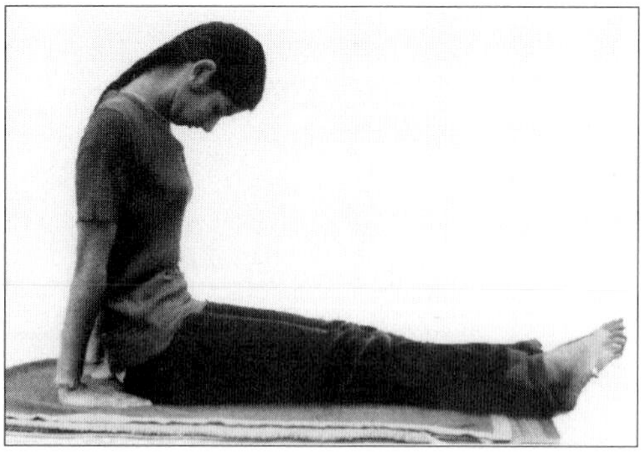

*Daṇḍāsana*

up to the sixth month. If holding your toes is not possible without bending forward too much, you may just keep your arms overhead and stay for six to twelve breaths. As a counterpose, exhale, and put your palms on the floor behind your back. Inhale and raise your trunk, keeping your legs spread. Exhale and return.

If one is capable of doing *śīrṣāsana* and *saravāṅgāsana*, *ūrdhvakoṇāsana* may be attempted. This posture has an added advantage in that, being an inverted posture, the legs become relaxed after a while in the position, and it will be possible to get a little more stretch of the thighs, groin, perineum, and pelvis. This posture should be done only up to the sixth month.

The above group of *āsanas* provide a necessary pelvic stretch and improve circulation; because of the accompanying long breathing, the *abhyāsī* is generally more relaxed and thus the stretching will be easier. The remaining *āsanas* and certain *niyamas* mentioned in yoga texts for pregnant women now follow.

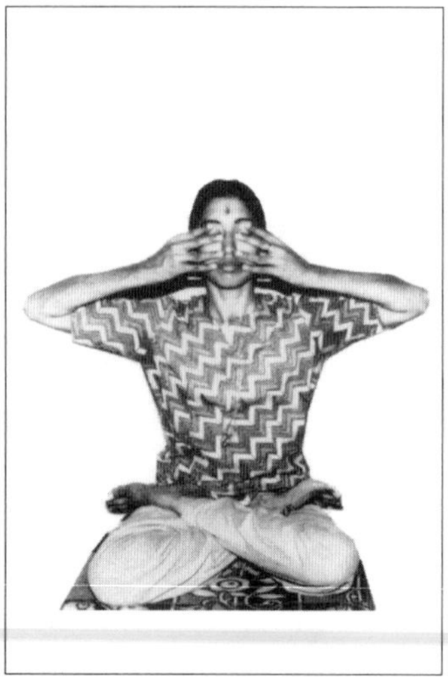

*Śanmukhīmudrā*

*Rakṣa prathaman caksurnertram*
*nāsam jihvām tadanutwanca*
*hṛdayam tundam nabhimyonim*
*tatastu rakṣat sakalam gātram.*

"Carefully protect the eyes, ears, nose, tongue, skin, heart, stomach, navel, and genitals. Because of such care [by the *yogābhyāsa*], the entire body is well protected." We have so far discussed yoga practices for proper fetal development and natural childbirth. Up to the sixth month, the two inverted postures and the *koṇāsanas,* along with their variations, were recommended as they are specifically useful for a good pelvic stretch. The *koṇāsanas* are generally said to be very helpful for strengthening the sex organs and can be employed as correctives and for proper development.

Apart from these *āsanas*, *vajrāsana* and *vīrāsana* are also helpful. Of the many sitting postures, *vajrāsana* is comparatively easy to do and combines grace and poise. It is a good posture for pregnant women to sit in comfortably, especially for doing *prāṇāyāma*. It helps to keep the back straight and derives its name from the fact that it makes the spine strong and supple. Unlike other sitting positions, which put considerable strain on the lower back, it helps to reduce the pressure on the abdomen for pregnant women. This and *vīrāsana* help relieve lower-back strain. Some of the variations, such as lifting the trunk on inhalation and back bending, help stretch the pelvis and make the spine supple.

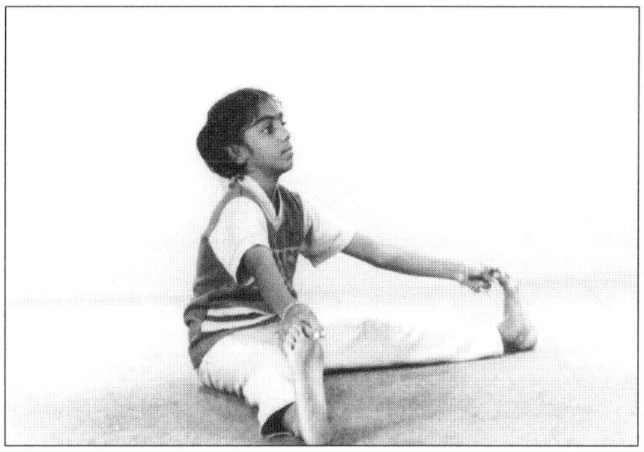

*Upaviṣṭhakonāsana*

Kneel and bend your legs, keeping knees, shins, and ankles together and stretched, with toes pointing outward, so that you sit on your heels with your shins on the carpet. Keep your palms on the knees. Stretch the back of your neck and place your chin a couple of inches below the neck for *jālandhara bandha.* Throw your shoulders back a little so that the shoulder blades draw closer to each other, forming a canal along the spinal column and opening up the chest. In this position, as a result of *jālandhara bandha*, a good stretch is obtained all the way down the spine. This is said to activate the *apāna* force, which has to be quite strong for natural childbirth.

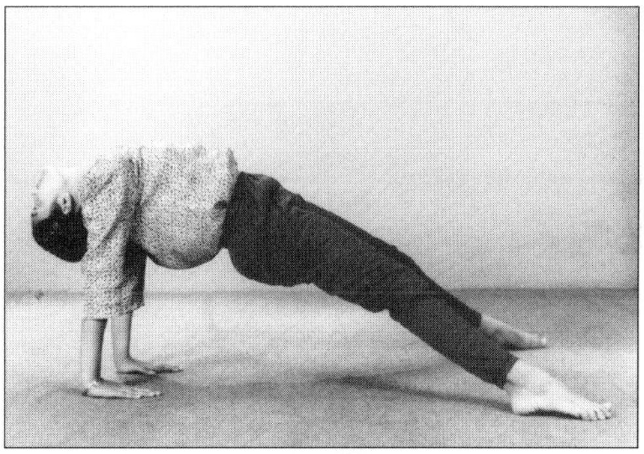

*Pūrvatāsana* in *upaviṣṭhakonāsana*

*Vajrāsana*, or spine posture, is believed to have been perfected by the sage Dadhīci, whose spine became a deadly weapon in the hands of Indra. A few *vinyāsas* in this posture, such as back bending and raising the trunk (in the kneeling position), will also be helpful. Forward bending, however, should be avoided. *Vīrāsana* is a bit more complicated and has been explained in chapter 12. These *āsanas* also help improve the vascularity of the lower extremities, the lumbosacral region, and the pelvic organs. Apart from these, Nāthamuni also suggests *bharadvājāsana,* which was explained in chapter 12. This *āsana* gives a spinal twist, without pressure on the abdomen. *Bharadvājāsana* is also helpful for expanding the chest, and with that the spine get a complete exercise. Nāthamuni suggests doing these *āsanas* regularly during pregnancy to facilitate natural childbirth:

*Daṇḍa padma bharadvāja*
*vīra vajra samānitu.*
*Āsanani sadā kuryuḥ*
*sudhīrga recapūrakaiḥ*

It should be noted that these *āsanas* are best performed with long and smooth inhalation and exhalation. According to the system of my *ācārya, āsanas* are to be

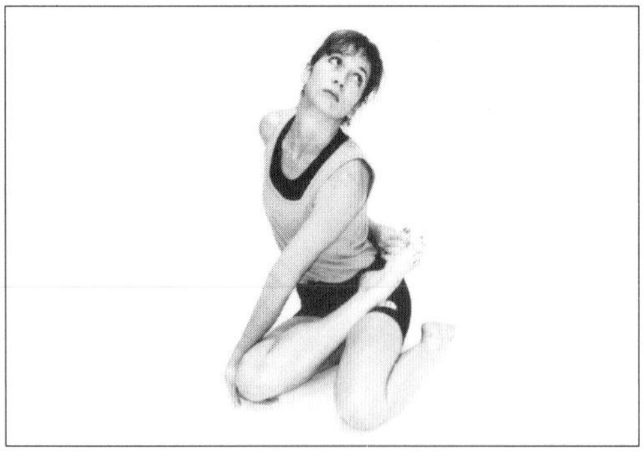

*Bharadvājāsana*

done with *vinyāsas* and coordinated long and smooth inhalations and exhalations. This tradition is handed down from Patañajali. The quotations from Nāthamuni are those that my *ācārya* dictated at different times in my classes.

Generally speaking, women who have been doing *āsanas* prior to becoming pregnant may continue to practice yoga during pregnancy, except for forward-bending exercises and certain *kriyās* like *kapālabhāti.* They should also refrain from doing *śīrṣāsana, sarvāṅgāsana,* and other more complicated inverted postures after the sixth month. Their diet should be nourishing, and they should create peaceful conditions at home. Moderate, carefully selected exercises such as those given above may be done for about half an hour per day to keep the body and mind fit to facilitate natural childbirth. A few precautions are necessary, however.

*Vegena dhāvanam, nātyam*
*ucchaiḥ ghoṣanam parityajet*
*garbhapāto vikārasca*
*śiṣūya antaiva na samśayaḥ*

"Running fast, dancing, and shouting in a high-pitched voice are to be avoided by pregnant women." These precautions are necessary, for violent movements such as these may lead to abortion, harm to the fetus, and even stillbirth. It is also necessary to take particular care to maintain harmony with one's husband *(patipriyā);* likewise, the husband should take care not to disturb the harmony of the expectant mother. In cases of sleep disturbance during pregnancy, which condition is quite common, it is suggested that the expectant mother regularly practice *ujjāyī prāṇāyāma,* while sitting in *padmāsana: Yadi nidrā vibhaṅgasyāth ujjāyī abhyāseth sadā.*

There are many variations in the practice of *ujjāyī,* and here the simplest, *anuloma ujjāyī,* is explained for practice by the *garbhinī* (expectant mother). Sit in any *āsana,* preferably *padmāsana.* Do the chin lock, *jālandhara bandha,* stretching the spine in the process. Both arms should be stretched with palms kept on the knees. The palms should be open and the fingers kept together. The elbows should not be bent. Breathe in slowly and evenly—the breath should be drawn in through both nostrils, but with a rubbing sensation in the throat that makes a hissing noise. The breathing sensation (the vibration), however, if done properly will be felt as far down as the diaphragm. The breath may be held for a few seconds *(mita kumbhaka)* or this may be dispensed with if it is difficult to do. Holding the breath is done by constricting the throat and not by closing the nostrils, as is done in other *prāṇāyāmas* such as *nāḍī śodhana*. The arms should remain outstretched. Bring the right hand to the nose with the fingers in *mṛgīmudrā* (thumb, little, and ring fingers kept straight and the other two fingers bent), and through each of the nostrils the inhalations and exhalations are alternately regulated. The exhalation should be done as slowly and evenly as possible. After the exhalation is completed, the right arm is brought back to its original position of being stretched, with the palm on the kneecap.

*Prāṇāyāma* should be practiced without *kapālabhāti* or *bhastrikā*, nor should it be interspersed with *uddīyāna bandha*. *Jālandhara bandha*, however, should be maintained since it is helpful in the control of *apāna vāyu.*

After the fifth month, a *garbhinī* should practice *prāṇāyāma* regularly. Two *prāṇāyāmas* that are recommended are *śītalī* and *nāḍī śodhana*. *Śītalī* is said to have a cooling effect on the system, and *nāḍī śodhana* removes toxins from the system. This last is a very important *prāṇāyāma* according to my *ācārya*, and in his *Yogañjali*, it is said that *nāḍīs* are the breeding ground for all disease, and *nāḍī śodhana prāṇāyāma* purifies the various *nāḍīs*.

In addition, the *garbhinī* should avoid all gossip and purposeless small talk *(vyartasamvada)* and delusion, and be careful not to let the mind go fickle *(cancala)* by letting in too many external influences. Daily *pūjā* or prayer *(parabhakti)* according to tradition and respect for one's *ācārya* will go a long way toward maintaining mental equipoise for an expectant mother.

Certain prenatal yogic exercises and *prāṇāyāmas* have been described so far, along with a few necessary restrictions *(niyama)*.

After childbirth, the regular practice of yoga may be started in about one month. The mother may start doing long, smooth *recaka* and *pūraka* (exhalation and inhalation), however, after ten days and for ten- to fifteen-minute stretches. The *kumbhakas* should be kept very short, two to five seconds. After one month, *āsanas* may gradually be practiced. Up to forty days, one may practice *āsanas* for fifteen minutes in the morning and evening. This may be increased to about half an hour until three months have passed. Thereafter, a practice taking three-quarters of an hour should be undertaken. This may be maintained up to the weaning of the child, when menstruation normally starts again. After the third month, medication used to be given for what is termed *garbhāśaya śuddhi*, or purification and regeneration of the uterus. Among the *āsanas* that normalize the uterus, specific mention should be made of *utkaṭāsana*, *sankatāsana*, and *karṇapīdāsana*. These *āsanas* massage the pelvic organs and improve vascularity, and thus help to cleanse the *garbhāśaya*.

When should girls take to yoga? They may start after their fifth year. However, they should be taught to practice *yama* and *niyama* along with *āsanas*, and they are usually not initiated into *prāṇāyāma* unitl their fourteenth year, or about the onset of puberty. The *āsanas,* however, can be done with regulated breathing. Since in the olden days girls were married before they became *rajasvalās* (pubescent), they could practice *prāṇāyāma* after marriage. From their eighteenth year they could take up *pratyāhāra* and *dhāraṇā* (meditation) on a *śubhāśraya* (object) or a pleasant *mūrti* (image of a deity), and these practices may be continued during the child-bearing years until age forty-five, or when the stage of menopause is reached. Then those who are inclined to become *brahmavādins,* or those spiritually inclined, may work on the other two *aṅgas* of *dhyāna* and *samādhi,* under the guidance of a guru. Or else they may continue with their daily *pūjā* culminating in *dhāraṇā.* All the other *aṅgas* may be observed and practiced regularly.

In a seminar on family planning organized by a voluntary organization, someone once remarked in jest that since yoga is mentioned these days as a cure-all, why not yoga for family planning? Yogis have studied this subject in some depth and have recommended *yogāsanas* that act as contraceptives for women. These are, however, very difficult postures that need to be practiced from an early age. Unless yoga is taught at a young age, its benefits, including the one under consideration here, will have a limited application. The culture of yoga practice, which is part of our heritage, should be inculcated early in life to derive the widest range of physical, physiological, psychological, mental, and spiritual benefits. Sage Nāthamuni's prescription for contraception is given in a capsule:

*Pāśāsanam yoganidrā*
*garbhapiṇḍañca bhadrakam*
*matsyendra āsanamityete*
*sarvagarbha nirodhakāḥ*

*Bahikumbhaka yuktiṛḥ*
*prāṇāyamasca samyutayaḥ*
*dhiaihi tribandhanaisca*
*bhaveyuḥ yadi nityaśaḥ*

"*Pāśāsana* (noose posture), *yoganidrā* (yogic reclining posture), *garbhapiṇḍa* (fetus posture), *bhadrāsana, matsyendra*—when these are mastered and practiced, conception will be prevented. Further, *prāṇāyāma* should be practiced regularly with emphasis on *bāhya-kumbhaka*, along with the three *bandhas, jālandhara, mūla,* and *uḍḍīyāna.*" These powerful *āsanas,* which work on the pelvic organs, provide the right amount of controlled pressure and twisting or squeezing of the uterus, and if aided by the *bandhas* in *bāhya-kumbhaka,* they should prevent, if properly done, the embedding of the fertilized ovum in the uterine walls.

For *pāśāsana,* start from *samasthiti* and keep the chin locked. Inhaling, raise both arms overhead, interlock the fingers, and turn the palms outward. On the next exhalation, press your feet and slowly twist your right side. Stay for a few breaths. Then exhale again slowly and deeply, lower your trunk, and bend your knees as in *utkaṭāsana*, except that your trunk should be at a right angle to your legs. In this position, exhaling completely, draw up your rectum and lower abdomen and place your armpit on the outer side of your right thigh, just below the knee. On the next exhalation, stretch your left arm and turn it around your right thigh. Then bend your elbow to take your forearm backward so that your left hand is near your left hip. Take a breath and maintain your balance. On the next exhalation, turn your right arm from the shoulder in the opposite direction behind your back to meet your hand, keeping your fingers interlocked. Stay for a few breaths. Then breathe in and exhale completely, drawing in your lower abdomen again and twisting a little more, holding your left wrist with your right hand. Turn and look over your right shoulder. Stay for a few breaths, raising your pelvic diaphragm on each exhalation. The inhalation will be short, but the exhalation will be long and smooth. On every exhalation tighten your grip, feeling greater pressure on the pelvic region and a mild twist in those organs. After a few breaths, return to *samasthiti* on inhalation.

Some of the *āsanas* that prepare one for *pāśāsana* are *utkaṭāsana*, *ardhamatsyendrāsana*, *pārśva-bhaṅgī* in *tāḍāsana*, *pārśva-uttānāsana*, and *marīcyāsana*. Long, smooth exhalation also helps in attaining the posture. This *āsana* applies tremendous pressure around the pelvis. It may be done lying down. *Āsanas* that help one perform *pāśāsana* are *paścima-uttānāsana*, *upaviṣṭhakoṇāsana*, *kūrmāsana*, and *karṇapīḍāsana*, as well as long and smooth exhalation. *Ekapāda* and *dvipādaśīrṣāsana* will also be helpful.

For *yoganidrā*, start with *samasthiti* and proceed to *uttānāsana* on exhalation. Then, holding the breath, jump back to *caturāṅgadaṇḍāsana*. Exhale, hold the breath, and jump forward to *daṇḍāsana*. Lie back on inhalation. Then, deeply exhaling, draw both legs overhead, bending your knees. Exhale and draw your left leg behind your left shoulder. Stay for a few breaths. On the next exhalation, draw your right leg farther up and slip it behind your right shoulder so that your ankles are

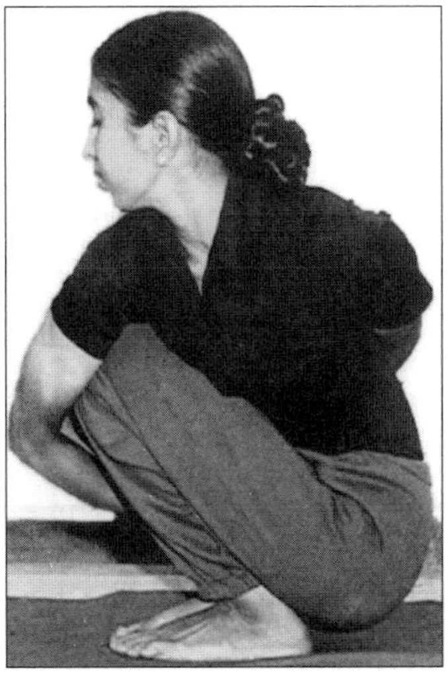

*Pāśāsana*

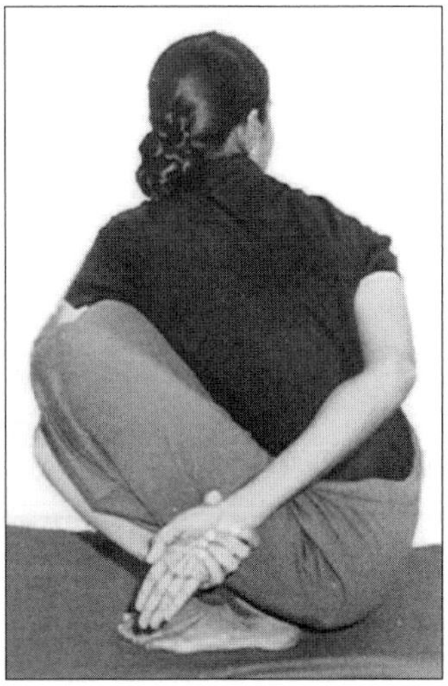

*Pāśāsana* (rear view)

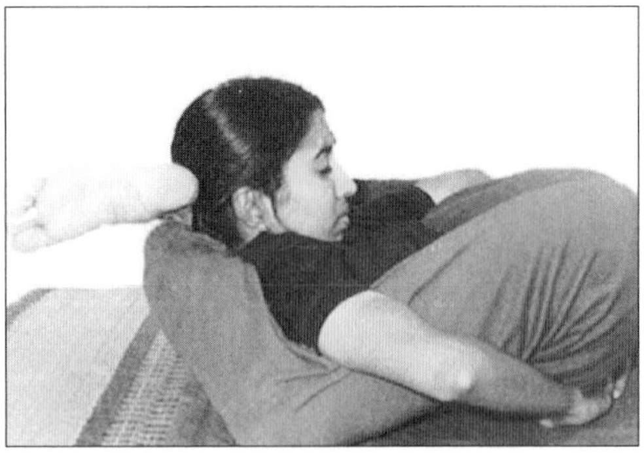

*Yoganidrā*

placed one on top of the other supporting your back. In this position, your back will be supported by your legs and ankles forming a base like a bed with the back resting upon it. Now slowly stretch your spine on exhalation, take your arms around your thighs, and clasp your right wrist with your left hand behind your back. Stretch your neck and try to straighten your spine. There is a peculiar, tremendous stretching of the pelvic as well as a fair amount of pressure. This posture, along with *dvipādaśīrṣāsana,* may be practiced for a period of time by those who are habitual aborters and then discontinued, which may help one in becoming pregnant. So long as these *āsanas* are practiced regularly, they act as contraceptives.

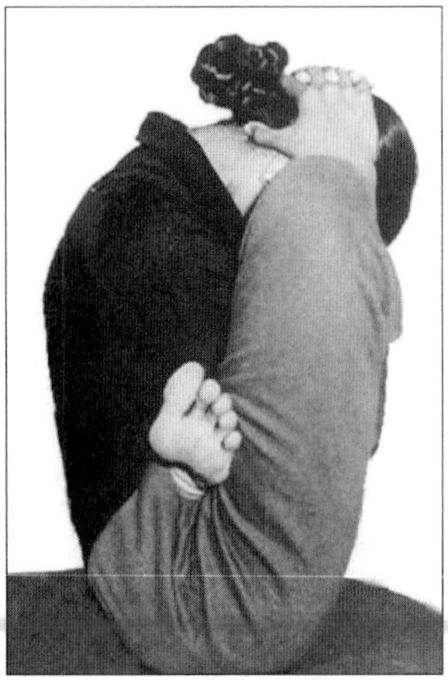

*Garbhapiṇḍāsana*

*Yoganidrā* is a great help, according to ancient wisdom, in preventing lung disease, tuberculosis, flatulence, and other abdominal diseases of the spleen, liver, and stomach. It helps to strengthen the *svādhiṣṭhāna* and *brahmaguha* ("cave of the heart") *cakras* for longevity. It controls *apāna vāyu,* and hence the pelvic organs get strengthened.

The *āsana* known as *garbhapiṇḍāsana* resembles a fetus. It is comparatively easy to follow. The procedure is the same up to *padmāsana.* Then slowly exhale, lean forward, and insert your hands—relaxing the shoulders—between your thigh and calf muscles until your elbows are through. Press the buttocks and, anchoring the coccyx, raise your lower extremities, lean forward, and hold the back of your head with your palms while exhaling deeply. As you exhale again, tighten your grip, straighten your spine, and draw your thighs close to your pelvis. Stay for a few breaths, made up of short inhalations and long, deep exhalations. Remain in this posture for a few breaths. Loosen the lock. Repeat with legs crossed, but changing the order of the bending of the legs for *padmāsana.* From *garbhapiṇḍāsana,* one may lie back to do *uttānakūrmāsana.* Both *āsanas* put a great deal of pressure on the pelvic organs.

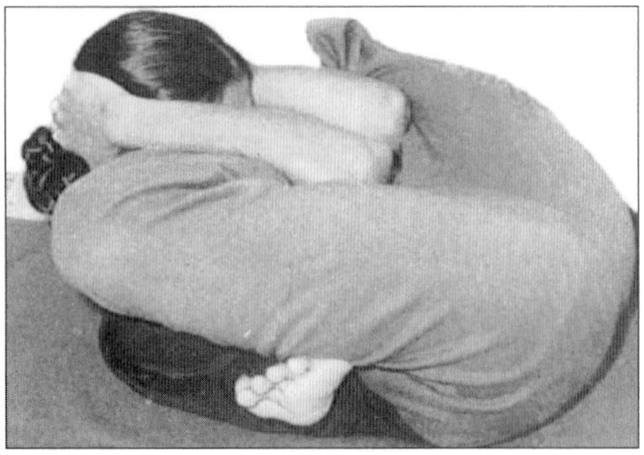

*Uttānakūrmāsana*

Among the *haṭhayogis* of the *nātha samapradāya*, Matsyendranātha, as his name indicates, was considered foremost among them. The *āsana* named after him is a masterpiece of *yogāsana* that shows the grace, poise, and strength of yoga and has great therapeutic value. *Āsanas* that help to prepare one for doing this posture are *ardhamatsyendrāsana*, *parivṛttaparśvakoṇāsana*, *pāśāsana*, *marīcyāsana*, and breathing practices that include long *recaka* and *uddīyāna bandha*.

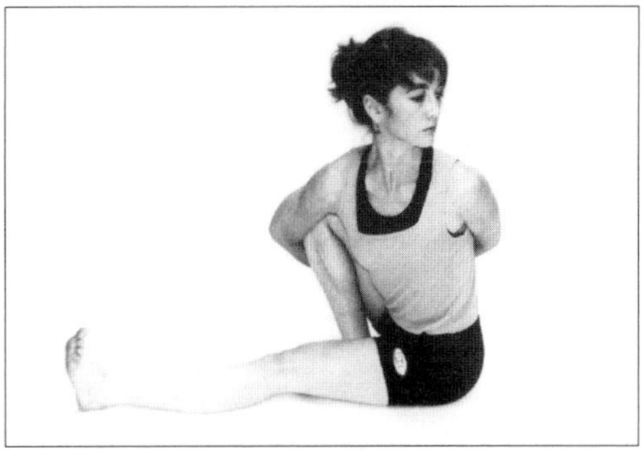

*Marīcyāsana (sthiti)*

Start from *samasthiti* and proceed to *daṇḍāsana*. Exhale and place your right leg on top of your left thigh, with your heel pressing the side of your navel. Stay for a breath. Draw your left knee up toward your body so that it is up to the chest, pressing your right heel against the abdomen in the process. On the next exhalation, slowly place your left foot outside your right knee and beside your right thigh! Stay for a few exhalations. On the next deep exhalation, anchoring your coccyx, twist your spine and turn your trunk toward your left side. This should be done smoothly so that your right armpit is outside your right knee. Pushing your chest forward, bring your right arm around and hold your left big toe. On the next exhalation, bring your left hand from behind and hold your right thigh near the groin. Stay for six breaths. On each exhalation, draw in the rectum and the lower abdomen and twist a little more, looking over your left shoulder. Then inhale and return step by step to *daṇḍāsana*. Repeat on the other side. It should be noted that in *matsyendrāsana*, unlike the previous two *āsanas,* there is also a twisting of the spine and pelvic organs, which is, to a certain extent, also experienced in *pāśāsana*. In *matsyendrāsana*, the heel is placed between the pubic bone and the iliac crest and with the crossing of the leg it is anchored by the side of the uterus, and in this posture the uterus is wrung, as it were. This is a very difficult posture to achieve and master, however. The other benefits of *matsyendrāsana* are mentioned in the *Haṭhayogapradīpikā:*

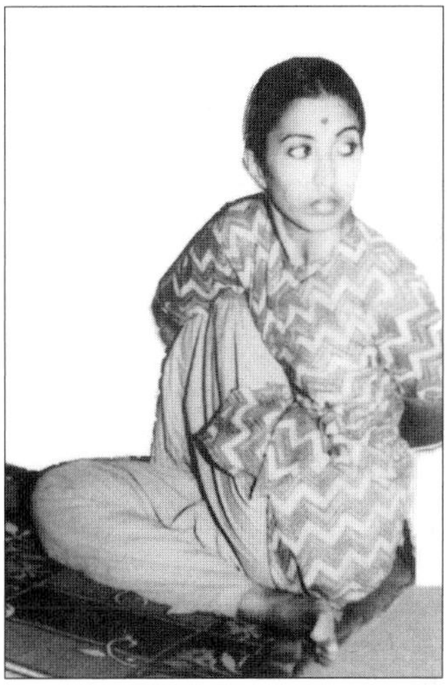

*Ardhamatsyendrāsana*

*Matsyendrapīṭam jaṭharapradīpam*
*pracanḍarugmaṇḍala khandanāstram*
*abhyāsataḥ kuṇḍalinīprabhodam*
*candrasthiram ca dadātipumsām.*

"*Matsyendrāsana* activates *jaṭharāgni* and thoroughly eradicates all chronic ailments. It activates *kuṇḍalinī* and gives mental steadiness." An anecdote is told about Matsyendra. Once, Lord Śiva, the Ādinātha, retiring to an uninhabited island

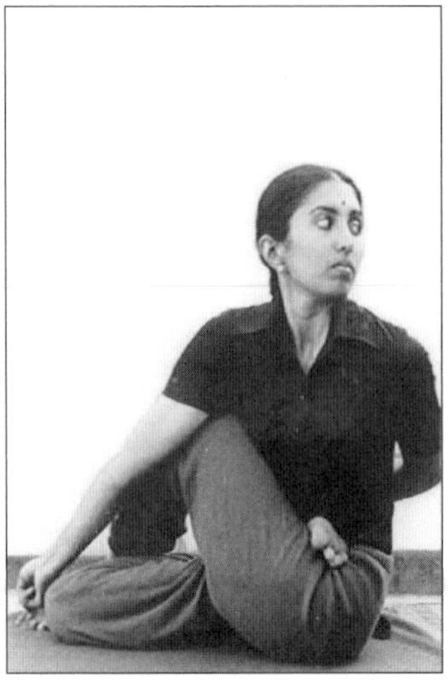

*Matsyendrāsana (purṇa)*

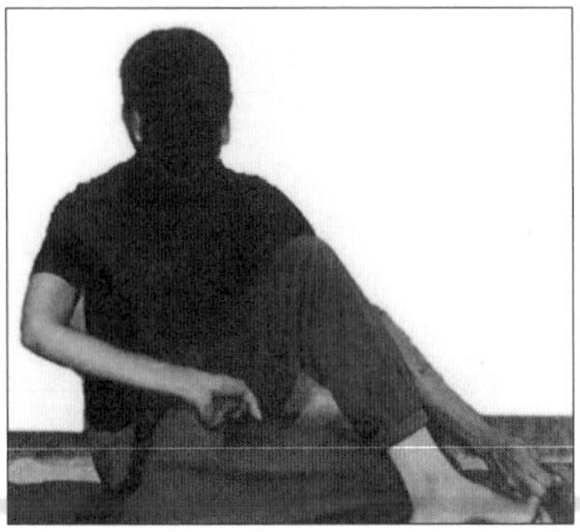

*Matsyendrāsana* (rear view)

and thinking it deserted, started tutoring his spouse Girijā on the secrets of *haṭhayoga.* A fish, remaining near the shore, started listening intently to those instructions. Thus it attained high concentration *(ekāgrata)* and remained steady in the waters with absolutely no movement. Noticing the fish, which was in *samādhi,* the Lord realized that yoga had been learned by the fish, and out of great compassion *(kripālu),* he sprinkled *(prokṣitavān)* water on the fish. With that the fish, known as Matsyendra, instantly attained its celestial body and was transformed into a *siddha,* thereafter becoming a great teacher of yoga. The *āsana* named after him is *matsyendrāsana* and resembles a fish that is twisting and beautifully poised.

The *āsanas* that can help prevent conception, it should be noted, do not work in all circumstances, the way a pill might work. Thus, unless one has been practicing yoga from a young age, these *āsanas* may not be of much practical value. But women not only can maintain good health, even as they follow the *gṛhāsta dharma* (the code of conduct for family life) as propounded by Manu, but they also can make use of yoga practice for *strīdharma* (the women's code of conduct). According to my *ācārya,* and apart from the above-mentioned *āsanas,* women can practice *marīcyāsana, ardhamatsyendrāsana, baddhakoṇāsana, baddhapadmāsana,* and *dhanurāsana* while exhaling, and the emphasis should be on exhalation while remaining in the postures. *Śīrṣāsana* with *uddīyāna bandha* and *ākuncanāsana* with *bāhya-kumbhaka* will help in family planning *(mitā santāna),* and will also help the mind to practice *dhyāna* later on. Needless to say, these *āsanas* should be practiced only under the guidance of a proper guru. These particular *āsanas* and *prāṇāyāmas,* which emphasize *bāhya-kumbhaka* and the three *bandhas,* especially *uddīyāna bandha,* are the very *āsanas* and *bandhas* to be avoided during pregnancy.

# 15 Yoga Texts

THERE ARE MANY FASCINATING WORKS on yoga found in *agrahārams* (communities) and certain households that are treasuries of yogic information, experiences, and instructions written by different yogis, *munis,* and *siddhās.* These works contain instructions about many unknown and lesser-known *āsanas (guptāsanas),* therapeutic practices, and meditative techniques. Except for a few, many of these manuscripts have not seen the light of the day. According to my *ācārya,* who himself did considerable research on these ancient works and evolved his *yogapaddhati* in part from them, it would be very rewarding for a research worker in yoga to investigate these texts. The present-day teaching of a few *āsanas,* assorted meditations, and other practices only skims the surface of one of the brilliant legacies of our ancient heritage.

A number of the texts have, however, been edited and printed. The most prominent of them all are Patañjali's *Yogasūtras* and the *Haṭhayogapradīpikā* of Svātmārāma. A brief description of some of the other, lesser-known works will be found in this chapter.

A very important text, useful from all angles, including therapy *(cikitsa),* is the *Yoga Rahasya* of Nāthamuni, a descendant of the great *nātha* group of yogis. I made an observation about the authorship of this book in chapter 1. Chapter 14 discussed some practical gynecological hints covered in this text.

Yoga encompasses a variety of disciplines, and therapy is certainly one of them. Many yogic texts prescribe a course of *āsanas* and *prāṇāyāma* for specific ailments, but the claims of some of them appear to be somewhat exaggerated, obscure, and incomplete. Further, different schools and teachers have developed their own combinations and methods, making claims that raise genuine doubts among the lay public and understandable resentment among medical men not subscribing to indigenous medicine. But one cannot deny that there is considerable scope for a dispassionate study of yogic texts, systems, and practices that brings to light the benefits of yoga for modern times. One has to approach the yogic texts with full faith, at least in the initial stages, since they are the works of great *ṛṣis*. And a *ṛṣi* is one who speaks the truth.

While on the subject of yoga's therapeutic value, it may be worthwhile to list some of the ailments that are supposed to respond to *yogāsanas* and *prāṇāyāma*.

1. *śirorogam:* different types of headaches. Though not all can be treated, some do respond to yoga.
2. *pīnaśayarogam:* diseases of the nose
3. *jvaram:* fever
4. *śūlam:* shooting pain, especially in the stomach
5. *bhagandram:* diseases of the generative organs
6. *gulma rogam:* diseases of the abdomen
7. *ārśa* on *guda rogam:* rectal disease, especially hemorrhoids
8. *śvayatu:* different kinds of inflammation
9. *śvāsam:* respiratory ailments, dyspnea, asthma, etc.
10. *chardhī:* vomiting liquids, blood
11. *akṣirogam:* ailments pertaining to the eyes
12. *athisaram:* diarrhea
13. *kuṣtam:* leprosy; *kusta* is said to be of two varieties—*sveta* or "white" and *kṛṣṇa* or "black." According to one school, eczema is a variation that may be dry or weeping.
14. *meharogam:* disease of sexual organs; STDs
15. *mūrca:* epilepsy
16. *apasmāram:* loss of memory
17. *nirnidrā:* sleeplessness or insomnia
18. *kampanam:* tremors
19. *ukkū:* stammering
20. *yakṛtu:* liver diseases; jaundice
21. *hṛdrogam:* heart palpitations; heart ailments

Yoga also recognizes mental or psychological diseases (treatment for which *siddhānta*, yoga practice including *prāṇāyāma* and *dhyāna*, is recommended). Mental illness is brought about by *kāma* (infatuation), *krodha* (anger), *bhaya* (fear), *dveṣa* (hatred), *lobha* (greed), *viṣādam* (confusion), *śoka* (sorrow), *asūyā* (intolerance), *avamānam* (guilt or loss of self-respect), *īrṣyā* (envy), *mātsaryam* (malice).

Apart from Patañali's *Yogasūtras*, the *Haṭhayogapradīpikā* is arguably the most authentic and exhaustive work on *haṭhayoga.* It consists of four chapters, or *upadeśas.* A detailed commentary by a sage called Brahmānanda and written in simple Sanskrit makes it a very useful reference work. The four *upadeśas* focus on *āsana, kumbhaka, mudrās,* and *nādānusandhānam,* or meditation on a mystical sound. The first three are *haṭhayoga* and the fourth is supposedly *rājayoga,* the main practice in which is *nādānusandhānam.* Other yoga postures that are not mentioned in the *Haṭhayogapradīpikā,* such as *vaśiṣṭāsana, dūrvāsāsana, kālabhairavāsana, sayaṇāsana, buddhāsana, marīcyāsana, bharadvājāsana, kaśyapāsana,* and *kauṇdinyāsana,* are named after great sages and indicate works by these *ṛṣis.*

The other main *haṭhayoga* texts are the Śiva Saṃhitā and the *Gheraṇḍa Saṃhitā,* and yet another important source of yogic information is the Upaniṣads. Twenty of the 108 Upaniṣads, starting from the Īśa Upaniṣad, for which Śrī Upaniṣad-Brahmayogin has written commentaries, are termed Yoga Upaniṣads and describe different kinds of yogas. The Śvetāśvatara and other major Upaniṣads such as Chāndogya (especially Dahara Vidyā, Bhūma Vidyā), are important ones for the yoga student.

The Śaṇḍilya Upaniṣad is from the Atharva Veda. The first chapter describes *aṣṭāṅgayoga,* but it follows the *haṭhayoga* authorities in prescribing ten *yamas* and ten *niyamas* for the first two *aṅgas.* (In Patañjali's *aṣṭāṅgayoga,* only five *yamas* and five *niyamas* are prescribed.) The eight *āsanas* described are the *svastika, gomukha, padma, vīra, siṃha, bhadra, mukta,* and *mayūra āsanas.* There are also interesting observations in the text about the locations of the *nāḍīs* and *cakras.* The fourteen *nāḍīs* described are *iḍā, piṅgalā, suṣumṇā, sarasvatī, varuṇa, pūṣā, hasthi-jihvā, yaśaśvini, visvodharā, kuhō, saṃkhinī, payaśvinī, alambuṣā,* and *gāndhārī.* The important *nāḍī śodhana prāṇāyāma* is described, followed by a description of *samantra prāṇāyāma.* The various *bandhas* and *mudrās* are then taken up, followed by discussion of the various kinds of visual attention *(dṛṣṭis).* The fifth *aṅga, pratyāhāra,* is presented in five different ways, based on different schools of yoga: The withdrawal of the senses is one; observing the self *(ātmabhāva)* in everything is the second form of *pratyāhāra;* renouncing the fruits of all prescribed activities is the third; total indifference to all things *(paraṅgmukhatvam)* is the fourth; and directing attention to the eighteen vital places in the body *(marmasthāna)* is the fifth kind of *pratyāhāra.* The sixth *aṅga—dhārāṇā—*is said to consist of five types. *Dhāraṇā* is focusing the mind and keeping it bound at a place, such as the heart region *(daharākaśa),* or in space, or on the worship of forms *(pañcamūrti dhāraṇā). Dhyāna* is of two kinds, *saguṇam and nirguṇam. Saguṇa,* according to the Sāṇḍilya Upaniṣad, is meditating on the form of the Lord *(mūrtidhyānam); nirguṇa* is meditating on the Self without any attributes, that is, beyond the three *guṇas. Samādhi* is the state of unity of *jīva* and *parama,* without distinction among the observed, observer, and observing *(triputī): Jivātma paramātma aikyavasthā triputirahita paramānandasvarupa śudhachaitanyatmika bhavati.* This is known as *asamprajñata samādhi.*

Other yoga texts that may be of interest include: Dhyānabindu Upaniṣad; Advayatāraka Upaniṣad; Śvetāśvatara Upaniṣad; Garbha Upaniṣad; *Yoga Kurantam* (as mentioned by my *ācārya*); *Vṛddha Sātāpatam;* Tejabindu Upaniṣad; *Gheraṇḍa Saṃhitā; Yoga Tārāvali;* Yogaśira Upaniṣad; Advitananda Upaniṣad; Triśikhibrāhmaṇa Upaniṣad; Śiva Saṃhitā; Brahmavidyā Upaniṣad; Yogaśikha Upaniṣad; Yogakuṇḍalī Upaniṣad; Nādabindu Upaniṣad; Darśana Upaniṣad; Amṛtabindu Upaniṣad; Yogacudāmanya Upaniṣad; Yogatattva Upaniṣad; *Śambhu Rahasya; Yoga Rahasya*; Sūta Saṃhitā; *Yoga Yājñyavalkya;* and *Yoga Vasiṣṭha.*

There are many other sources for information on yoga. The Purāṇas contain many valuable hints. Some Tantric texts are also good sources, as are the Vaiṣṇavite, Śākta, and Śaivite Upaniṣads. With the renewed interest in yoga, there is plenty of scope for both practice and research in yoga.

Let us look at the yogis' view of the human body. One text says: "At the time of birth, the body is naturally composed of *vāta, pitta,* and *kapha.* But later on, if the appropriate *vāyus* do not flow properly in the different *nāḍīs*, then diseases result, leading to death." Even though there are many medicines for the treatment of different ailments, it is also necessary that the *prāṇas* flow in the *nāḍīs* without let or hindrance. If the *vāyu sancāra* (flow of vital energy) is not proper, then medications will be of no avail. The specific *aṅga* of yoga, *prāṇāyāma,* is therefore very important in the treatment of diseases. And for success in *prāṇāyāma*, the cause of the accumulation of dross, or *mala,* in the body, that is, the three *doṣas*, should not be in excess. Any excess is easily discerned by such symptoms as tremor, heavy and shallow breathing (as against fine and deep breathing), pain in the joints, glandular inflammation, and digestive disorders. These conditions prevent the proper flow of the *vāyus,* leading to more serious ailments and a shortening of the life span. In order to do *prāṇāyāma* regularly, it is necessary to practice the various *āsanas* with the necessary *vinyāsas*, accompanied by coordinated breathing and *kriyās* to clean the *nāḍīs.*

The macrocosm is made up of three *guṇas*, as described in the philosophical systems of Sāṃkhya, Vedānta, and Yoga, and so is the body. Yogis divide the body into three parts according to the *guṇas*, the *sattvic, rajasic,* and *tamasic.* The head, which is the *sattvic* part, contains the perceptive organs, or *jñānendriyas.* These are the eyes, nose, ears, and tongue. This *sattvic* part helps the individual toward understanding of correct living *(dharma)* and discrimination between good and evil. The *jñanendriyas*, remaining in their respective positions in the head, help the mind. *Sattva*—the quality yoga attempts to bring out as the dominant *guṇa* in the individual—is known by brightness *(prakāśa)* and lightness *(laghutva),* as is said in the *Sāṃkhya Kārikā* of Īśvarakṛṣṇa: *Sattvam laghu prakasakam istam.*

The nature of *rajas* is activity, and the *rajasic* part, which is between the head and navel, helps the *sattvic* and *tamasic* parts in their respective natures. The *tamasic* portion has the properties of heaviness *(gurutva)* and obstruction or screening *(āvarana)*. The none-too-desirable *tamasic* quality becomes the predominant one through lack of yogic practices, eating the wrong types of food, and so on, in both obese and lean body types. Such people complain about heaviness in their lower extremities. According to yogis, when *tamas* predominates, dross accumulates in the lower abdomen and clogs the *nāḍīs* with *mala*, thus preventing the proper *vāyu sancāra* in the *nāḍīs*. The lower abdomen is the part of the body where the *nāḍīs* converge and, if not taken care of, becomes the breeding ground of all ailments. Yogic science, by the judicious use of *āsanas*, the *bandhas*, and appropriate *prāṇāyāmas*, makes the *agni tattva* (fire element) in the body active, which helps to remove the *malas*.

Certain specific yogic exercises are recommended to help bring out *sattva* in the *sattvic* part and to reduce the effect of *tamas* in the *tamasic* part of the body. For instance, the following exercises help the *sattvic* part and give the *abhyāsī* good memory, power of concentration, intelligence, and long life:

1. Among *āsanas*, *śīrṣāsana* and its many variations or *vinyāsas*.
2. Among *mudrās*, *mahāmudrā* performed with long inhalations and exhalations on both sides of the body.
3. Among the *bandhas* and *jālandhara bandha*, both while practicing *prāṇāyāma* and *āsanas*, or wherever appropriate.
4. Among the *prāṇāyāmas*, *nāḍī śodhana*.
5. Among the *kumbhakas*, *ujjāyī* and *sūryabheda*.

The *rajasic* part of the body is kept healthy, strong, and active by a few specific exercises. Practiced regularly, these help to prevent weakness of the heart and to improve circulation:

1. Among the *āsanas*, *sarvāṅgāsana* and its *vinyāsas*.
2. Among the special postures, *vasiṣṭhāsana*.
3. Among the *bandhas*, *uddīyāna bandha;* this should be practiced at the appropriate stage of breathing, even in *āsanas* such as *sarvāṅgāsana*.
4. Among the *kriyās*, *kapālabhāti kriyā* or *bhastri*.
5. Among the *prāṇāyāmas* or *kumbhakas*, *śītalī prāṇāyāma*.

The *tamasic* part is cleaned and kept in good condition by the following *āsanas*. When this part is kept well exercised by yogic *āsanas*, one feels extremely light and supple, and hence young.

1. *Paścimatānāsana,* or the posterior-stretching posture, helps stretch the muscles and joints in the lower extremities.
2. *Matsyendrāsana,* a masterful *āsana* of grace, poise, strength, and efficiency, along with its variations, helps massage the lower abdomen as well as squeeze the ankle, knee, and hip joints.
3. *Baddhapadmāsana* helps reduce heaviness around the vulnerable lower abdomen.
4. *Marīcyāsana,* named after Marīci Mahāṛṣi, and its variations help reduce the lower abdomen, hips, and thighs.
5. *Jaṭharaparivṛiti* helps the hips and cuts to size the sides of the body and the legs.
6. Among the *kumbhakas, nāḍī śodhana, ujjāyī,* and *sūryabheda.*

The above lists are general. The yoga therapist can prescribe many other *āsanas* and *vinyāsas* in standing, sitting, and lying-down positions, including twisting movements. Though some may doubt the efficacy of these *vinyāsas,* each variation has been found to have particular applications for some diseases and conditions, in the same way that medical science prescribes different medicines for various ailments in different parts of the body. In fact, yogic science has numerous fundamental and hybrid *āsanas* and *prāṇāyāmas* for the eradication of different ailments in different parts of the body for different kinds of people.

Bodily functions are maintained by the ten *vāyus,* and it is necessary to know their location and function. These *vāyus* should be strong and the *nāḍīs* in fine fettle for one to enjoy good health. The ten *vāyus* consist of five *mukhya* (important) *vāyus*—*prāṇa, apāna, samāna, udāna,* and *vyāna*—and five that are less important—*nāga, kūrma, kṛkara, devadatta,* and *dhanañjaya.* Of the first five, *prāṇa* and *apāna* are the most important, and it is their integration that is *haṭhayoga.* According to yogis, *prāṇa vāyu* is the chief of all. The station of *prāṇa* is *hṛdaya* (the heart). Its function is to draw fresh air from the outside and keep the body's *agni tattva* active, so as to remove dross from the body and increase longevity. By the practice of stipulated activities such as *yogāsanas* and *prāṇāyāma,* the *prāṇa*'s influence extends through the appropriate *nāḍīs* to the face *(mukha),* nose *(nāsika),* chest *(hṛnmadhya),* navel *(nābhi),* and even to the toes *(pādaṅguṣṭha). Apāna* is the *vāyu* next in importance. Centered in the rectal region *(gudhasthāna),* it acts to excrete, and its influence (by correct living and practice) extends to the abdomen *(udara),* testes *(vṛṣaṇa),* hips, thighs, and generative organs. This whole area is called the house of *apāna,* or *apāna nilaya. Vyāna,* as its name indicates, permeates the whole body and helps to maintain the tissues, marrow, *medhas* (brain), and so on. It helps the flow of blood and other fluids in their various conduits *(nāla).* Its range is mentioned particularly as being around the ears, neck, eyes, and head. *Udāna,* remaining in the gullet *(kanṭha)*, helps remove the *doṣa* of excess *kapha* and helps control the instrument of speech, and hence modulation *(dhvanī)* of the voice. It is said to keep the various joints *(sandhi)* in proper working condition. *Samāna vāyu*, remaining in the center of the body (the navel region for humans), acts as the great homogenizer of food and subsequently metabolizes with the right functioning of *jaṭharāgni*. The *vāyus* thus maintain bodily functions, provided they are strong and the 72,000 *nāḍīs* that act as their pathways are not obstructed with roadblocks. Of the remaining five *vāyus*, *nāga* is the belcher; *kūrma* does the job of periodic blinking, thereby protecting the eyes; *kṛkara* controls sneezing, thus keeping the nasopharynx free of dust and phlegm; *devadata* helps one yawn when the intake of *prāṇa vāyu* is low; and *dhanañjaya* maintains the body's temperature within the specified limits and keeps the body warm for up to four hours after death. *Vāyus* and *nāḍīs* have to work in unison for the proper functioning of the various organs. Hence it is necessary to know the location, function, and sphere of activity of the *vāyus*, as well as the location and pathway of important *nāḍīs*, in order to take appropriate remedial action.

Yoga philosophy also mentions a few other bodily principles that should be clearly understood by the *abhyāsī*. The principle of fire, or *anala*, is said to be in the shape of a triangle *(trikoṇa)* having its flame always pointing upward. It is in the region of the *nābhi*, or navel. This is a very important principle, especially for *kuṇḍalinī* arousal and for both physical health and the supernatural experiences mentioned in many yogic texts. Just as the body is divided according to the *guṇas*, so it is also divided into five regions based on the subtle aspects of the five *bhūtas*, or elements. The body is made up of these five principles, and the goal is to reduce the *pṛthvī tattva* and increase the other *tattvas*. Special *dhāraṇās* are mentioned for locating the centers of these principles in the body, and each has its special locale. *Pṛthvī*, or the earth principle, is from the feet to the knees *(pādādijānuparynatam);* the stretch from the knees to the rectum is called the region of water, or *ap;* the rectum to chest *(hṛnmadhya)* region is called *vahnisthāna*, or fire region; the area from midheart to the middle of the eyebrows *(bhrumadhya)* is the *vāyu*, or air, region; and from there to the top of the head *(mūrdhantam)* is the *ākāśasthāna*, or the region of ether (or space). There are variations in these divisions among various scholars.

Yogic texts also refer to the eighteen different vital points in the body called *marmasthāna*, which were determined by the Aśvins, the physicians of the gods. As recorded in the Yoga Upaniṣad:

> *Padaṅguṣṭha gulpha jhanghā*
> *jānūru pāyu meḍra nābhi hṛdaya*
> *kanṭakūpa tālu nasikāsinetram talu nasikasinetram*
> *bhrūnmadhya lalāta mūrdhni sthānam*

These vital *sthānas* are the two big toes; the backs of the heels; the skin; the knees; the groin; the rectum; the perineum (and generative organ); the navel; the heart; the gullet; the upper palate; the nose; the eyes; between the eyebrows; the forehead; and the top of the head. Thus, in examining a patient, the following aspects are observed by yogis:

1. The two big toes
2. Both joints above the heels
3. Both knee joints
4. The thigh joints
5. The *sīvanī nāḍī* below the genitals
6. The genitals
7. The navel
8. The heartbeat
9. The tone of speech and the throat
10. The pit below the throat *(kaṇṭa kūpa)*
11. Breathing
12. The muscle between the eyebrows
13. The tongue, its color and movement
14. The face and expression
15. The head and its movements
16. The temperature at the top of the head

The approach to yoga these days may be classified in three ways. First, Yoga is treated as a Vedic philosophy based on the sūtras of Patañjali. It deals with all aspects of *samādhi*—its prerequisites and ramifications—and culminates in the realization of the distinctive natures of both *prakṛti* and *puruṣa,* or indwelling consciousness. This realization leads to *kaivalya* or *mokṣa,* according to Yoga philosophy.

Second, yoga is treated as an art and as a complete physical culture *(sarvāṅga sādhana).* The many *āsanas* and their variations, along with coordinated breathing, are what make it an art, and it is considered one of the sixty-four arts *(kalās* or *vidyās).* This physical culture itself is fascinating to many. Third, yoga is considered to be a therapy for many ailments, and as both curative and especially preventive. Naturally the therapeutic approach *(cikitsa krama)* will be distinctly different from that of the student of yoga who approaches it as an art or a philosophy. Many texts talk about the benefits of certain *āsanas*, *prāṇāyāmas*, *mudrās*, *bandhas*, and so on. According to Āyurveda, those diseases that are chronic and that cannot be cured *(asādhya)* or completely eradicated by medicine alone can and should be treated with *yogāsanas* and *prāṇāyāmas.*

Finally, certain texts talk about yoga practice being structured according to one's age. These sources divide people according to their stage of life and suggest different approaches. Those approaches are called *śṛṣṭi*, *sthiti*, and *laya*. Certain *āsanas* and *vinyāsas* should be done during the age of growth *(śṛṣṭi)*, others during middle age, when there is neither growth nor decay, and still others during the period of decay, called the *laya krama*.

# 16 Antaraṅga Sādhana

IN PREVIOUS CHAPTERS MANY GROUPS of *yogāsanas* and *prāṇāyāmas* have been explained, along with their benefits. While these *haṭhayoga* practices offer many physical and physiological benefits, Patañjali would urge aspirants to go beyond them and work toward the transformation of the mind *(citta pariṇāma)* itself. This practice, known as *antaraṅga sādhana,* helps create qualitative and permanent changes in the *citta* by means of practice, and these changes increase and successively strengthen the *saṃskāras* (habits) of *nirodha, samādhi,* and *ekāgrata,* to the exclusion of the distracted *(vyuthita) saṃskāras. Prāṇāyāma* helps to reduce the painful and distracting tendencies of *citta* when it leans toward becoming predominantly *sattvic.* Such a *sattvic* mind also becomes capable of concentrating and holding onto subtle objects.

Many of us stop with *āsanas* and *prāṇāyāma.* While by themselves these offer many benefits, such as physical health and sufficient mental clarity to carry on one's day-to-day work, other psychological experiences and the ultimate spiritual experience require further rigorous practice. Since we usually return to our normal way of thinking after practicing these first two aspects of *sādhana,* the senses will continue to distract the mind. Alternating between rudimentary *yogābhyāsa* and sensual activities, we may wonder about the real efficacy of *yoga sādhana.*

*Pratyāhāra,* the fifth *aṅga* of yoga, helps prevent this backward slide. The main antagonist to further *yogābhyāsa* is the indulgence through the sensual objects that lead again to passion and delusion. Practicing *yamaniyama, āsana,* and *prāṇāyāma* leads to mental clarity, and the influence of the *indriyas* on the mind is greatly reduced. There is also a better awareness of the spotless *sattvic* aspect of *citta,* and the *indriyas* also become *sattvic,* merging, as it were, with the *citta sattva;* that is, as the *citta* is given other, subtler *tattvas,* the *indriyas* do not cause any interference.

*Pratyāhāra,* some suggest, is a result of *āsana* and *prāṇāyāma,* while others say it is also a specific practice. *Śaṇmukhīmudrā,* a simple exercise mentioned earlier, helps strengthen the *pratyāhāra* habit. But a fundamental decision about what object, or *tattva,* should be used for contemplation by the now free *sattvic citta* needs to be made. On this question, there are as many views as there are schools. For instance, *haṭhayogis* refer to *nādānuśaṅdhāna,* or listening to the *anāhata* (which literally means the "unstruck sound," or the sound produced without the rubbing of two objects) made possible by *śaṇmukhīmudrā,* and this should be attempted. The third chapter of the *Yogasūtras* is devoted exclusively to the technique of concentration, the *tattvas* to be used for concentration, and the benefits, or *siddhis,* that accrue to the *abhyāsī.* The technique itself consists of three stages, but taken as one it is called *saṃyama,* or *antaraṅga sādhana.* The three parts—*dhāraṇā, dhyāna,* and *samādhi*—represent the different stages of realization, each succeeding the other.

In Patañjali's first chapter, the various aspects of *samādhi* are described in detail. In the second chapter, the prerequisite practices for making the mind fit for *dhāraṇā* are described. In the third chapter, for the sake of creating interest and also for those so inclined, certain *siddhis* are described along with the means for their attainment. Going back to the question of what should be the object of contemplation, Patañjali is delightfully vague so as to accommodate different groups of *antaraṅga abhyāsīs*—whether devotees, religious people, *bhairāgis, jñanis,* or *siddhās.* The commentaries and the Purāṇas, however, offer some specific guidelines. Even though by means of the five steps from *yama* to *pratyāhāra* the basic obstacle that is the restlessness of the *citta* is greatly reduced, since the *citta* is basically wandering and unsteady *(manascancalam asthiram),* without conjoining with an object it does not become steady; hence the need for the support provided by an object *(āśraya).* But we have excluded, by means of *bahiraṅga sādhana,* those contacts that produce painful bondage. Thus it is necessary to find the support *(āśraya)* of that object (whether form, thought, or feeling) that, without being the cause of a slide back to bondage, would progressively lead the *abhyāsī* to *kaivalya* (there are very many names given to this ultimate state of *citta*) through stages of superior enlightenment.

Such an object is called a *śubhāśraya.* If the mind, in contacting an object that does not cause it to suffer restlessness and subsequent bondage *(bandha),* that object or support is known as *śubhāśraya.* This *śubhāśraya* can be of two kinds, *bāhya* (outer) and *antara* (inner). It has been the practice to start with *bāhya dhāraṇā.* Focusing the mind on a charming *mūrti* (statue) of the Lord, made of *pañcaloha* (five-metal alloy) and, according to the *āgamas,* fortified by the mantra, is *bāhya dhāraṇā.* When a devotee, however, by repeated practice, has the *citta vṛtti* of the enchanting form of the Lord, even without the aid of the *vigraha* (icon), then it becomes *antara dhāraṇā. Bhakti* is not merely the unrestrained emotion of love, but the channeling of the *citta* toward the *divya* form of the Lord so that the *bhakta* has it always in his *citta* to the exclusion of all other thoughts, or *vṛttis.*

The yogis, however, suggest other kinds of *antara dhāraṇā* that will be equally helpful to *bhaktas, jñanis,* and *bhairāgis.* Focusing attention, as is taught by the sages, on such centers in the body as the navel *(nabhi cakra),* the heart region *(hṛdaya puṇḍarīka),* the crown of the head *(sahasrāra),* the tip of the nose *(nasāgra),* the tip of the tongue *(jihvāgra),* and between the eyebrows *(bhrūmadhya)* is also *antara dhāraṇā,* which when developed to *dhyāna* and *samādhi* leads to various *siddhis.* The Viṣṇu Purāṇa states:

*Prāṇāyāmena pavanam*
*pratyāhārena ca indriyam*
*vaśīkritya tataḥ kuryāt*
*tatsṭānam subhāśrye.*

"Having brought [the neurological forces] under control by *prāṇāyāma,* the senses by *pratyāhāra,* one should resort to contemplation on a peaceful principle for mental stability." According to the Viṣṇu Purāṇa, *antara dhāraṇā* is firmly fixing the enchanting form of the Lord in one's mind, and this practice of *dhāraṇā* should be done until *dhyāna* takes place. The Śrīmad Bhāgavata and many other Purāṇas describe this practice in detail. The differences among *dhāraṇā, dhyāna,* and *samādhi* are subtle, but these have also been described in yogic texts and the Purāṇas. When the *citta,* having taken to a *śubha* object, continues to remain submerged in the *vṛtti* without switching to another, that state of the mind is called *dhyāna vṛtti.* Even though *dhāraṇā* is also a *citta vṛtti* on a single object, there is considerable effort in warding off other, intruding *vṛttis.* In *dhyāna,* without effort, the mind stays with the object, this according to the Viṣṇu Purāṇa.

In *dhyāna,* the distinction between the meditator *(dhyāta)* and the object of meditation *(dhyeya)* remains. But when the distinction between the *dhyāta* and *dhyeya* vanishes and only the object shines in its full glory, then this is *samādhi,* or, more specifically, *samprajñata,* or *sabīja, samādhi.* The technical term used by yogis for *antaraṅga sādhana* is *saṃyama.* One more pertinent observation may be made. The *antaraṅga sādhana* produces its own changes in the *citta*: It is said that *citta* is but the remainder of previous *saṃskāras (saṃskāra śeṣam hi cittam);* the more powerful *saṃskāras* replace the weaker *saṃskāras (prabalena durbalasya bādhaḥ),* an observation that is common knowledge.

Because of repeated sensory (and sensual) experiences, our *citta* has *saṃskāras* that are of an outgoing nature *(vikṣipta).* Because of their *vāsanās* (subtle residues), people repeatedly go for such experiences. In addition, a strengthening of such *saṃskāras* takes place by repeated indulgence. But it is possible to change this situation through the type of practice that is detailed in the science of yoga. The *antaraṅga sādhana* produces mutations in the brain. The *vyutthita citta,* full of outgoing *saṃskāras,* is replaced by *nirodha saṃskāra,* which refuses to respond to external stimuli. Then the *saṃyama* produces a *samādhi pariṇāma,* or a mental transformation, that allows one to remain in one object to the exclusion of all other *citta vṛttis,* including the feeling of a separate individual identity. When this state is continued, the *citta* becomes completely transformed and can remain with one *vṛtti* only, which is called *ekāgrata pariṇāma.* Just as it is difficult to make the *vyutthita* or wandering *citta* stop to even start the practice of yoga, when this final *citta pariṇāma* or *sabīja samādhi* is achieved, the *citta* transformation becomes so complete that it is equally difficult to disturb such a concentrated mind. The Upaniṣads, Purāṇas, and Smṛtis praise such states. It is the contention of yoga that such stages of transformation are possible, and that they are mechanical processes attainable by right practice—and by practice alone.

Vyāsa's commentary on Patañjali refers to a number of places or objects for such *saṃyama,* each one leading to its own *siddhis,* supernormal powers, and possessions. Every *citta* has the capacity for such transformation and such accomplishment.

It is said that by *saṃyama,* or deep concentration, on the distinction between word *(śabda),* the object referred to by the word *(artha),* and the formation of the mind *(pratyaya),* one can understand the languages of all species. By *saṃyama* on one's basic tendencies *(saṃskara),* one can understand one's previous births; if *saṃyama* is focused on moods *(pratyaya),* mind reading becomes possible.

By developing the tendencies—to the extent of *saṃyama*—of friendship, compassion, satisfaction, and indifference to those who are, respectively, contented, suffering, righteous, and unlawful, one acquires enormous mental strength. By *saṃyama* on the principle of light, known as *jyotiṣmatī vṛtti,* one's range of vision increases to long distances and fine objects. *Saṃyama* on the sun is said to bring knowledge of the universe. *Saṃyama* on *candra* (moon), if one does yogic *sādhana,* leads to knowledge of the galaxies. *Saṃyama* on the Pole Star provides the key to the motion of the stars and the galaxies. Nearer home, within oneself, by *saṃyama* on the navel region *(nābhi cakra)* one comes to know one's anatomy *(kāyavyūha).* Concentration on the inside of the throat (near the glottis) leads to control of the physiological functions of thirst and hunger. A *nāḍī* called *kūrma* is identified as the bronchial area; concentrating on that, steadiness of mind (breath) accrues. By *saṃyama* on *brāhmarandhra* (the top of the head), one communicates with *siddhapuruṣas* (yogis who have attained *siddhis*).

All people have intuitive knowledge, but in some it is more manifest and more frequent. It is called *prātibhā*, or "superior clarity of mind," which is indicative. By concentrating and developing this intuitive power, everything comes to be known. By concentrating on one's own heart region, as described in such *vidyās* as *dahara vidyā,* one understands one's own mind. The *citta* is of *triguṇas,* but the *puruṣa* is pure consciousness. By concentrating on this distinction, one gets to know the real nature of one's own self. The *saṃyamas* referred to so far are concerned with specific principles that lead to various kinds of knowledge *(samprajñāta).* But *saṃyama* can also be used to realize the nature of *puruṣa.* There are other yogic feats possible that involve channeling the active Śakti *(kriyā rūpa śākti).* The Śrīmad Bhāgavata catalogs *siddhis* in a different way, however, and always with *bhakti* on the Lord.

*Citta* by nature has the capacity for subtlety, but owing to the particular *dharmādharma* of an individual, it remains confined to one's body. The above *saṃyamas* help to loosen the knots *(granthi)* that cause the bondage. Hence, these yogic exercises literally remove all restrictions of the *prakṛti,* allowing the mind to discover the means to transcend such physical restrictions and enter into another body *(para śarīra āveśa).* This ability is still achieved by many practitioners, even in the present day.

Just as the sense organs act on external matters, the five major *vāyus* are the causes of the *abhyantara vṛtti,* or physiological activities, such as respiration, circulation, and so on. Through mastery of a *vāyu* called *udāna* one is able to fly like a hovercraft over water, brambles, and marshy land. One becomes lustrous like the *devas* with the conquest and voluntary control of *samāna.* Through *saṃyama* on the ear, which is a *sattvic* evolution of the *ahaṃkāra* principle and the *tamasic* evolution of *ahaṃkāra,* which is space *(ākāśa),* and their relationship (which is sound), one can hear the subtlest of sounds. Such hearing is called *divya śrotram.* It may be extended to other *indriyas* by concentration on their corresponding *karaṇa* (instrument), *bhūta* (medium), and *tanmātra* (effect). Other *siddhis* include levitation and *animādhisiddhis* (eight supernatural abilities), grouped as *bhūtasiddhis.* It will suffice to say that practice with faith in the *śāstras* and proper guidance from a guru will lead to the development of these *siddhis.* The limit to such powers is Lordship or Īśvaratva. Having, by *saṃyama,* suppressed the *rajas* and *tamas* aspects from the *citta,* and if one repeatedly resorts to *saṃyama* on the distinction between *prakṛti* and *puruṣa,* then, as Īśvara, one receives the power to create worlds and gain knowledge of *trikāla* (past, present, and future).

The one *dhyāna* that is necessary and sufficient is *bhagavad dhyāna.* When Īśvara is meditated upon, His form constantly kept in mind, all the *siddhis* are given by Him. This contention obviates the need for different kinds of *saṃyama.* The repetition of the Śrīnivāsa mantra to Viṣṇu and Lakṣmī, goddess of fortune, is said to give both *iha śukha* and *para śukha* (happiness here and bliss beyond). According to Śrī Śaṅkarācārya, the repetition of the mantra *brahmaivāham nasamsāri muktoham* gives the eightfold *siddhis.* Obviously this is only a sop for gaining *ātmajñāna.*

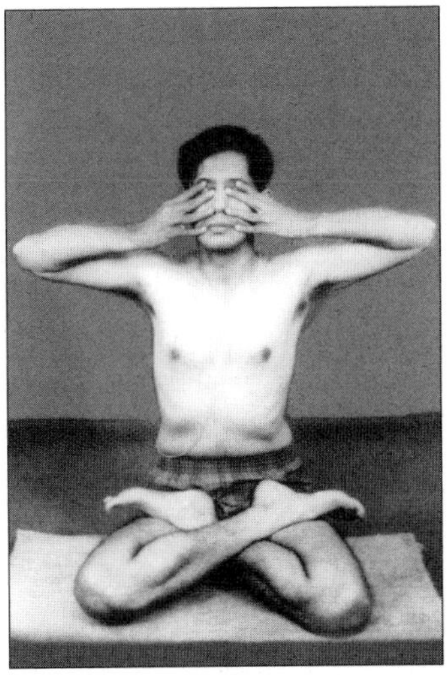

*Śaṇmukhīmudrā* for *saṃyama*

Whether one is a *siddha,* a *bhakta,* or a *jñāni,* yoga is a necessary practice for success. The *siddha* has to resort to *saṃyama* to attain the *siddhis,* and *saṃyama* is a yogic process. A *bhakta* has to do *bhagavad dhyāna* to achieve *parābhakthi,* which, as mentioned in various Purāṇas is facilitated by yoga. A Vedantin, who seeks the identity of the individual soul with *paramātman,* or the merging of the two apparently different phenomena, also has to meditate constantly on the *mahāvākya* (great formula), *"Tat tvam asi"* ("Thou are that") through *nididhyāsanam,* or intense concentration, which again is a yogic discipline. A *bhakta,* a *jñāni,* or a *siddha* is basically a yogi. *"Tasmāt yogi bhavārjuna,"* Lord Kṛṣṇa exhorts Arjuna—"become a yogi." Yoga is a means for both *iha* and *para śukham* (happiness here and hereafter).

# 17 Freedom

*SAMYAMA,* OR *ANTARAṄGA SĀDHANA,* CAN LEAD TO various superior accomplishments and in the third chapter of his treatise Patañjali indicates the parameters and principles *(tattvas)* to be contemplated in order to achieve them. As in the sūtra on *āsana* practice, he does not detail the methods needed to achieve them, and one needs to refer to other texts or approach experienced *siddha* yogis for such guidance. Achieving *siddhis* as they are popularly understood, however, is not the real goal to a yogi. The ultimate *siddhi*, according to Patañjali, is the direct perception of the Self and the final dissolution of the *citta* into its basic constituents, namely, the three *guṇas.* So *kaivalya* is the mother of all *siddhis* (if one looks at it as a *siddhi,* or accomplishment), and the *sādhana,* or practice, directed at this *siddhi* is called *ati-antaraṅga sādhana* (a practice beyond all internal practice, or *antaraṅga sādhana*).

Not all *siddhis* arise by virtue of the yogi's *saṃyama.* For some people, *siddhis* are innate—present from birth—possibly owing to *saṃskāras* acquired in previous births that come to fruition in the present birth. This kind of *siddhi* is known as *janmaja*, which means "arising from birth itself." The *japa* of specific mantras can also produce some *siddhis,* and there are sages who are adept at that practice, which is known as *mantrāja siddhi,* or extraordinary accomplishment arising out of mantras. Some herbs are found to produce *siddhis* and several Purāṇic stories tell of feats brought about by the use of herbs, mostly by *asuras,* or demons. This kind of *siddhi* is known as *ouṣadhija siddhi.* Some *tapasvins,* or those who do penance, also are known to achieve *siddhis.* One example we have already seen is in the story of Nandikeśvara, who by great *tapas* on Lord Śiva attained sainthood in his present birth. These are known as *tapoja siddhis,* or extraordinary accomplishments arising out of *tapas*. Finally are those *siddhis* that are the result of *saṃyama* or *samādhi* by a yogi, which are known as *samādhija siddhi*. How do these *siddhis* happen, and why for some and not for ordinary folk? The answer given by Patañjali is very simple, and may even appear simplistic. Since for both *siddhās* and ordinary mortals *prakṛti* (nature) is the common cause, it follows that extraordinary transformation becomes possible if one develops the power to understand *prakṛti* and change its course. The situation is like the farmer who allows the water to flow to different fields by closing and opening different bunds. The strong karmas done by the yogi have the power to alter the *prakṛti* elements to produce results that appear out of the ordinary. So a yogi is even able to create different *cittas* and exhaust past karmas by experiencing the results of residual karmas through them.

But none of this leads to *kaivalya*, the ultimate goal. Not even all the possible *siddhis* of *prakṛti* will deliver the yogi from the cycle of birth and death if he does not reach the state of *kaivalya*, according to the yogis of the Vedic order. For to achieve all the *siddhis*, even though he may understand *prakṛti* in all its ramifications, he still has to have *avidyā*, or a misconception, about the Self in the form of the I-exist feeling *(asmitā mātrāt)*. Thus the yogi with the locus of the pseudo-self can still control several minds and work out or exhaust his residual karmas. Now the important differences among the various kinds of *siddhās*, like the born *siddha*, the mantra-proficient *siddha*, the herb- or drug-induced *siddha*, the penance-driven *siddha*, and the yogi *siddha*, come into view. Among all the *siddhās*, only those who are proficient in *saṃyama*, or yogic concentration, can progress to *kaivalya*, not only by exhausting past karmas *(karmāśayas)* but also by not producing fresh residual karmas, which then leads to the cessation of future births. As a corollary it may be said that the actions of the yogi who has attained *kaivalya* are neither good *(dharma)* nor bad *(adharma)*, they are neither white nor black. But for other *siddhās* actions are of three kinds, purely *dharmic*, out-and-out *adharmic*, or despicable, and those that are mixed, as we discussed in chapter 5. The four kinds of activities, according to Patañjali, are those that are good, those that are bad, those that are mixed, and those that are neither good nor bad. People who do purely good activities—those who selflessly serve all beings—or who perform activities that are ordained by the scriptures get to become angels. Those that are hell-bent on doing *adharmic* acts are hell-bound, and will suffer. But almost all human actions are mixed *(miśra)*, being thus partly *dharmic* and partly *adharmic*. Several examples can be cited. Giving a large donation to a social cause is a *pūrta* or a *puṇya*. It produces good results for the donor in this or in a future birth. But if the wealth gotten and donated was obtained through ill means, then it is clear that the subject will experience both good and bad effects. But if one studies the *śāstras*, the suffering from bad acts appears to be more severe than are the good effects of doing a *puṇya*. To trivialize it, any happiness that may accrue in donating a million rupees to a good cause may not even be comparable to one-sixteenth the part of the suffering one will experience by, say, stealing goods worth a million rupees with a collar that is white or blue. Hence all human activities are mixed. Robbing Peter to give charity to Paul has a mixed result, and on balance may possibly be a liability.

But the action of a yogi who has attained *kaivalya*, that is, an action performed without desire or malice (*rāga* and *dveṣa*), which is possible only if the basic confusion about the Self has been cleared by yogic contemplation, does not produce any *karmāśaya* that in turn produces any future experience, either way. But all other karmas—including *siddhis*—that remain unproductive for the time being in a latent form *(karmāśaya)*, invariably produce results in the future, whether here or hereafter. So as long as there is the root cause of *avidyā*, people act to satisfy the pseudo-self, which action produces results in the future, and all the unripe actions are encased by *avidyā* in the repository of *citta*. Objects that can excite the ego through the senses sustain the cycle of experiences. But once the *karmāśaya* are made ineffective by removing the root cause, called *avidyā*, or spiritual misconception, then the yogi will not indulge in either *dharmic* or *adharmic* activities, and the remaining *karmāśayas* tend to lose their potency for future trouble in the form of experiences.

How does experience take place at all? According to yogis, when the *citta* relates to an object, it undergoes changes in that it takes the form of the object itself. Whenever a change *(pariṇāma)* takes place, the *citta* is said to know, but if the *citta* does not undergo a change, then it has not known the object—even though the eyes may have seen it. But as far as the *puruṣa* is concerned, the modifications in the *citta* resulting from objects are constantly and invariably seen or experienced by it. If the *puruṣa*, like the *citta*, also undergoes changes, then it itself may not know when there is a change. This is incongruous, and hence one can intuitively know or infer that there has to be a nonchanging conscious principle that always *(sada)* knows *(jñāta)* whatever picture is created in the *citta*. This understanding is central to both Sāṃkhya and Yoga, that there is a distinct *puruṣa* that is immutable, and only that principle should be known as Self *(pratyak ātma)*. Why? Because the Self is that which is innermost, subtle, conscious, and without a second.

Having been convinced by several arguments *(anumāna)*, the *citta* realizes that the Self that should be called "I" is really the nonchanging experiencer and not the I-feeling or ego that is experienced. When this gets established in the *citta*, the yogi tends to contemplate more and more the true nature of the real Self. Having realized that the Self, or *puruṣa*, does not require anything at all to be and remain satisfied, since it has no desire whatsoever, the *citta* slowly veers around to the view that it has really nothing to do, and its constant endeavors hitherto have no relevance. It slowly recognizes that the pressures to satisfy the pseudo-self are never ending. Having realized the nature of the Self and the pseudo-self, the *citta* slowly gravitates toward a state of equilibrium of the *guṇas* in which state it savors the continuous flow of peace that comes when the feverish activity arising out of the wrong impressions *(avidyā)* about the Self slows down. Then the *saṃskāra* (habits) of not engaging in frivolous and feverish ego-satisfying activities goes on increasing and, as if in a balance, the *citta* gravitates more and more toward the *nirodha* state. In the practice of *nirodha,* or nonengagement, in moment after moment the *citta* stays in a state of *nirodha,* and the three *guṇas* reach a state of equilibrium. There are no *sattvic,* or pious, activities. There are no *tamasic,* or sinful, impulses and activities. Nor are there *rajasic,* or forceful and violent, outbursts. This state of *citta* continues, and then all that remains in the *citta* is nothing but *nirodha saṃskāras.* So *nirodha* does not force the *citta,* but shows the *citta* the way of *nirodha,* which is Patañjali's yoga system. The yogi in that state remains there until death takes over, when even the *sāmānya vṛttis* of the *citta* cease. Since he has no residual *karmāśayas*—because they have been either used up or made ineffective by the removal of *avidyā*—he is not born again, never born again. When the *citta* remains in the state of *nirodha* continually, this is called *kaivalya,* or aloneness, or freedom. Freedom from what? Freedom from the self-imposed compulsions to satisfy the self-locus, the pseudo-self, the *ahaṃkāra.* It can be viewed as freedom for the *puruṣa* as well, even though it is always free, only the disturbed mind does not think so. One is no longer required to see the various activities of the *citta,* which has been resolved into its basic constituents. Yoga is therefore also the freedom of the mind, by the mind, for the mind, and from the mind itself. The *citta* is no more a slave to an assumed master. The Self is free, as free as ever.

Patañjali wonders for whom is the freedom. It is for both the Self and especially the mind. Then there is no master, no servant. There is only freedom, absolute and permanent.

# Glossary

| | |
|---|---|
| *abhāva* | nonexistence |
| *abhiniveśa* | fear, especially of death; an affliction *(kleśa)* of the mind |
| *abhyāsa* | practice |
| *abhyāsī* | practitioner |
| *ācārya* | teacher, who guides by example |
| *adharma* | disorder, sin, nonpiety |
| *adhikāri* | fit person |
| *adhomukha* | downward; facedown |
| Ādiśeṣa | the serpent king; acting as couch to the Lord, Ādiśeṣa incarnated as Patañjali |
| Āditya | lit., "son of Aditi"; sun |
| Advaita | nondualism; a philosophy based on the theory that the individual soul and the supreme being are one and the same in their essential characteristic. The dualism is only apparent; being unreal. |
| *agni* | one of five principal elements *(bhūtas),* fire; energy |
| Ahalyā | wife of the sage Gautama, revered as one of the seven chaste women in mythology |
| *aham* | I |
| *ahaṃkāra* | self, viewed as doer, agent |
| *ahiṃsā* | eschewing violence; highest yogic injunction (don't) |
| *airāvata* | white elephant of Indra, the celestial king |
| *aiśvarya* | riches; supernatural powers, synonymous with *vibhūti, siddhi* |

| | |
|---|---|
| *ākāśa* | one of five principal elements *(bhūtas);* space; ether |
| *akliṣṭa* | favorable |
| *ānanda* | bliss |
| *ananta* | infinite; cap., a name of Viṣṇu |
| *aṅga* | part, limb |
| *annamayakośa* | the physical body; lit., "the sheath made of food" |
| *antaḥkaraṇa* | the "internal organ" or brain |
| *antaḥ-kumbhaka* | holding the breath in |
| *antaraṅga* | internal part or aspect; of the mind, *citta* |
| *antarāya* | inpediments to spiritual progress. Patañjali lists nine of them—one physical and eight mental. |
| *anya, anyata* | other, different |
| *āpaḥ, ap* | one of the five principal elements *(bhūtas),* water; liquid. |
| *apāna* | one of five *prāṇas;* physiological force operating in the lower part of the body |
| *aparigraha* | nonaccumulation of wealth and possessions; eschewing illegal gratification |
| Āpastambha | a sage *(ṛṣi)* who codified laws *(dharma)* in *sūtras* (aphorisms) and work on *dharma;* lit., "one who stops the flow of water" |
| *apavarga* | renunciation; roll back |
| *apsarā* | celestial damsel, dancer |
| *āraṇyaka* | lit., "of the forest"; portions of scriptures (Vedas) chanted in the forest |
| *ardha* | half, partial |
| *artha* | meaning of word; wealth; goal |
| *aruṇa* | lit., "one without any debts"; one who gives, one who releases one from debts; the sun, since it always gives warmth and light |
| *āsana* | yogic posture |
| *asmitā* | I-exist feeling; a fundamental, cognizable *kleśa* (mental affliction) |
| *asparśa yoga* | lit., "untouched" or "untainted"; yoga of Advaitins to achieve liberation *(mokṣa)* |
| *aṣṭāṅgayoga* | eight-part or eight-step yoga |
| *asteya* | nonstealing; another yogic injunction, one of the yamas |
| *asura* | nonangelic being; a demonic individual |
| *aśvamedha* | horse sacrifice performed by emperors; the mantras may be merely chanted for benefits on specific days in the month; the highest Vedic rite |

| | |
|---|---|
| *ātma* | self; lit., "that which (1) enjoys" or "experiences"; (2) "pervades"; (3) "acquires" *(karmas)* |
| *avatāra* | incarnation |
| *avidyā* | misconception, mistaken impression, or misunderstanding, especially about the true nature of Self. The most fundamental mental affliction *(kleśa),* according to yogis. |
| Āyurveda | lit., "science of life"; an ancient, established system of therapy and a healthy way of life |
| *baddha* | bound; restrained |
| *bahiraṅga sādhana* | practice of the first five aspects of eight-part yoga |
| *bāhya-kumbhaka* | holding the breath "out" after exhalation and before inhalation |
| *bandha* | locking, or pulling up, a group of muscles |
| Bhagavad Gītā | Song of Lord Kṛṣṇa. A discourse on Yoga and Vedānta to Arjuna in the battlefield. It is a part of the great epic *(itihāsa),* the Mahābhārata, written by Vyāsa. |
| *bhakti* | devotion, sublime love toward the supreme being |
| Bhaktisūtra | a classic work of Nārada on *bhakti* methods. |
| *bhaktiyoga* | yoga of devotion. Integration of the individual soul with the supreme through love, devotion. An important aspect of both the Bhagavat Gītā and the Yogasūtras. |
| Bharadvāja | a famous sage |
| *bhastrikā* | bellows, breathing; a breathing exercise resembling the forced blowing of air |
| *bhāṣya* | commentary; elucidation of a basic text |
| *bhūloka* | earth; world |
| *bhūta* | (1) being; (2) one of the five principal elements—space, air, fire, water, and earth |
| Brahmā | creator; one of the trinity |
| *brahmacarya* | (1) the student stage of life; (2) a vow of celibacy; (3) a yogi's vow not to transgress the institution of marriage |
| Brahman | lit., "that which has (or appears to have) grown into the universe"; pure consciousness, the substratum of the entire universe |
| *buddhi* | intellect; an aspect of the internal organ *(antaḥkarana),* or brain |
| *cakra* | active centers functioning along the spine |

| | |
|---|---|
| Camakam | a chapter in the Yajur Veda listing the boons sought from Rudra. Usually recited after chanting Rudram, perhaps the most popular Vedic chant of Śiva. |
| *candra* | moon; the left nostril |
| Candraśekhara | crescent crested; Lord Śiva |
| Caraka | author of a treatise *(Caraka Saṃhitā)* on Āyurveda, and believed to be Patañjali |
| *carita; caritra* | story; history or life history |
| Cidambaram | lit., "space of consciousness"; a temple city in south India where Lord Śiva is believed to have performed the celestial dance |
| *cikitsa* | medicine |
| *cit* | pure consciousness, the immutable individual Self in yoga |
| *citta* | lit., "that which appears to have consciousness"; mind, brain, the internal organ |
| *citta vṛtti* | fluctuation of the mind |
| *dakṣiṇa* | right side |
| *ḍamaru* | hand-held drum |
| *darśana* | exposition; there are six *darśanas* or schools of philosophy: Vaiśesika, Nyāya, Mīmāṃsā, Sāṃkhya, Yoga, and Vedānta |
| *deśa* | place, position; a place in the body where breath is controlled in prāṇāyāma |
| *deva* | angel; a god usually associated with an aspect of nature |
| Devī | Mother goddess |
| Devī Māhātmya | a revered Sanskrit work of 700 verses narrating the exploits of Devī (goddess). It is also known as Candi and Durgā-sapta-śatī. |
| *dhāraṇā* | lit., "to support"; an activity of the mind when an attempt is made to repeatedly hold a thought or object in mind, the first stage of meditation; retention, memory |
| *dharma* | order; essential characteristic; law; a manifestation of *sattvic* quality |
| Dhātupāṭha | a text giving the meaning (in Sanskrit) of Sanskrit roots |
| *dhyāna* | lit., "to think repeatedly," especially of a higher principle; meditation; *bhagavad dhyāna* is "meditation on the Lord" |
| *dhyātā* | the yogi or devotee who does the meditation |
| *dhyeya* | the object of meditation |
| *draṣṭṛ* | the observer; another technical name for the Self in yoga |

| | |
|---|---|
| *dṛśya* | the observed, referring to the entire *prakṛti* in all its manifestations, including the ego |
| *duḥkha* | lit., "vitiated" *(du),* "internal environment" *(kham);* mental pain; suffering |
| *dveṣa* | hatred, a *kleśa* or mental affliction |
| *dvipāda* | two feet; two legs |
| *eka* | one |
| Ekāgni Kāṇḍa | chapter in the Vedas containing mantras of Vedic ceremonies performed with one fire "location." Contains the whole mantras of Vedic initiation *(upanayana)* and wedding, including vows *(vivāha).* |
| *ekāgra* | one-pointedness; a state of mind achieved by repeated sustained practice of appropriate yoga, transforming the *citta (pariṇāma)* |
| *ekapāda* | one leg |
| *ekatatva* | one principle; the Lord |
| *gaṇa* | servants of Śiva, also known as *sivagaṇa* |
| *gāṇapatya* | system of worship of Gaṇapati; one of the six orthodox systems of worship *(ṣanmata)* |
| Gaṇeśa | also Gaṇapati; lit., "leader of *gaṇas"* (the elephant-headed deity) |
| *garbha nirodha* | contraception |
| Garuḍa | of the eagle family, vehicle of Lord Viṣṇu |
| *ghanapāṭha* | an involved chanting method of Vedic mantras and hymns |
| Goṇikā | mother of Patañjali |
| Govinda | lit., "cowherd"; another name for Lord Kṛṣṇa |
| Govudapāda | an Advaitin, said to be an incarnation of Lord Śiva; author of a masterpiece, called *Māṇḍūkya-kārikā,* an independent commentary to Māṇḍūkya Upaniṣad, on Advaitic lines |
| *granthi* | knot; there are three knots in the spine blocking the upward movement of the esoteric *kuṇḍalinī* |
| *guṇa* | a constituent of *prakṛti.* The three *guṇas* are *sattva, rajas,* and *tamas.* |
| guru | teacher, "heavy" with knowledge; planet Jupiter; heaviness, a manifestation of *tamas* |

| | |
|---|---|
| Hariharaputra | son of Śiva and Viṣṇu in his female form as the enchantress (Mohini) |
| *hastavinyāsa* | variations of hand positions in a yogic posture |
| *Haṭhayogapradīpikā* | classic yoga text by Svātmāramā |
| *himālaya* | lit., "the abode of ice" or "snow"; the great mountain |
| Hindu | follower of ancient Indian religion, lit., "one who eschews violence" |
| *homa* | minor fire sacrifice to propitiate Vedic gods |
| *hṛdaya* | heart |
| Indra | head of *devas* (angels) |
| Indrāṇī | Indra's consort |
| *indriya* | one of the five senses |
| *iṣṭa devatā* | one's chosen, favorite deity |
| Īśvara | Lord; one who is everywhere; in yoga, the prime, preeminent preceptor; pure, unfettered consciousness |
| Īśvarapraṇidhāna | surrender to the Lord; Yoga of devotion; a *niyama* of aṣṭāṅgayoga; an aspect of *kriyāyoga;* a principal means of freedom *(kaivalya)* |
| *itihāsa* | lit., "how it was," history; an epic. The Rāmāyaṇa and Mahābhārata are *itihāsas.* |
| *jālandhara bandha* | chin lock, useful in *ujjāyī prāṇāyāma;* said to prevent nectar *(amṛta)* dripping from the head, which is subsequently consumed by gastric fire |
| *japa* | repetition of a mantra |
| *japakrama, japavidhāna* | an elaborate method of doing *japa* |
| *jñāna* | wisdom |
| *jñānayoga* | a yoga relying on sharp uncompromising intellect and yogic practice, to realize the unchanging, absolute, underlying principle of the universe (Brahman) |
| *jīva* | lit., "the living principle"; individual soul |
| *jīvana* | living; life |
| *jīvana prayatna* | effort of life; breathing |
| *kalā* | art; there are sixty-four of them, including yoga |
| *kāla* | time |
| *kāma* | pleasure, enjoyment |

| | |
|---|---|
| Kāmākṣi | lit., "one who confers boons to Her devotees with the grace of Her glance"; the presiding deity in a famous temple in Kānci |
| *kāṇda* | a portion; a section of the Veda |
| *kaivalya* | lit., "aloneness"; the acme of yogic practice; freedom of soul and mind |
| *Kālidāsa* | lit., "a servant or devotee of Kāli," the energetic black goddess, and an aspect of Śakti. A great Sanskrit poet *(mahākavi)* |
| *kapālabhāti* | an active, repetitive upward movement exercise of the pelvic diaphragm, abdominal muscles, and the diaphragm for forcible exhalation; lit., "that which makes the skull (face) shine" |
| *kārikā* | a detailed commentary |
| karma | action; the karma theory is a basic premise on which all Vedic philosophies, including Yoga, rest |
| *karmāśaya* | action that is yet to fructify |
| *karmayoga* | action without fear or desire for the results; doing prescribed duties; one way of escaping from the cycle of *saṃsāra* (transmigration) |
| *kāvya* | great literary work |
| *kleśa* | affliction |
| *kriyā* | activity |
| *kriyāyoga* | yoga practice mentioned by Patañjali for the purification of mind, body, and senses |
| *kumbhaka* | breath holding; in or out |
| *kuṇḍalinī yoga* | yogic practice based on the arousal of the energy (Śakti) in the form of a coiled serpent and subsequent merger with the Śiva principle in the *sahasrāracakra* |
| *kūrma* | tortoise |
| *kūrma nāḍī* | a pathway in the lower part of the neck |
| *kūṣmāṇda homa* | a Vedic rite for purification from the effects of doing forbidden acts |
| Lakṣmī | goddess of beauty and wealth, consort of Lord Viṣṇu |
| Lalitā | a form of Śakti or mother |
| *langhana* | to diminish; to reduce |
| *langhana kriyā* | moving while exhaling or holding the breath out |
| *layayoga* | to merge with a superior principle |
| Mahābhārata | an epic *(itihāsa)* written by Vyāsa, which contains the |

| | |
|---|---|
| | famous Bhagavad Gītā and Viṣṇu Sahasrānama (1,000 names or mantras of Viṣṇu) |
| Mahābhāṣya | lit., "the great commentary"; a work of Patañjali (at the bidding of Śiva) on Sanskrit grammar |
| *mahākāvya* | a great work of literature |
| *mahāmudrā* | lit., "the great seal," a yogic energy-channeling exercise |
| Mahānārāyaṇa Upaniṣad | the last chapter of the Yajur Veda (Kṛṣṇa) containing several oft-used Vedic mantras |
| *mahat* | lit., "great principle"; the universal mind. The first manifestation of *prakṛti.* |
| *manas* | mind |
| *mano-vāk-kāya* | the three principal instruments of human activity, the mind, speech, and body |
| Maṇḍūkya Upaniṣad | Upaniṣad of the Atharva Veda giving an esoteric interpretation of the sacred syllable OM |
| mantra | a syllable, a short passage, or hymn that is usually repeated mentally. A mantra has a deity whose name or attribute the mantra is and a sage or seer who discovered it. Sometimes a meter such as *gāyatrī,* is also associated with it. |
| *mārjāla* | cat |
| Mārkaṇḍeya | a great devotee of Śiva; the Pūraṇa (mythology) associated with him contains the famous Devī Māhātmya |
| Mīmāṃsā | lit., "discussion"; a philosophy vouching for the efficacy of the Vedic rites |
| *mitā santāna* | family planning |
| *mokṣa* | liberation |
| *mṛgīmudrā* | a hand gesture resembling a deer running; used to control the nostrils while doing *prāṇāyāmā.* |
| *mūḍha* | lit., "covered"; a mind that is dull or dark, the effect of a predominance of *tamas* |
| *mudrā* | gesture of happiness; sealing or blocking some portion of a passage to redirect energy |
| *mūla* | root; original |
| *mūla bandha* | rectal lock |
| *mūlagrantha* | original religious and spiritual texts, namely, the Vedas |
| *nāda* | sound, usually pleasing |
| *nāḍī* | a passage, usually of *praṇic* energy |
| *nāḍī śodhana* | a *prānāyāma* for cleaning the *nāḍīs* |
| Nāgarāja | serpent king; another name for Ādiśeṣa |

| | |
|---|---|
| Nandikeśvara | the bull vehicle of Śiva; lit., "the blissful one" |
| Narasiṃha | an incarnation of Lord Viṣṇu, in the form of man-lion |
| *nātya* | dance |
| *nidrā* | sleep |
| *nirnidrā* | insomnia |
| *nirodha* | total stoppage or cessation of mental activity or the thought train in a yogi; the highest level *(bhūmi)* of *citta* |
| *nītī* | justice |
| *nitya sūri* | eternally enlightened; the first beings of creation who escaped the clutches of *avidyā* |
| *nivṛtti* | reactive effort to avoid or escape from what is considered undesirable, namely, *saṃsāra* |
| *nivṛtti śāstra* | a school of philosophy purporting to teach how to escape permanently from pain, rebirth, for example, Yoga, Vedānta |
| *niyama* | a prescribed duty |
| Nyāya | justice; law; logical thinking; one of the six orthodox philosophies relying on one's intellect |
| Nyāyācārya | an expert logician of the Nyāya Śāstra |
| OM | the first Vedic mantra; name of the Lord; according to Vedānta, the syllable represents the creation, sustenance, and dissolution of the universe; it also represents the stages of waking, dreaming, and sleeping. The unmanifest sound represents the transcendental stage of the mind *(turīya)* or the period of quiet between creations *(pralaya).* |
| Omkāra | the word OM |
| *pada* | lit., "word"; Sanskrit grammar |
| *pāda* | foot; quarter; a chapter in a book |
| *pādāṅguṣṭha* | big toe |
| *paddhati* | system |
| *pañcāgni vidyā* | an Upaniṣadic dissertation about the transmigration of the soul from one birth to another through five transformations (five fires) |
| Pāṇini | a grammarian who wrote the Pāṇini sūtras, based on the inspiration he had by watching the dance of Śiva |
| *parāmātma* | supreme soul |
| *pārāyaṇa* | recitation of religious texts |

| | |
|---|---|
| *pariṇāma* | transformation of mind *(citta)* due to yogic practice |
| *parivṛtta* | turned around |
| *pārśva* | the side |
| *paścima* | back of the body |
| Patañjali | incarnation of Ādiśeṣa, author of *Yogasūtras* and works on grammar and Āyurveda |
| *paurāṇika* | an expert speaker on Purāṇas (mythology) |
| *pradhāna* | primary, original; name for the state of total involution of the universe or the complete state of equilibrium of the three *guṇas* |
| Prahlāda | lit., "the totally blissful one"; son of the demon king Hiranyakaśipu. Prahlāda was a great devotee of Lord Nārāyaṇa/Viṣṇu. |
| *prajñā* | thorough and correct knowledge, arising out of yogic practice |
| *prakṛti* | matter; see *pradhāna* |
| *pramāṇa* | means of attaining right knowledge |
| *prāṇa* | life energy/force |
| *praṇava* | lit., "greatest praise"; name of Īśvara; the OM syllable |
| prāṇamayakośa | lit., "the sheath made of prāṇa" |
| *prāṇāyāma* | fourth step in *aṣṭāṅgayoga;* yogic breathing exercises; control and regulation of breath |
| *prasārita* | stretched out |
| Praśna Upaniṣad | one of the ten prominent Upaniṣads, written in the form of questions *(praśna)* and answers about the ultimate reality (Brahman) |
| *pratikriyā* | counterposture; movement to an involved *āsana* or *vinyāsa* |
| *pratyāhāra* | lit., "starving the senses," that is, of their stimuli such as sound and taste |
| *pratyakṣa* | direct perception |
| *pratyaya* | ideas, mental content; attitude |
| *pravṛtti* | proactive effort to obtain or retain what one considers desirable |
| *pṛṣṭāñjali* | back salute |
| *pūjā* | worship |
| *puṇya* | good; virtuous |
| Purāṇas | mythological works; eighteen Purāṇas are well known, such as the Viṣṇu Purāṇa, Śiva Purāṇa, and the Bhagavaa Purāṇa |

| | |
|---|---|
| *puruṣa* | the indwelling principle, pure consciousness, the soul |
| *pūrva* | front of the body |
| *rāga* | lit., "attachment"; desire, an affliction *(kleśa);* opposite of *dveśa* |
| *rajas* | one of the three *guṇas;* the active, or energy, constituent of nature |
| *rājayoga* | yoga of enlightenment |
| Rāmāyaṇa | the story of Rāma, an incarnation of Viṣṇu, the most popular epic. Several versions are available in India and south Asia; Vālmīki's version in 24,000 verses is the most authentic. |
| *recaka* | controlled exhalation as practiced by yogi |
| *ṛṣi* | lit., "one who sticks to truth"; a seer of mantras |
| *ṛtam* | truth, straightness |
| *rūpa* | form |
| Sadāśiva | lit., "ever peaceful"; Lord Śiva, name of an Advaitin yogi from deep south India |
| *sādhaka* | seeker; aspirant; yoga practitioner |
| *sādhana* | correct sustained practice that leads to accomplishment |
| *sādhya* | achievable; goal |
| *sahasranāma* | a devotional work of 100 mantras praising the same deity, usually found in the Purāṇas |
| *sahasrāra* | thousand- (or countless-) petaled center; the abode of Śiva in the microcosm |
| Śākta | system of worship of Śakti; one of the six orthodox systems of worship |
| Śakti | goddess of power |
| *samādhāna* | constant focus of the mind |
| *samādhi* | union; completion |
| *samāhita citta* | mental balance and contentment |
| *samāna* | the *prāṇa* that helps digestion |
| *samantraka* or *sagarbha prāṇāyāma* | *prāṇāyāma* done with mantras or imaging the form of a deity |
| *sāmānya* | general activity (association) of the mind |
| *samāpatti* | focusing the mind |
| *samasthiti* | balancing correctly on both feet—correct standing position; also the starting position of doing *āsanas* as per *vinyāsakrama* |

| | |
|---|---|
| *samāvartana* | a ceremony performed by a student at the end of his Vedic studies and before taking to family life |
| Sāṃkhya | lit., "thoroughly researched exposition"; one of the six orthodox systems of philosophy, subscribing fully to the theory of karma but balking at the premise of a creator/god |
| *sampradāya* | tradition |
| *samsāra* | phenomenal existence |
| *saṃskāra* | residual or latent impression of past experience |
| *saṃtoṣa* | contentment; one of the *niyamas* |
| *saṃyama* | constraint |
| *saṃyoga* | correlation, integration |
| *sandhyāvandana* | prayers and oblations to Vedic gods according to the prescribed method, done at dawn, midday, and dusk every day |
| *sannyāsa* | renunciation; the fourth stage of life |
| *sarva* | all |
| *sarvāṅga* | the whole body |
| *śāstra* | an orthodox subject; scriptures |
| *śāstrīyayoga* | traditional yoga |
| *sattva* | one of the three *guṇas*, the most beneficial to the individual in spiritual pursuit. It manifests as order, right conduct, piety, clarity of mind, lightness of body, and extraordinary achievements. |
| *satya* | lit., "that which never changes"; truth, the essence |
| *śauca* | cleanliness; one of the *niyamas* |
| Sāyāṇa | Vedic commentator on all four Vedas |
| *sāyujya* | integration of the individual soul into the supreme |
| *siddhi* | accomplishment, supernatural powers; one of the results of yoga practice |
| *sloka* | a verse of a text |
| *Smṛti* | lit., "what is remembered"; sanskrit texts containing teachings of ancient sages |
| *sthiti* | stability; steadiness |
| *Subrahmaṇya* | son of God (Śiva) |
| *sukha* | happiness, joy, comfort |
| *sukhaprasava* | hassle-free childbirth |
| *sūkta* | hymns and short prayers to the Vedic gods |
| Sundara Kāṇḍa | a section of the Rāmāyaṇa of about 3,000 verses recited over seven days for several benefits |

| | |
|---|---|
| *sūryanamaskāra* | sun salutation; a sequence of twelve *vinyāsas* and *āsanas* that can be done with appropriate mantras |
| sūtra | a succint way of writing and presenting a subject in a cogent way, like a string of beads |
| *svādhyāya* | recitation and study of the scriptures |
| *svara* | note or pitch in chanting |
| *tamas* | a *guṇa*, associated with laziness, heaviness, bondage, darkness, disorder, inpurity, delusion, and chaos |
| *tāṇḍava* | vigorous celestial dance, especially of Lord Śiva |
| *tanmātra* | lit., "that alone"; pure aspect of sound, touch, form, taste, and smell |
| *tapas* | lit., "to heat" and burn away dross; austerity; an aspect of *kriyāyoga* and a *niyama* |
| *taṭākamudrā* | abdominal lock in a lying-down position; pond gesture |
| *tattva* | principle or element |
| *udāna* | lit., "moving up"; one of the five *prāṇas* associated with upward movement to organs of the head |
| *uddīyāna bandha* | abdominal lock |
| *ujjāyī* | yogic breathing method with a constriction in the throat, making a hissing noise; lit., "uplifting" |
| Umā | the goddess Śakti, consort of Śiva |
| *ūrdhvamukha* | facing upward |
| Upaniṣad | Vedic texts specially giving the methods of realization of the Self |
| *upāsana* | devotional practice; formal meditation. Upaniṣads give several methods of *upāsana* of Brahman, the ultimate reality. |
| *upaviṣṭha* | seated |
| *uttāna* | a stretch |
| *uttarasānti* | peace invocation chanted at the end of lesson or function |
| *utthita* | raised, extended |
| *vairāgya* | desirelessness; a state of mind of dispassion |
| Vaiśeṣika | an early orthodox philosophy, giving perhaps the first atomic theory of the universe |
| Vāruṇa | Vedic god of rain |
| Vāsukī | mythological serpent, used as rope to churn the milky ocean |

| | |
|---|---|
| Veda | the basic Hindu scripture. The Vedas give the knowledge of actions that bring what is favorable and remove what is not. |
| Vedānta | one of the six orthodox philosophies based on the Vedas |
| *vidyā* | specific body of spiritual knowledge or practice |
| *vikalpa* | imagination; the third type of *vṛtti* |
| *vikṣepa* | distraction; an obstacle to attaining one-pointedness |
| *vikṣipta* | distracted |
| *vinyāsa* | different positions, or variations, of classic yogic postures; art |
| *vinyāsakrama* | a logical and well-planned sequence of movements and positions in one or more yogic postures or posture sequences; usually performed making use of appropriate breathing sequence while doing the movements; yoga as an art form |
| *viparīta karaṇi* | a term used for inverted yoga postures; especially a simple version of the shoulder stand |
| *viparyaya* | confusion; mistaken impression about an object |
| Viṣṇu | lit., "all pervading"; sustainer of the universe; one of the trinity |
| *vitarka* | (1) counterargument; (2) counter-thought; (3) objects (gross) that are discernible to the senses |
| *viveka* | discernment |
| *viveki* | one capable of discernment |
| *vṛtti* | activity, function of the *citta;* fluctuations of consciousness |
| *vyāyāma* | exercise |
| *yajña* | ritual |
| *yama* | (1) self-control, don'ts for a yogi; (2) cap., god of death |
| *yamaniyamas* | yogic don'ts and dos |
| yoga | (1) union; (2) concentration; (3) cessation of endless train of thoughts; cap., one of the six traditional philosophies |
| *yogābhyāsa* | practice of yoga |
| *yoganidrā* | (1) a yogic posture resembling lying in a hammock (2) a state of nonactivity of the supreme before creation |
| Yogeśvara | Lord of Yoga; name attributed to Lord Kṛṣṇa and sometimes Lord Śiva |
| *yogī śvara* | foremost yogi |

# Index